W

Ar

Manual

Second edition

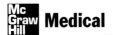

Medical

First edition published 2000
Reprinted 2000
Second edition published 2004
Text © 2004 Anthony Padley
Illustrations and design © 2004 McGraw-Hill Australia Pty Ltd
Additional owners of copyright are named in on-page credits.

National Library of Australia Cataloguing-in-Publication data:
    Padley, Anthony.
    Westmead pocket anaesthetic manual.
    2nd ed.
    ISBN 0 074 71486 4.

    1. Anaesthetics – Handbooks, manuals, etc. 2. Anaesthesia –
    Handbooks, manuals, etc. I. Westmead Hospital. II. Title.

617.96

Published in Australia by
McGraw-Hill Australia Pty Ltd
Level 2, 82 Waterloo Road, North Ryde NSW 2113
Acquisitions Editor: Thu Nguyen
Production Editor: Rosemary McDonald
Editor: Joy Window
Proofreader: Tim Learner
Designer (cover and interior): Lara Scott, Unhinged Productions
Illustrator: Lorenzo Lucia
Typeset in Stone Informal 7.5/10 by Lara Scott, Unhinged Productions
Printed on 65 gsm matt art by 1010 Printing Limited, Hong Kong

The McGraw·Hill Companies

Westmead Pocket Anaesthetic Manual

Second edition

Anthony P. Padley

The **McGraw·Hill** *Companies*

Sydney New York San Francisco Auckland
Bangkok Bogotá Caracas Hong Kong
Kuala Lumpur Lisbon London Madrid
Mexico City Milan New Delhi San Juan
Seoul Singapore Taipei Toronto

This manual is dedicated to my loving wife Tracey
and to our three wishes that came true: Max,
Angus and Hugo.

Contents

CONTENTS

C

Westmead Pocket Anaesthetic Manual

F

G

H

I

M

N

CONTENTS

R

CONTENTS

T

U

V

Preface to the Second edition

The practice of anaesthesia can be described as long periods of tranquillity punctuated by brief periods of sheer terror. It is to help deal with these often sudden and unforeseen potential, or actual, life-threatening events that this manual is intended.

The *Westmead Pocket Anaesthetic Manual Second Edition*, like the first edition, aims to provide a vast array of essential anaesthetic knowledge in a convenient, rapid access alphabetic format. This information is packaged in a compact, pocket-sized book designed for 'carry everywhere' use. In this new edition of the manual over 70 new topics have been added, reflecting the many advances in anaesthetic practice over the past 4 years. All other topics have been extensively revised and expanded where necessary. Of necessity, several topics of lesser importance in the first edition have been deleted due to space restrictions.

Overall, this edition contains over 450 entries covering crisis management, drugs, regional anaesthesia and other procedures, the anaesthetic implications of many medical conditions and anaesthesia for specific surgical problems. There are also included many guidelines on topics such as endocarditis prophylaxis, equipment and monitoring issues and interpretation of investigations such as blood tests and respiratory function studies.

Exciting advances in anaesthesia covered in this second edition include new equipment such as the LMA ProSeal, Univent tubes, the M-entropy awareness monitor and biphasic defibrillators.

Many new drugs are also evaluated, including the most recent antiplatelet medications, COX2 inhibitors and the haemostasis agent NovoSeven.

This edition places a stronger emphasis on obstetric anaesthesia with topics such as cardiomyopathy of pregnancy and discussion of the anaesthetic implications of diseases such as Eisenmenger's syndrome in the pregnant patient.

There is in this edition, compared with the first, a more detailed discussion of complications of anaesthetic procedures such as epidural block with percentage risks quoted where possible. This will be of great assistance to anaesthetists attempting to provide patients with informed consent in our ever-worsening medico-legal environment.

Acknowledgments

I would like to thank the anaesthetic consultants and registrars of Westmead Hospital for their invaluable advice and assistance. In particular I would like to thank Associate Professor Peter Klineberg for his support and encouragement. My thanks also go to my father, Terence Padley, for proofreading this manual, to Dr Mark Cooper for his cardiological expertise, and to Lorraine Koller, Deputy Director of Pharmacy at Westmead Hospital.

Criticisms, comments and suggestions are welcome for subsequent editions of this book and can be e-mailed to anthonypadley@bigpond.com or posted to PO Box 2748, North Parramatta, NSW 1750, Australia.

Disclaimer

Considerable care and effort has gone into ensuring that drug dosages and other information in this book is accurate. However, the user is advised to check drug doses carefully. The author shall not be responsible for any errors in this publication.

List of abbreviations

AAA	abdominal aortic aneurysm
ABG	arterial blood gas
ACE	angiotensin converting enzyme
AEC	airway exchange catheter
AED	automated external defibrillators
AF	atrial fibrillation
ALS	advanced life support
AP	anterior–posterior
AS	aortic valve stenosis
ASD	atrial septal defect
ATE	arterial thromboembolism
AV	atrioventricular
BIS	Bispectral Index (a type of EEG monitor)
BLS	basic life support
BLM	bleomycin
BMI	body mass index
BPF	bronchopleural fistula
bpm	beats or breaths per minute (depending on context)
BSL	blood sugar level
C	cervical vertebra
CABG	coronary artery bypass grafting
CEA	carotid endarterectomy
CCF	congestive cardiac failure
CNS	central nervous system
COMT	catechol-amino transferase
CO	carbon monoxide
COX	cyclo-oxygenase
CP	cervical plexus

CPAP	continuous positive airway pressure
CPP	cerebral perfusion pressure
CPR	cardiopulmonary resuscitation
CS	Caesarean section
CSF	cerebrospinal fluid
CT	computerised tomogram
CVA	cerebrovascular accident
CVS	cardiovascular system
CXR	chest X-ray
DA	dopamine receptor
DC	direct current
DIC	disseminated intravascular coagulation
DLT	double lumen tube
DTA	distal thoracic aorta
DVT	deep venous thrombosis
ECC	external cardiac compression
ECG	electrocardiography, electrocardiograph
EDBP	epidural blood patch
EDLA	extended duration local anaesthetic
EEG	electroencephalograph
EF	ejection fraction
EMLA	eutectic mixture of local anaesthetic agents
ET	endotracheal
FBC	full blood count
FDP	fibrin degradation products
FEV_1	forced expiratory volume in the first second
FFP	fresh frozen plasma
FGF	fresh gas flow
FiO_2	fractional concentration of inspired O_2
FOB	fibre-optic bronchoscope

FVC	forced vital capacity
G6PD	glucose-6-phosphate dehydrogenase
GA	general anaesthesia
GCS	Glasgow coma score
GEB	gum elastic bougie
GTN	glyceryl trinitrate
5-HT$_3$	5 hydroxytryptamine 3 (receptor)
HOCM	hypertrophic obstructive cardiomyopathy
HRT	hormone replacement therapy
ICP	intracranial pressure
ICS	intercostal space
ICU	intensive care unit
IDDM	insulin-dependent diabetes mellitus
IM	intramuscular
IO	interosseous
IOP	intra-ocular pressure
IPPV	intermittent positive pressure ventilation
IV	intravenous
JW	Jehovah's Witness
KCl	potassium chloride
L	lumbar vertebra
LA	local anaesthetic
LBBB	left bundle branch block
LD	loading dose
LFTs	liver function tests
LMA	laryngeal mask airway
LMWH	low molecular weight heparin
LV	left ventricle
min	minute

MAC	mean alveolar concentration (of anaesthetic drug in O_2 preventing movement in response to a painful stimulus in 50% of subjects)
MAP	mean arterial pressure
MCL	midclavicular line
MET	metabolic equivalent
MG	myasthenia gravis
MH	malignant hyperthermia
MI	myocardial infarction
MOA	monoamine oxidase
MRI	magnetic resonance imaging
N	Newton
NDNMBD	non-depolarising neuromuscular blocking drug
NG	nasogastric
NIDDM	non-insulin-dependent diabetes mellitus
NMS	neuroleptic malignant syndrome
NR	normal range
N/S	normal saline
NSAIDs	non-steroidal anti-inflammatory drugs
OCP	oral contraceptive pill
OSA	obstructive sleep apnoea
PA catheter	pulmonary artery catheter
PCA	patient-controlled analgesia
PCEA	patient-controlled epidural analgesia
PDPH	postdural puncture headache
PDE III	phosphodiesterase inhibiting (drugs)
PE	pulmonary embolus
PEA	pulseless electrical activity
PEEP	positive end-expiratory pressure
PEFR	peak expiratory flow rate

PONV	postoperative nausea and vomiting
PV	per vaginam
PVR	pulmonary vascular resistance
rFVIIa	recombinant activated Factor VII
Rh	Rhesus factor
RSI	rapid sequence induction
s	second
S	sacral
SA	sinoatrial node
SAB	subarachnoid block
SAH	subarachnoid haemorrhage
SB	sternal border
SBE	subacute bacterial endocarditis
SVC	superior vena cava
SVR	systemic vascular resistance
SVT	supraventricular tachycardia
T	thoracic vertebra
TBSA	total body surface area
TBV	total blood volume
TCP	transcutaneous cardiac pacing
TVA	total intravenous anaesthesia
TL/TR	therapeutic level/therapeutic range
TOE	transoesophageal echocardiography
U	units
UEC	urea, electrolytes and creatinine
URTI	upper respiratory tract infection
USA	United States of America
VF	ventricular fibrillation
VT	ventricular tachycardia
VTE	venous thromboembolism
WCC	white cell count

Aa

Abdominal Aortic Aneurysm Repair

Topics Covered in this Section
▶ Elective Open Abdominal Aneurysm Repair
▶ Endoluminal Abdominal Aortic Aneurysm Repair
▶ Ruptured Abdominal Aortic Aneurysm Repair

See also *THORACO ABDOMINAL AND THORACIC ANEURYSM REPAIR*.

Elective Open Abdominal Aortic Aneurysm (AAA) Repair

▶ *Morbidity and Mortality of Elective AAA Repair*

The overall mortality rate for elective surgery is about 2–5%, usually due to cardiac events such as myocardial infarction.[1] Peri-operative renal failure is another serious complication, usually due to acute tubular necrosis secondary to renal ischaemia.[2] The incidence of renal failure with infrarenal cross-clamping is 3–5% and up to 17% with suprarenal cross-clamping.[3]

▶ *Anaesthetic Aims*

1 Maintain optimal intravascular volume and cardiovascular stability throughout the peri-operative period.
2 Prepare for potentially massive blood loss.
3 Prevent/detect/treat myocardial ischaemia. Ischaemic heart disease is usually present.
4 Maintain renal function. There is often underlying renal disease.

▶ *Patient Assessment and Preparation Prior to the Day of Surgery*

1 Evaluate cardiovascular function and optimise management of cardiovascular disease. See *CARDIOVASCULAR PERI-OPERATIVE RISK PREDICTION FOR NON-CARDIAC SURGERY and CARDIO-VASCULAR INVESTIGATIONS.*

2 Organise pre-donated autologous blood or cross-matched homologous blood.

3 Consider commencing the patient on β blocker therapy such as atenolol to decrease the incidence of cardiac events in the first 6 months after surgery.[4] See *ATENOLOL.*

▶ *Pre-operative Management*

1 Prepare for potentially massive blood loss using such equipment as a cell saver, Alton Dean rapid infusion systems, rapid infusion device catheters and pulmonary artery catheter introducer sheaths. See *RAPID INFUSION CATHETER EXCHANGER SET and BLOOD LOSS ASSESSMENT AND INITIAL MANAGEMENT.*

2 Establish appropriate monitoring including arterial line, triple lumen central venous line or pulmonary artery catheter and 5 lead ECG monitoring with ST segment analysis (see *ST SEGMENT ANALYSIS*). Also monitor urine output and body temperature. Transoesophageal echocardiography has an increasingly important monitoring role.

3 Consider utilisation of a thoracic epidural sited at about the T8–9 level for intra-operative and postoperative analgesia.

4 Maintain body temperature with devices such as an upper body Bair Hugger. The *legs must not be actively warmed* while the aorta is clamped, as this will worsen the effects of leg ischaemia.

5 Prepare an infusion of glyceryl trinitrate (50 mg in 250 mL 5% glucose) to be used as a vasodilator.

▶ *Intra-operative Management up to the Time of Cross-clamping*

1 Aim for the smooth induction of anaesthesia with cardiovascular stability using, e.g. fentanyl, propofol or thiopentone and rocuronium.

2 Maintain anaesthesia with O_2, N_2O and isoflurane or sevoflurane.

3 Provide prophylactic antibiotic 'cover' such as cephazolin 1 g IV.

4 Initiate strategies to attempt to protect renal function, including the following:

(a) Maintain optimal intravascular volume.

(b) Give mannitol before cross-clamping. The optimal dose of mannitol is unclear from the literature but 10–25 g would appear to be reasonable.[5,6] Mannitol may be helpful by attenuating the reduction in renal cortical blood flow due to cross-clamping and reducing renal cell oedema due to ischaemia.[7] Its osmotic diuretic effects increase glomerular filtration rate which may help 'flush' tubular debris from nephrons, reducing tubular obstruction.[7] Mannitol may also be useful as a scavenger of oxygen free radicals.

(c) Frusemide may be of benefit by decreasing the resorption of solute, thus reducing cellular metabolic activity and giving some protection against cellular ischaemia. In addition frusemide may stimulate prostaglandin E_1 release, improving renal blood flow.[7]

(d) Although it has been suggested that dopamine has renal protective effects, there is no conclusive evidence that dopamine is useful for the prevention of renal failure.[8] Fenoldapam is a new, experimental highly selective dopamine 1 receptor agonist. This drug causes a significant increase in renal blood flow and decreases renal vascular resistance, and may be of use in aortic surgery in the near future.[2]

5 Give heparin prior to clamping of the aorta. Discuss the heparin dose with the surgeon.

6 Give sufficient IV fluid to maintain pulmonary capillary wedge pressure at 10–15 mmHg and a urine output of $\geq$ 60 mL/h.[7]

▶ *Physiological Effects of Aortic Cross-clamping*

These effects depend in part on how proximally the aorta is clamped. The haemodynamic responses include:

(a) an increase in systemic vascular resistance with increased left ventricular end diastolic wall stress

(b) increased mean arterial pressure

(c) no significant change in heart rate[3]

(d) increase in cardiac preload, especially with supracoeliac cross-clamping but it may decrease or not change.[7] This effect depends on several factors such as prevailing sympathetic tone.[7] With infracoeliac cross-clamping there are inconsistent effects on preload.[5] Compression of the inferior vena cava and other factors may interfere with blood volume redistribution and preload.

(e) probable increase in filling pressures (central venous pressure, pulmonary capillary wedge pressure) in patients with significant coronary artery disease, and decrease in patients without coronary artery disease[7]

(f) possible decrease in cardiac output and stroke volume

(g) increase in systemic vascular resistance and decrease in cardiac output with increased duration of aortic cross-clamping[3]

(h) a 75% increase in renovascular resistance and a 30% decrease in renal blood flow due to infrarenal cross-clamping.[3]

Strategies to Minimise the Physiological Effects of Cross-clamping

1 Aim for slightly reduced filling pressures for the half hour prior to clamp placement.[9]
2 Vasodilator therapy, e.g. glyceryl trinitrate (GTN) infusion, can reduce or reverse the decrease in cardiac output due to the increase in afterload resulting from cross-clamping.
3 GTN is particularly indicated if there is myocardial ischaemia or hypertension during cross-clamping.
4 If more aggressive afterload reduction is required, commence sodium nitroprusside.
5 If mean arterial pressure cannot be maintained, commence inotropic support. If impaired myocardial contractility is suspected, consider a dobutamine infusion.[10]
6 The greatest blood loss usually occurs at the time when the aneurysm is open and there is back bleeding from the lumbar arteries.[7]

Physiological Effects of Unclamping the Aorta

1 Systemic vascular resistance is suddenly decreased with a decrease in mean arterial pressure. Reactive hyperaemia of the lower body and washout of accumulated vasodilator substances contributes to the fall in mean arterial pressure. This effect begins after 10 s and a maximal response occurs 15 min after unclamping.[4]
2 Accumulation of myocardial depressant substances may occur.

Strategies to Minimise the Physiological Effects of Unclamping

1 Prior to unclamping, fluid load the patient to a central venous pressure (or pulmonary capillary wedge pressure) of ≈ 16 mmHg or at least slightly greater than pre-clamping pulmonary capillary wedge pressure.[9]

2   Replace blood loss appropriately. See *BLOOD LOSS ASSESSMENT AND INITIAL MANAGEMENT* and *BLOOD TRANSFUSION*.

3   Cease vasodilator therapy prior to unclamping.

4   Releasing the clamp gradually may allow for smoother cardiovascular control. Consider reapplying the clamp if sustained hypotension occurs. Inotropic support may be required.

Endoluminal Abdominal Aortic Aneurysm Repair

▶ *Preparation for Surgery*

Preparation for potentially massive blood loss must be made. Positioning on the operating table must be extremely precise and requires the assistance of the radiographer.

Anaesthetic requirements include:

1   rapid infusion catheter (7 or 8.5 Fr)

2   intra-arterial blood pressure monitoring

3   central line or pulmonary artery catheter insertion (recommended by some authors)[11]

4   5 lead ECG monitoring

5   urinary catheter, temperature probe

6   warming blanket over upper body.

▶ *Induction and Maintenance Phase*

1   Aim for cardiovascular stability as for an open procedure. Haemodynamic stability is significantly greater with endoluminal repair compared with open repair.[12]

2   The patient must be heparinised at the time of femoral or iliac artery instrumentation.

3   Stent grafts are usually self-expanding. Some require balloon dilatation to obtain an endo-seal. During the phase of balloon inflation or placement of the self-expanding graft, hypotension may be required.[11] This is to reduce the force pushing the stent distally. Hypotension can be achieved by increasing the inspired

concentration of sevoflurane, boluses of propofol, a glyceryl trinitrate infusion or use of a thoracic epidural.[11]

Ruptured Abdominal Aortic Aneurysm Repair

Between 30% and 60% of patients with ruptured abdominal aortic aneurysm die before reaching hospital.[13] Of the patients who survive to hospital admission, about 50% die in the peri-operative period.[14]

▶ *Principles of Management—Pre-anaesthetic Phase*

1   Transfer the patient to the operating theatre with minimal delay. Diagnostic procedures should be kept to a minimum. The aggressiveness of initial fluid resuscitation prior to surgery is a controversial issue.[13] Some clinicians argue that fluid resuscitation leads to more bleeding, and that a systolic BP of 50–70 mmHg should be accepted and maintained with minimum transfusion of blood or colloid.[14,15] Other researchers believe a more conventional approach should be taken, aiming for a mean blood pressure of around 65 mmHg.[13]

2   After ensuring a clear airway and ventilation the next priority is the insertion of several large bore IV cannulas so that adequate intravascular resuscitation can occur. See *BLOOD LOSS ASSESSMENT AND INITIAL MANAGEMENT—Anaesthesia in the Presence of Severe Blood Loss.*

3   Cross-match blood as soon as possible.

4   Obtaining intra-arterial blood pressure monitoring is the next priority. Other invasive pressure-monitoring devices can be placed after the aorta is clamped.

▶ *Induction and Maintenance of Anaesthesia*

1   Request that the surgeon surgically prepare and drape the patient prior to induction of anaesthesia. This is to minimise the time from anaesthesia to the application of the aortic clamp.

2   There is no evidence to support one choice of anaesthetic agent over another, as long as the drugs are used appropriately to

minimise cardiovascular instability.[13] A rapid sequence induction should be used but recommended induction agents include combinations of fentanyl, thiopentone (in small doses), etomidate and ketamine. One or more of these drugs is combined with a rapidly acting muscle relaxant such as rocuronium or suxamethonium. Rapid attainment of aortic cross-clamping is the next priority, to reduce haemorrhage. When bleeding is controlled and the patient stabilised, ongoing management is as described for elective repair.

See also *THORACOABDOMINAL AND THORACIC AORTIC ANEURYSM REPAIR.*

Abruptio Placentae

Description
This condition is defined as the separation of the placenta from its attachment to the decidua basalis prior to delivery of the foetus, resulting in haemorrhage. It occurs in 0.66% of deliveries[16] and accounts for 15–20% of all perinatal deaths.[17] About 90% of abruptions are mild to moderate and well tolerated by foetus and mother.

Symptoms and Signs
1   Severely painful unrelenting uterine contractions with incomplete uterine relaxation.
2   Non-reassuring foetal heart trace/foetal death.
3   Concealed or revealed blood loss, which may cause various degrees of shock.
4   Coagulopathy, DIC.

Anaesthetic Management
1   Ensure the patient has adequate airway and ventilation.
2   Resuscitate the patient's intravascular volume with appropriate fluids (crystalloid, colloid, blood). See *BLOOD LOSS ASSESSMENT AND INITIAL MANAGEMENT.*

3 Identify and treat coagulopathy.

4 Consider invasive monitoring such as CVP and direct arterial blood pressure measurement.

5 Aim for a urine output of 0.5–1 mL/kg/h and a haematocrit of 30%.

6 Delivery may be vaginal in mild cases, or in some cases of foetal death.

7 Epidural or spinal anaesthesia can be used cautiously in controlled situations where the patient is cardiovascularly stable and has been fully resuscitated, there is not significant foetal distress, and coagulopathy is not present.[17]

8 For patients with coagulopathy or uncontrolled haemorrhage or foetal distress, GA will usually be required.[18] See *CAESAREAN SECTION* (CS).

Activated Clotting Time (ACT)

Tests the intrinsic and common clotting pathways. Used for such purposes as monitoring heparin therapy during cardiac surgery. NR for ACT 90–120 s. For full heparinisation aim for ACT > 400 s, preferably > 500 s.

Activated Factor VIIa (NovoSeven)

See *RECOMBINANT ACTIVATED FACTOR VII.*

Activated Partial Thromboplastin Time (APTT)

Tests the intrinsic clotting pathway. NR 25–30 s. Prolonged APTT occurs with heparin therapy and a decrease in the activity of clotting factors V, X, XI, XII and fibrinogen. See *HEPARIN.*

Acute Dystonic Reaction

See *DYSTONIC REACTION, ACUTE.*

Acute Fatty Liver Of Pregnancy

See *FATTY LIVER OF PREGNANCY, ACUTE.*

Acute Intermittent Porphyria

See *PORPHYRIA.*

Adenosine

Adenosine is a naturally occurring purine nucleoside which is used therapeutically as an anti-arrhythmic and hypotensive drug. Adenosine acts mainly at the SA and AV nodes, by stimulating adenosine receptors. It causes reduced automaticity in the SA node and slowed conduction through the AV node.

Indications

1   Used for reverting paroxysmal supraventricular tachycardia (SVT) to sinus rhythm.
2   Useful in the management of supraventricular and broad complex tachycardia associated with Wolff-Parkinson-White syndrome.
3   Used to help diagnose supraventricular dysrhythmias by providing transient AV nodal block to enable the atrial rhythm to be clearly visualised on ECG.
3   Has also been used to provide temporary asystole. One report describes the use of adenosine 48 mg to provide asystole for 35 s to enable the repair of a massively bleeding ruptured subclavian artery.[19]

Dose in Adult for SVT

6 mg IV given as rapidly as possible, flushed through with 20 mL of N/S. If no effect after 2 min, give 12 mg, then 18 mg if SVT persists.[20] A brief period of asystole lasting up to 15 s is common.

Dose in Child for SVT

0.05 mg/kg IV, increase by 0.05 mg/kg every 2 min to a maximum of 0.25 mg/kg

Dose for Controlled Hypotension

40 µg/kg/min up to 500 µg/kg/min

Contraindications

Adenosine is contraindicated in patients with:

1 asthma
2 sick sinus syndrome and second and third degree heart block unless a pacemaker is present.

Notes

1 Adenosine may cause bronchospasm and profound bradycardia with ventricular excitability.
2 Patients on xanthines (e.g. theophylline) that block adenosine receptors may require an increased dose of adenosine.
3 Patients with denervated hearts, or who are taking dipyridamole or carbamazepine may have an exaggerated response to adenosine, and a reduced dose should be used.
4 The effects of adenosine last 20–30 s.

Adrenaline

Catecholamine sympathomimetic drug. Agonist at α and β adrenergic receptors. The degree of stimulation of the various receptors depends on the dose. In adults β-1 and β-2 actions predominate at doses less than 2 µg/min. α and β actions occur at doses 2–10 µg/min. Predominantly α actions occur at doses greater than 10 µg/min.

Indications

Adrenaline is used in the treatment of:

1 cardiac arrest
2 anaphylaxis
3 low cardiac output states
4 as a vasoconstrictor to reduce bleeding at the site of surgery and to increase the duration of local anaesthetic agents
5 to reduce upper-airway obstruction secondary to inflammation
6 bronchospasm.

Dose

▶ IV Infusion

Add 6 mg of adrenaline to 100 mL N/S (60 µg/mL). The usual dose range for inotropic support is 0.01–0.1 µg/kg/min. Start at 5 mL/h, titrate to clinical effect.

▶ IV Bolus Dose

Depends on the situation. Do not give a dose > 10 µg in an adult except in extremis.

▶ Adult Cardiac Arrest

1 mg IV boluses

▶ Paediatric Cardiac Arrest

10 µg/kg IV (0.1 mL/kg of 1:10 000 solution). If a second dose is required, give 100 µg/kg IV. See *CARDIAC ARREST*.

▶ Adult Anaphylaxis

0.1–0.5 mg IV boluses (≈ 1 mL of 1:10 000 solution) over 5 min or 0.3–0.5 mg IM if no IV access, or if anaphylaxis is not immediately life-threatening.

▶ Paediatric Anaphylaxis

5–10 µg/kg IV (0.05–0.1 mL/kg of 1:10 000 solution), or, if no IV
access, 10 µg/kg (0.01 mL/kg of 1:1000 adrenaline) IM. Repeat
dose 20 minutely × 3 if required.

See *ANAPHYLAXIS/ANAPHYLACTOID REACTIONS.*

Table A1 Rate of adrenaline infusion (6 mg in 100 mL N/S) in mL/h for 70 kg patient

Dose	mL/h
0.01 µg/kg/min	0.7
0.05 µg/kg/min	3.5
0.1 µg/kg/min	7

▶ Dose via Nebuliser

Useful for the treatment of croup and postextubation stridor.
Administer 0.5 mL/kg of 1:1000 adrenaline up to 5 mL.[21] 1 mg is
reported to be effective in the adult.[22]

▶ Adding Adrenaline to LA Solutions

For a solution containing 1:200 000 adrenaline, add 0.1 mL of
1:1000 solution (100 µg) to 20 mL of LA.

▶ Topical Adrenaline (Used as a Vasoconstrictor)

Use the 1:10 000 solution. Apply liberally to the site, e.g. to skin graft
donor site. There is very little systemic absorption of topical adrenaline.[23]

Note: Adrenaline is inactivated if mixed with sodium bicarbonate.

Adrenergic Receptors

These are divided into α1, α2, β1 and β2 adreno-receptors.

α1 Adreno-receptor Stimulation Effects

Positive inotropy and arterial and venous vasoconstriction.

α2 Adreno-receptor Stimulation Effects

1 Decreased noradrenaline release from sympathetic nerve endings (presynaptic action).
2 Decreased sympathetic outflow (central action).

β1 Adreno-receptor Stimulation Effects

1 Positive inotropy and chronotropy.
2 Increased renin release.

β2 Adreno-receptor Stimulation Effects

1 Vasodilatation of skeletal muscle, coronary and splanchnic vascular beds.
2 Relaxation of bronchial smooth muscle.
3 Insulin and glucagons secretion.

Air Embolism

See *GAS EMBOLISM, VENOUS*.

Airway Anaesthesia

See *AWAKE FIBRE-OPTIC INTUBATION*.

Airway Exchange Catheters (AEC)

Description

These devices are very useful for the following situations:

1 Trial of extubation in intubated patients who are difficult to intubate

2 Changing ET tubes in intubated patients who are difficult to intubate

AECs consist of long, narrow tubes with multiple openings at the tracheal end and a connection at the proximal end for jet ventilation, circuit ventilation or bag ventilation.

Directions for Use

1 Insert the airway exchange catheter through the endotracheal tube, aligning the distance markers.
2 Remove the proximal connector from the AEC.
3 Extubate the patient over the AEC, ensuring that the tip of the AEC remains well within the trachea.
4 If required, the patient can be oxygenated via the AEC either by providing supplementary oxygen to the spontaneously breathing patient or by jet ventilation in the paralysed patient.
5 If re-intubation is required, railroad an endotracheal tube over the AEC using optimal patient positioning and laryngoscopy to assist the intubation.[24]
6 If the tip of the endotracheal tube 'catches' at the level of the laryngeal inlet, rotate the ET tube 90° counterclockwise.[24]
7 There is a significant risk of barotrauma if jet ventilation is used.

Airway Fire

See *TRACHEOSTOMY, ELECTIVE.*

Airway Haemorrhage

See *HAEMOPTYSIS, MASSIVE.*

Albumin Solution

Intravenous colloid solution derived from pooled human plasma. It is sterilised by heat treatment and ultrafiltration, and the risk of disease transmission is extremely low.[25] A stabiliser such as sodium caprylate may be added. Albumin has a molecular weight of 69 000 (69 kDa) and is used for:

1   plasma volume expansion
2   treatment of hypoalbuminaemia
3   plasma exchange therapy.

Presented as a 4% solution and a 25% solution in isotonic saline. The 25% solution is hypotonic but hyperoncotic, and is used to provide albumin in situations where patients may be unable to cope with a fluid and/or electrolyte load, e.g. renal failure. The half-life of albumin in the plasma is > 24 h.

Note: Some studies have suggested that the use of human albumin solution in the resuscitation of critically ill patients is associated with an increased mortality.[26] However, the SAFE study reported that there was no increased morbidity with the use of 4% albumin for intravascular resuscitation of critically ill patients compared to N/S.[27]

Alfentanil

Potent short-acting opioid with a peak effect 1 min after injection. Duration of action ≈ 10 min.

Dose for Spontaneously Breathing Patient

7 µg/kg IV bolus, maintenance dose 2–3 µg/kg IV at 10–15 min intervals

IV Bolus and Infusion Dose for Controlled Ventilation Patients

Procedures lasting 10–30 min: 20–40 µg/kg
Procedures lasting 30–60 min: 40–80 µg/kg
For procedures lasting longer than 60 min, use an infusion of 0.5–1 µg/kg/min.

Dose for Reducing the Hypertensive Response to Intubation

20–50 µg/kg IV. Effects last 30–45 min. See *HYPERTENSIVE RESPONSE TO INTUBATION (ATTENUATION OF)*.

Allergic Reaction Prevention

Required for situations such as radiological contrast studies in patients with a history of allergy to contrast media. Although reactions cannot always be prevented, pretreatment does appear to reduce the incidence and severity of reactions.[28]

Suggested Drug Regime for Reducing Risk of Allergic Reaction

1   Prednisone 25 mg PO night before and morning of procedure.
2   Promethazine 25 mg PO night before and morning of procedure.
3   Cimetidine 400 mg PO the night before and the morning of procedure.

In Addition

Have equipment and drugs ready to deal with an allergic reaction. See *ANAPHYLAXIS/ANAPHYLACTOID REACTIONS*.

Note: Allergic reactions are more common with older ionic contrast agents compared with newer agents, and more common with venography compared to arteriography.

Aminophylline

Methylated xanthine derivative used to treat bronchospasm.

Loading Dose

5 mg/kg over 20 min followed by an infusion of 0.5 mg/kg/h. Mix 500 mg aminophylline with 500 mL N/S. For a 70 kg man give a bolus of 350 mL over 20 min, then run an infusion at 35 mL/h.

Note: Do not give a loading dose if the patient is on oral theo-phylline. TR 10–20 µg/mL.

Amiodarone

Iodinated benzofuran drug that is a predominantly class III anti-arrhythmic drug. The pharmacology of amiodarone is extremely complex. Amiodarone is useful for the treatment of

1 tachydysrhythmias, in particular recurrent ventricular tachy-cardia and fibrillation, atrial fibrillation and atrial flutter
2 ventricular fibrillation resistant to DC cardioversion. Amio-darone is currently the drug of choice for this indication.[29,30]

Dose for Treatment of Tachydysrhythmias Not Associated with Cardiac Arrest

▶ *IV Dose (Adult)*

5 mg/kg in 250 mL 5% glucose IV over 20 min to 2 h, then 10–15 mg/kg IV in 500 mL 5% glucose over 24 h. (Infusions of amio-darone over longer periods than 2 h must be contained in glass or polyofine bottles and a non-PVC giving set, because amiodarone absorbs to PVC.) Give preferably via a central line as the drug carrier is highly irritant. Amiodarone is not compatible with normal saline.

▶ *Oral Dose*

200–400 mg 8 h. After 1 week reduce the oral dose to 200–400 mg daily.

Dose for Shock Resistant VF or VT Associated with Cardiac Arrest or Pre-Arrest

▶ *IV Dose (Adult)*

300 mg in 20 mL 5% glucose IV bolus over 1–2 min. If the initial dose is ineffective give a second dose of 150 mg IV.

Precautions/contraindications

1 Patients on amiodarone given metoprolol or propranolol may suffer severe bradycardia, cardiac arrest or ventricular fibrillation.[31]

2 There is an increased risk of severe cardiac dysfunction including dysrhythmia for patients on amiodarone exposed to inhalational anaesthetic agents.[31]

3 Amiodarone is contraindicated in patients with iodine hypersensitivity, pregnancy or thyroid dysfunction.

Amniotic Fluid Embolus (AFE)

Pathophysiology

This syndrome is due to amniotic fluid components entering the maternal circulation and producing a potentially fatal reaction with severe hypoxia, cardiovascular collapse and coagulopathy. Both obstruction and vasoconstriction are thought to be present in the pulmonary vasculature. Mortality is high (> 80%)[32] with about 50% of deaths occuring in the first hour.[33] The incidence is between 1:8000 and 1:80 000 pregnancies. The diagnosis is a clinical one and other causes of sudden collapse, e.g. anaphylaxis, must be considered. There is no specific test for AFE although the presence of foetal squames in the pulmonary circulation/alveoli is suggestive. There are no specific risk factors for AFE except pregnancy itself.[34]

Clinical Manifestations

Most episodes of AFE occur during labour, particularly during the first stage.[34] Typically there is:

1 dyspnoea, bronchospasm, cyanosis
2 headache, loss of consciousness, seizure
3 disseminated intravascular coagulopathy and haemorrhage
4 hypotension, tachycardia
5 cardiopulmonary arrest.

If the patient survives the initial episode subsequent complications may include non-cardiogenic pulmonary oedema, renal failure and permanent brain damage.

Management

Treatment involves the following:

1 protecting the airway and optimising ventilation
2 maintaining intravascular volume with appropriate fluids including blood
3 providing circulatory support with inotropes
4 correct coagulopathy (see *DISSEMINATED INTRAVASCULAR COAGULATION (DIC)*).
5 See also *CARDIAC ARREST*.
6 Deliver the foetus immediately if resuscitation is not successful within 5 minutes. This is in the best interest of the patient and foetus.

Amrinone

Bipyridine derivative phosphodiesterase III inhibitor useful for its positive inotropic and vasodilator actions. It is indicated for the treatment of low cardiac output states of cardiac cause.

Dose

Mix 100 mg in 250 mL N/S (not glucose). Give LD of 750 µg/kg ($\approx$ 130 mL in 70 kg patient). Follow this with an infusion of 5–20 µg/kg/min ($\approx$ 50–200 mL/h in 70 kg patient).

Advantages

1 Cardiac output increases without a significant increase in myocardial O_2 consumption. There is little increase in heart rate.
2 Amrinone has positive lusiotropic effects (aids myocardial relaxation).

3 Amrinone's pulmonary vasodilator action is useful in the setting of pulmonary hypertension and right ventricular failure.

Disadvantages

1 Vasodilation may result in hypotension.
2 Amrinone can cause thrombocytopenia if used for more than 24 h, due to the metabolite n-acetyl amrinone.
3 High doses may cause tachycardia.

Anaphylaxis/Anaphylactoid Reactions

Topics Covered in this Section
▶ Pathophysiology
▶ Clinical Manifestations
▶ Treatment: First Line Therapy
▶ Treatment: Second Line Therapy
▶ Investigations
▶ Special Points

Pathophysiology

Anaphylaxis (Type 1 hypersensitivity reaction) results from an IgE mediated degranulation of mast cells and basophils in response to a triggering agent such as a drug. These cells release vasoactive subtances, histamine being the most important. The pathophysiological basis of anaphylactoid reactions is less clear. An offending substance such as a drug causes degranulation of mast cells and basophils through a non-immunological mechanism. The clinical manifestations of anaphylactoid and anaphylactic reactions are indistinguishable and the treatment is identical. The incidence of anaphylaxis is about 1:6000–1:20 000 anaesthetics.[35] Anaphylaxis is most frequently due to muscle relaxants (69%), especially suxamethonium and rocuronium.[36],[37] Vecuronium and pancuronium are the next most frequent, followed by atracurium.[35] Antibiotics account for about 8% of anaphylactic reactions under anaesthesia.[37] Latex is the second most common cause of anaphylaxis after NMBDs (12.1%).[37]

Clinical Manifestations

These reactions range from being mild to fatal and are associated with:

1   rash, erythema
2   soft tissue swelling (with potential airway compromise)
3   bronchospasm
4   hypotension and circulatory collapse
5   cardiac arrest.

Treatment: First Line Therapy

1   Eliminate possible initiating substance, e.g. stop blood transfusion, remove contact with latex.
2   Ensure adequate airway and ventilation. Emergency intubation may be required.
3   Notify the surgeon and discontinue surgery and anaesthesia if feasible.
4   *Adrenaline* is the drug treatment of choice. It is indicated in patients with circulatory compromise, airway swelling and/or breathing difficulties. For life-threatening anaphylaxis administer adrenaline intravenously if IV access is immediately available.[38]

    Adult dose: Give 50–100 µg IV over 5 min. Give higher doses if the patient is in extremus (0.1–0.5 mg). If ongoing adrenaline is required, commence an adrenaline infusion (6 mg in 100 mL N/S). See *ADRENALINE*. If IV access is not available or the reaction is not immediately life-threatening, give 0.3–0.5 mg IM, repeating after 5–10 min if required.[38]

Paediatric dose: 5–10 µg/kg IV (0.05–0.1 mL/kg of 1:10 000 adrenaline) or 10 µg/kg IM (0.01 mL/kg of 1:1000 adrenaline). Repeat dose 20 minutely × 3 if required.

A noradrenaline infusion should be added to adrenaline if adrenaline alone is ineffective.[39]

Patients on β blocker drugs may be resistant to adrenaline. Adrenaline dosages may need to be increased or other inotropes added.[37]

5 *Intravenous fluids*: give IV N/S if hypotension is present. Large volumes may be required (2–4 L).[38] Colloids (e.g. gelatin solutions) can be used in addition to, or instead of, crystalloids but there is no evidence of improved outcome.[39]

6 If the patient becomes pulseless initiate external cardiac compression regardless of ECG rhythm.
See *CARDIAC ARREST*.

7 Treat bronchospasm (see *BRONCHOSPASM*).

8 *Glucagon. Adult dose*: 1–2 mg IV every 5 min may be of benefit in patients unresponsive to adrenaline.[38]

9 Histamine 2 receptor (H_2) blocking drugs, e.g. cimetidine 300 mg PO, IM or IV, may be helpful in protracted anaphylaxis.

Treatment: Second Line Therapy

1 *Promethazine*: 0.2 mg/kg IV ($\approx$ 20–50 mg, max. 100 mg), or other suitable antihistamine drug.

2 *Hydrocortisone*: For an adult give 200 mg every 6 h (child— 10 mg/kg).

Organise ongoing management in the ICU.

Investigations

1 Serum tryptase 1 h after the reaction. The normal value is 5 µg/L and an elevated value (> 25 µg/L) is strongly indicative of an anaphylactic reaction having occurred.[37]

2 Refer to an appropriate clinic for further testing after a period of 4 weeks. Useful investigations at this time include:
   (a) skin tests (intradermal and prick tests)
   (b) allergen-specific IgE testing (RAST).
   The aim of testing is to identify which drugs are 'safe' or 'unsafe'. The patient should carry a relevant letter and should wear a 'MedicAlert' bracelet. Information should be added to the letter each time the patient has an anaesthetic or other relevant drug for the first time.

Special Points

1 Patients on histamine 2 receptor blocking drugs such as ranitidine may suffer A–V node block in the presence of massive histamine release.

2 Anaphylactic shock may be exacerbated in patients on β receptor blocker drugs, which increase histamine release.

3 In patients who die from presumed anaphylaxis, serum tryptase and detection of drug reactive IgE antibodies in blood taken after death can help confirm or exclude diagnosis of an allergic reaction.[40]

Ankle Blocks and Innervation of the Foot

The foot is innervated almost entirely by the sciatic nerve, except for the skin on the medial side of the lower leg and foot and the arch of the sole. These areas are innervated by the saphenous nerve. This is a branch of posterior division of the femoral nerve. Sciatic branches are the:

1 *sural nerve*, which supplies the skin on the back of the lower leg and lateral foot

2 *medial plantar nerve*, which innervates the skin on the medial sole of the foot and the plantar surface of first three and a half toes

3   *lateral plantar nerve*, which supplies the lateral sole
4   *superficial peroneal nerve*, which supplies the medial side of the great toe and most of the dorsum of the foot
5   *deep peroneal nerve*, which innervates the skin between the great and second toe.

Ankle Block Technique

Requires five separate injection sites.

▶ *1 Tibial Nerve Block*

This nerve is also referred to as the medial popliteal or posterior tibial nerve. It gives rise to the medial and lateral plantar nerves and the medial calcaneal nerve. The nerve runs behind the medial malleolus, crossing the posterior tibial artery posteriorly.

(a) Place the patient prone with the ankle supported on a pillow. Insert a 22 G needle, just behind the pulsation of the posterior tibial artery. The nerve lies adjacent to the artery. Direct the needle 45° anteriorly, seeking paraesthesia in the sole of the foot.[41]

(b) If paraesthesia is obtained inject 5 mL of LA (e.g. lignocaine 2%). If paraesthesia is not obtained, inject 10 mL of LA in a fan-like pattern between the posterior tibial artery and the achilles tendon.

▶ *2 Sural Nerve Block*

The nerve runs behind lateral malleolus. Insert the needle into the groove between the lateral malleolus and the calcaneus. Inject 5 mL of LA.

▶ *3 Saphenous Nerve Block*

This nerve runs in front of the medial malleolus. Infiltrate LA around the long saphenous vein just anterior to the medial malleolus.

▶ *4 Deep Peroneal Nerve Block*

Insert the needle just lateral to the anterior tibial artery (which continues on as the dorsalis pedis artery) at the distal end of the tibia at the level of the skin crease. Inject 5 mL of LA.

▶ *5 Superficial Peroneal Nerve Block*
Infiltrate a ridge of LA from the anterior tibia to lateral malleolus, using ≈ 10 mL of LA.

Anticholinergic Crisis

See *MYASTHENIA GRAVIS.*

Anticholinergic Syndrome

See *CENTRAL ANTICHOLINERGIC SYNDROME.*

Anticoagulation Therapy and Surgery

Topics Covered in this Section
▶ Patients with a history of deep venous thrombosis/pulmonary embolus
▶ Patients with a history of acute arterial embolism within 1 month of surgery
▶ Patients at risk of acute arterial embolism without mechanical heart valves
▶ Patients with mechanical heart valves
▶ Patients with recurrent DVT/PE
▶ Warfarin and emergency surgery
▶ Warfarin and minor surgery
▶ Anticoagulant therapy and regional anaesthesia

The following recommendations are based on balancing the risk of peri-operative anticoagulation with the risk of thromboembolism.[42] Patients on warfarin fall into three main groups:

1   patients with a history of deep venous thrombosis/pulmonary embolus
2   patients with atrial fibrillation ± arterial embolism, e.g. CVA
3   patients with mechanical heart valves.

The anticoagulant management of these patients on warfarin is discussed by dividing them into the categories described below.

Patients with Deep Venous Thrombosis/Pulmonary Embolus

In patients on warfarin *without* DVT or PE within *3 months of surgery*:

1   Cease warfarin 4 days before surgery. Use subcutaneous heparin or low molecular weight heparin (LMWH) in prophylactic doses. See *DEEP VENOUS THROMBOSIS (DVT) PROPHYLAXIS*.

2   Measure INR on the day before surgery. If INR < 1.5, it is safe to proceed with surgery. If INR > 1.5 consider giving vitamin K 1 mg IV. This will take 8–12 h to be effective. See *WARFARIN*.

3   Recommence warfarin without a loading dose on the evening after surgery, or the next day, and continue prophylactic doses of heparin subcutaneously until the patient is fully warfarinised.

In patients on warfarin *with* a history of DVT or PE *within 1 month of surgery*:

1   Surgery should be avoided in the first month after DVT/PE but, if this is not possible, admit the patient and cease warfarin therapy.

2   When INR < 2.0 fully heparinise the patient. Keep the APTT > 2–3 × normal (APTT NR = 25–30 s). Alternatively use LMWH in full anticoagulation doses, i.e. enoxaparin sodium (Clexane) 1 mg/kg or dalteparin sodium (Fragmin) 100 U/kg 12 h.

3   Cease the heparin infusion 6–8 h before surgery, or give the last dose of LMWH at least 24 h before surgery.

4   Recommence the heparin infusion no sooner than 24 h after major surgery and even longer if the risk of bleeding is considered high. Recommence the heparin infusion *without a bolus*, at

the expected maintenance infusion rate. See *HEPARIN, UNFRAC-TIONATED AND LOW MOLECULAR WEIGHT HEPARINS*. If LMWH is used do not recommence until at least 24 h after surgery and even longer if the risk of bleeding is high.

5   Continue heparin or LMWH until resumption of warfarin therapy and INR > 2.

In patients on warfarin for a DVT or PE between more than 1 month but less than 3 months before surgery:

1   Cease warfarin 4 days before surgery. When INR < 2.0 give prophylactic doses of heparin or LMWH.

2   Postoperatively anticoagulate the patient as for DVT or PE within 1 month of surgery.

Patients with a History of Acute Arterial Embolism Within 1 Month of Surgery

For patients on warfarin for acute arterial embolism (e.g., patients with AF and CVA) within 1 month of surgery:

1   Elective surgery should not be undertaken.

2   For urgent surgery cease warfarin. When INR is < 2.0 fully heparinise the patient or give LMWH in full anticoagulation doses.

3   Cease heparin infusion or full dose LMWH prior to surgery as described above for DVT/PE within 1 month of surgery.

4   Postoperatively recommence full heparin/LMWH anticoagulation when it is safe to do so and restart oral warfarin.

Patients at Risk of Acute Arterial Embolism Without Mechanical Heart Valves

This group includes patients with atrial fibrillation on prophylactic warfarin. These patients do not require pre- or postoperative full heparinisation therapy. Treat as for patients with history of no DVT/PE within 3 months prior to surgery (including the use of subcutaneous prophylactic heparin).

Patients with Mechanical Heart Valves

If these patients have not had an acute arterial embolism within the last month, neither pre- nor postoperative full dose heparinisation is required. Treat as for patients on warfarin without DVT/PE within 3 months of surgery including the use of prophylactic doses of heparin or LMWH.

Patients with Recurrent DVT/PE

Unless DVT/PE within the last 3 months, treat as for patients with mechanical heart valves.

Warfarin and Emergency Surgery

See *WARFARIN*.

Warfarin and Minor Emergency

In many cases patients having minor surgery can be left on their usual warfarin therapy without interruption. These procedures include tooth extractions and cutaneous surgery.[43,44]

Anticoagulant Therapy and Regional Anaesthesia

See *EPIDURAL ANAESTHESIA, Anticoagulant Therapy and Epidurals.*

Aortic Valve Incompetence (Chronic)

Chronic aortic valve incompetence (AI) is usually much better tolerated than aortic valve stenosis. Chronic AI results in left ventricular dilatation and hypertrophy, eventually leading to left ventricular failure with reduced exercise tolerance and dyspnoea. An ejection fraction of < 55% and atrial fibrillation are associated with increased risk of cardiac morbidity and mortality.[45]

Management Aims During Anaesthesia
(Chronic AI only)

1   Avoid bradycardia as this can result in acute left ventricular overload. A mild tachycardia may be beneficial.

2 Avoid increases in systemic vascular resistance, which can result in an increase in the regurgitant fraction and left ventricular failure. Afterload reduction may be beneficial.

3 Maintain myocardial contractility. Avoid drugs that are myocardial depressants.

4 Give appropriate antibiotic prophylaxis to prevent bacterial endocarditis.

See *BACTERIAL ENDOCARDITIS PROPHYLAXIS*.

Aortic Valve Stenosis (AS)

Aortic stenosis results in a fixed resistance to left ventricular ejection and left ventricular hypertrophy. Severe valvular heart disease is a major predictor of significant cardiovascular risk for non-cardiac surgery.[46] Patients with suspected severe aortic stenosis should be referred to a cardiologist for assessment and/or aortic valve replacement. However, several studies have shown that patients with even severe AS tolerate non-cardiac surgery reasonably well, with a lower mortality than that quoted for aortic valve replacement (which is ≈ 4%).[47]

Clinical Picture

Symptoms include:

1 dyspnoea, especially on exertion

2 angina due to the hypertrophied myocardium being vulnerable to ischaemia

3 syncope, usually with effort, due to the heart being unable to maintain adequate output and blood pressure during the period of vasodilatation associated with exercise

4 sudden death.

Examination and Investigation Findings

1 A pulse pressure < 30 mmHg suggests severe disease.

2 CXR may show left atrial enlargement and dilatation of the

aortic root. Pulmonary oedema can occur acutely.

3 ECG may show LV hypertrophy, LV strain pattern and LBBB.

4 Echocardiography will help evaluate disease severity through measurement of parameters such as valve area and transvalvular pressure gradient (see Table A2).

Table A2 Aortic valve area as an indication of AS severity[48]	
Severity of AS	Aortic valve area
Normal valve area	2.5–3.5 cm^2
Mild AS	> 1.5 cm^2
Moderate AS	0.8–1.5 cm^2
Severe AS	< 0.7 cm^2

A transvalvular pressure gradient across the aortic valve greater than 50 mmHg is consistent with severe disease. A transvalvular gradient of < 20 mmHg indicates mild disease.

Management Aims During Anaesthesia

1 Maintain sinus rhythm to preserve the contribution of atrial contraction to preload. Always have a defibrillator immediately available.

2 Ensure adequate preload and maintain normovolaemia.

3 Maintain systemic vascular resistance as a decrease may result in a decreased mean arterial pressure with decreased coronary blood flow and subsequent myocardial depression. A vicious cycle can thus be created as myocardial depression leads to further decreases in coronary blood flow and cardiac output.

4 Avoid bradycardia, which may result in decreased cardiac output and overdistension of the left ventricle.

5 Avoid tachycardia, which can result in decreased left ventricular filling and ejection.

6 Consider invasive monitoring, including use of an arterial line and a PA catheter. CVP measurement may be an unreliable measure of preload in patients with reduced left ventricular compliance.

7 Give appropriate antibiotic prophylaxis to prevent bacterial endocarditis. See *BACTERIAL ENDOCARDITIS PROPHYLAXIS*.

8 Treat hypotension with a vasoconstrictor agent. Use ephedrine if heart rate is low or metaraminol if heart rate is high.

9 If cardiac arrest occurs, external heart massage may be ineffective and internal heart massage should be considered early.

Aortic Stenosis and Obstetric Anaesthesia

Management of obstetric patients with aortic stenosis is a complex issue and must be individually tailored to each patient. Ideally a multidisciplinary approach should be instituted with the involvement of obstetricians, cardiologists and anaesthetists, and with progressive assessment of the patient's cardiac function throughout pregnancy. The issue of whether regional anaesthesia or general anaesthesia is used is highly debatable.[49,50] The skill and experience of the anaesthetist, rather than the type of anaesthetic, is the critical factor.

Apgar Score

See *NEONATAL RESUSCITATION*.

Aprotinin

Naturally occurring serine protease inhibitor which inhibits trypsin, plasmin and plasma and tissue kallikreins, thus inhibiting fibrinolysis and promoting haemostasis. It is the most potent of the antifibrinolytic drugs.[51]

Uses

Reduction of blood loss during operations such as in cardiac,[52] orthopaedic,[53] vascular, liver and prostate surgery.

Dose

▶ *Adult*

Loading dose $1–2 \times 10^6$ kallikrein inhibition units (KIU) IV slowly, followed by an infusion of $0.25–0.5 \times 10^6$ KIU/h until the bleeding stops.

Arrow MAC 2 Lumen Central Venous Access Device

The MAC is a 2 lumen central venous access kit from Arrow International. The device provides multilumen, large bore, central venous access and is inserted in an identical way to a pulmonary artery catheter introducer sheath, using a Seldinger technique. The distal lumen of the MAC is 9 Fr and there are two large side lumens of 12 G each. A MAC-compatible triple lumen central line can be passed through the MAC and locked into place with a luer lock fitting. Alternatively a PA catheter can also be inserted through the MAC.

Arterial Blood Gas (ABG) Analysis

NR of Arterial Blood Gas Values

pH	7.36–7.44
PaO_2	85–100 mmHg (11.3–13.3 kPa)
$PaCO_2$	36–44 mmHg (4.8–5.9 kPa)
Bicarbonate*	22–26 mmol/L
Standard bicarbonate†	22–26 mmol/L
Base excess‡	0 ± 4

*This is the plasma bicarbonate concentration calculated from the pH and pCO_2 values using the Henderson Hasselbalch equation.

†This is the bicarbonate concentration when $PaCO_2 = 40$ mmHg and the blood is fully oxygenated at 37°C.

‡Defined as the amount of strong acid needed to titrate 1 L of fully saturated blood at 37°C to a pH of 7.4 when the $PaCO_2$ is 40 mmHg.

'Rules of Thumb' for ABG Interpretation[54]

1 If $PaO_2 + PaCO_2 > 140$ mmHg the patient is receiving supplemental oxygen.

2 PaO_2 decreases with age:

$$PaO_2 \approx 100 - \frac{age}{3}$$

3 With a respiratory acidosis, for every 10 mmHg increase in $PaCO_2$, bicarbonate increases by 1 mmol/L acutely and by 3–4 mmol/L chronically.

4 With a respiratory alkalosis, bicarbonate decreases by 2.5 mmol/L per 10 mmHg fall in $PaCO_2$, down to a minimum of 18 mmol/L.

Table A3 Direction of changes in pH, $PaCO_2$ and bicarbonate in certain pathological conditions

Pathological state	pH	$PaCO_2$	Bicarbonate	BE
Metab acidosis	↓	↓	↓	-ve
Metab alkalosis	↑	↑	↑	+ve
Resp acidosis	↓	↑	↑	+ve
Resp alkalosis	↑	↓	↓	-ve

5 With a metabolic acidosis, the $PaCO_2$ is usually within ± 5 mmHg of the last two digits of the pH value down to a pH of 7.15.

6 In a metabolic alkalosis, the $PaCO_2$ is usually within ± 5 mmHg of the last two digits of the pH value up to a pH value of 7.60.

Arterial Injection

See *INTRA-ARTERIAL INJECTION*.

ASA (American Society Of Anesthesiologists) Grading[55]

I   Healthy patient
II   Mild systemic illness
III Severe systemic illness that is not incapacitating
IV   Severe systemic illness which is a constant threat to life
V   Patient moribund and unlikely to survive 24 h with or without surgery
E   Emergency surgery
T   Trauma

Aspiration, Prevention and Treatment

Patients at Risk

1 Pregnant patient. Aspiration risk may begin as early as 12th week and continues until 2–3 days postdelivery. See *PREGNANCY AND NON-OBSTETRIC SURGERY—ANAESTHETIC CONSIDERATIONS*.

2 Obese patients. See *BODY MASS INDEX AND OBESITY*.

3 Patient with history of reflux and/or hiatus hernia.

4 Patient with a full, or potentially full, stomach due to such situations as:

(a) inadequate pre-operative fasting. See *FASTING PRE-OPERA-TIVELY*.

(b) less than 6 h between the time of a significant injury (e.g. limb bone fracture) and time of last solid food

(c) emergency abdominal surgery.

5 Many other pre-existing illnesses, such as burns and decreased level of consciousness, can predispose to aspiration.

Strategies to Prevent Aspiration and/or Minimise its Effects

1 Adequate fasting pre-operatively. See *FASTING PRE-OPERATIVELY*.

2 Ranitidine 150 mg PO the night before and the morning of surgery.

3 Sodium citrate 0.3 M 30 mL PO 'on call' to operating theatre.

4 Consider metoclopramide 10 mg IV or IM to increase the rate of gastric emptying and increase lower oesophageal sphincter tone.

5 Placement of a nasogastric tube and sucking out of gastric contents prior to induction of anaesthesia. This is strongly recommended in patients with intestinal obstruction and/or abdominal distension.

6 Use of 'rapid sequence induction' technique. See *RAPID SEQUENCE INDUCTION*.

7 Extubate patient in the lateral position when the patient is 'awake' and able to protect his or her own airway.

Management of Aspiration

This is a life-threatening emergency.

1 Put patient immediately in left lateral position with 30° of head down tilt ('tilt and turn') and vigorously suck out the pharynx and larynx. Apply cricoid pressure immediately unless patient is actively vomiting. See *RAPID SEQUENCE INDUCTION*.

2   Intubate the patient and suck out the trachea with 'Y' catheter suction tube (the appropriate size suction catheter = 2 × the ET tube internal diameter).

3   Do not allow the patient to desaturate during suctioning. Ventilate with 100% oxygen.

4   If there is clinical/radiological evidence of airway obstruction by aspirated material, perform bronchoscopy and remove the obstruction. Bronchial lavage may be helpful.

5   Decide whether:
    (a) aspiration is significant or not. The lower the pH of the aspirate and the greater the volume, the greater the potential for lung injury. Patients are at risk if pH of aspirate < 2.5 and volume aspirated is > 25 mL.[56]
    (b) Decide whether surgery should be abandoned.
    (c) If surgery is abandoned, or at the time surgery is completed, decide whether patient should remain intubated or should be extubated.

6   Anticipate/treat bronchospasm. See *BRONCHOSPASM*.

7   Give antibiotics if there is aspiration of feculent material, otherwise only give antibiotics if evidence of infection (fever, leukocytosis) develops. For contaminated aspirate consider penicillin or clindamycin, plus gentamicin ± metronidazole.[57,58]

8   Insert a nasogastric tube and empty the stomach.

9   Commence/continue antacid therapy (e.g. H_2 blocker drug).

10 In patients who have aspirated and who are to remain intubated and ventilated, consider early application of PEEP.[58]

Asthma

Pre-operative Preparation of the Asthmatic Patient

1   Optimise the patient's antiasthma medication and continue therapy up to the time of surgery.

2 If the patient is asymptomatic, tests of respiratory function are usually not required. If the patient is suffering from an acute exacerbation of their asthma, elective surgery should be postponed because of the increased anaesthetic risk.[57] If optimal condition of the patient is in doubt, or the patient has moderate to severe asthma, lung function tests are indicated. The most helpful are spirometry, in particular forced expiratory volume in 1 second (FEV_1), forced vital capacity (FVC), peak expiratory flow rate (PEFR), and arterial blood gas analysis. For adults, a PEFR of < 120 L/min, FEV_1 of < 1 L, and hypercapnia are indicative of severe disease.[60,61] With severe asthma, FEV_1 will usually be less than 50% of FVC.

3 If the patient has been on steroid therapy for a significant period of time, steroids must be continued and extra steroid dosage given to cover the stress of surgery. See *STEROID 'COVER'*. For patients with moderate to severe asthma, consider initiating a course of steroid therapy to cover the peri-operative period, e.g. *prednisone* 40 mg daily started 3 days prior to surgery, or *hydrocortisone* 1–3 mg/kg IV daily.[62]

4 Cancel elective surgery if the patient is suffering from an acute URTI or chest infection. Wait for 2–3 weeks after clinical recovery before elective surgery.[63]

5 Always consider regional anaesthesia.

Premedication

If premedication is required consider pethidine and promethazine ± a bronchodilator. Avoid histamine-releasing drugs and, at least on theoretical grounds, histamine 2 receptor antagonists such as cimetidine.[64]

Induction

Suitable drugs include propofol and ketamine. Thiopentone may cause increased airway constriction.[61] Prior to intubation, the patient should be deeply anaesthetised. Consider lignocaine 1–2 mg/kg IV to help prevent bronchoconstriction.[63] Topical lignocaine is not effective and may induce bronchoconstriction in asthmatics.[65] Avoid intubation if possible. LMA is tolerated much better than intubation in asthmatics.[66]

Maintenance

Sevoflurane, isoflurane and halothane cause bronchodilation. Sevoflurane is probably the inhalational agent of choice.[64] Desflurane can cause bronchoconstriction and should be avoided in the asthmatic.[64] Use a non-histamine-releasing neuromuscular blocking drug such as rocuronium.

Treatment of Intra–operative Bronchospasm

See *BRONCHOSPASM*.

Emergency

Extubate the patient 'deep' if possible. If patient must be extubated awake consider lignocaine 1–2 mg/kg IV 5 minutes before extubation.

Postoperative Management

1 Restart patient's anti-asthma therapy as soon as possible after surgery.
2 Consider chest physiotherapy, e.g. incentive spirometry.

Analgesic Considerations

▶ *Opioids*

It is probably preferable to use non-histamine-releasing opioids such as fentanyl.[60] Morphine does cause some histamine release and is traditionally avoided.[61] All opioid drugs may cause respiratory depression.

▶ *Non-steroidal Anti-inflammatory Drugs (NSAIDs)*

An acute exacerbation of asthma can be precipitated by NSAIDs, especially in patients who are hypersensitive to aspirin.[67]

Note: Do not give asthmatic patients β blockers or aspirin.

Atenolol

Selective β1 adreno-receptor blocker useful for the treatment of hypertension, angina and tachydysrhythmias. The routine use of atenolol (or other β blockers) in patients at risk of cardiac complications may significantly reduce the cardiac-related morbidity and mortality associated with major surgery.[4] *Manufacture of IV atenolol in Australia ceased in June 2003*. At the time of writing IV atenolol is still being manufactured in the USA.

Dose for Hypertension

▶ *Adult*

2.5–10 mg IV. Give in 1 mg/min increments.

Oral dose: 50–100 mg/day

▶ *Child*

0.05 mg/kg/dose IV every 5 min until desired response, maximum of 4 doses.

Oral dose: 1–2 mg/kg 12–24 h.

▶ *Dose for Reduction of Cardiac Mortality Peri-operatively in 'At Risk' Patients*

5–10 mg IV 30 min before induction and in the recovery room postoperatively. Then give 50–100 mg 12 h for 1 week. Withhold atenolol if bronchospasm, cardiac failure, 3° heart block, heart rate < 55 bpm or systolic blood pressure < 99 mmHg.[4]

Atracurium

Bisquaternary non-depolarising neuromuscular blocking drug with an intermediate duration of action. Main features include minimal cardiovascular effects (can cause some hypotension due to hista-mine release).

Degrades spontaneously due to Hofmann degradation. Can be used in the presence of liver/renal failure.

Dose
0.3–0.5 mg/kg IV lasts ≈ 20–25 min; for subsequent doses give 0.15 mg/kg, lasts ≈ 20 min.

Infusion Dose
0.5 mg/kg/h (titrate infusion rate to twitch response). Stop infusion ≈ 10 min before planned emergence.

Note: Accumulation of the metabolite laudanosine with prolonged use of atracurium (days) can potentially result in seizures.[68]

Atrial Fibrillation (AF), Acute
Identify and Treat Cause if Possible
The most common causes are:[69]
1 ischaemic and valvular heart disease
2 hypertension
3 thyrotoxicosis
4 pneumonia
5 electrolyte and acid base disturbances

Patients Requiring Immediate Treatment
These can be defined as patients with heart rate > 150 bpm, chest pain or evidence of shock.[70] Cardioversion may also be required urgently if there is severe aortic stenosis or hypertrophic cardio-pathy.
1 Seek urgent expert assistance.
2 Heparinise the patient.
3 Provide DC cardioversion under sedation or anaesthesia.[70] If a monophasic defibrillator is used, give 25–100 J initially.

The shock must be synchronised with the QRS complex. Up to 200 J may be required. Biphasic defibrillation is more effective than monophasic shock and requires less energy.[71] Start with 70–100 J.

4 Correct possible causes or exacerbating factors, e.g. hypokalaemia.

5 If cardioversion fails or AF recurs, give amiodarone. See *AMIODARONE*.

6 Repeat cardioversion after amiodarone and if this is not successful or AF recurs consider a second dose of amiodarone.

Patients Not Requiring Immediate Treatment Known To Have AF < 24 h

Seek expert advice. Patients without CVS compromise can be treated with:

1 heparin ± warfarin

2 amiodarone for rate control and chemical cardioversion (flecainide 100–150 mg over 30 min is an alternative[70]).

Consider DC cardioversion if chemical cardioversion is unsuccessful or the patient may suffer eventual compromise from AF. Do not cardiovert if there is digoxin toxicity or a history of sick sinus syndrome or bradycardia.[69]

Patients Known To Have AF > 24 h

Treat patients with suboptimal perfusion or structural heart disease with:

1 heparinisation

2 amiodarone

3 DC cardioversion in 3–4 weeks. Do not cardiovert without either 3 weeks of anticoagulation or exclusion of intracardiac thrombus by transoesophageal echocardiography. Continue anticoagulation for 4 weeks after successful cardioversion.

Low risk patients can be treated as follows:

1 If ventricular rate is 100–150, provide rate control with β blockers or verapamil or diltiazem.
2 Treat with heparinisation, warfarin and DC cardioversion in 3–4 weeks (or earlier after intracardiac clot excluded by TOE) as described above. Consider chemical cardioversion with e.g. amiodarone but with the same precautions as for electrical cardioversion.

Atrial Fibrillation, Chronic

For patients with chronic AF the aim is to control ventricular response either chronically or acutely. The optimal ventricular rate for patients in AF is 90 bpm.[69]

Therapy for Slowing Ventricular Response to AF

▶ *Digoxin*

Oral dose adult: Give loading dose of 0.5–1 mg, followed by 0.25–0.5 mg every 6 h to a maximum dose of 1.5–2 mg in the first 24 h. Usual maintenance dose in adult is 62.5–250 µg/day depending on such factors as age and renal function.[72]

IV dose adult: Loading dose 500 µg over 30 min, repeat after 6 h if required. Give up to ≈ 20 µg/kg total LD.

Oral dose child: 15 µg/kg loading dose, then 5 µg/kg dose 12 h.

IV dose child: 15 µg/kg over 30 min, then 5 µg/kg 6 h later, then 5 µg/kg dose 12 h.

Note: Peak effect occurs at ≈ 2 h. TR 1–2 ng/mL.

▶ *Verapamil*

Adult: 1 mg/min IV to a total dose of 15 mg.

▶ *β blocker*

E.g. esmolol or metoprolol (see entries).

▶ *Anticoagulation with warfarin*

Anticoagulation with warfarin is usually required with chronic AF due to the risk of stroke.

Atrial Flutter, Acute

With atrial flutter the heart rate is often exactly 150/min due to an atrial rate of 300 with a 2:1 heart block. This rate can thus be a clue for the diagnosis.

Electrical Cardioversion

Will be required urgently if there is cardiovascular compromise. Use monophasic synchronised shock starting with 25–50 J in the adult, or a biphasic shock of 25–50 J. Atrial overdrive pacing may also be effective. Patients may be converted to sinus rhythm or AF (see above).[73]

Chemical Cardioversion

Acute atrial flutter is usually unresponsive to drug therapy.[69] Ibutilide appears to be the most effective drug.[73]

Drugs to Slow the Ventricular Rate

These drugs are the same as those used for chronic AF.

Atropine

Anticholinergic drug which acts as a competitive antagonist at muscarinic receptors. Used:

1 for drying airway secretions
2 to treat bradycardia by opposing vagal tone
3 to counter the muscarinic stimulatory effects of the acetyl-cholinesterase inhibitor drugs.

Dose

For treating bradycardia in adults and children, give 15–20 µg/kg IV or IM. In adults 3 mg causes complete vagal blockade. To counteract the muscarinic effects of neostigmine, give atropine 1.2 mg in adults and 20 µg/kg in children.

Note: Atropine can induce anticholinergic syndrome (see *CENTRAL ANTICHOLINERGIC SYNDROME*).

Awake Fibre-optic Intubation

1 Premedicate with a drying agent e.g. atropine 0.6 mg IM 30 min before procedure.

2 Sedate with agents such as midazolam, fentanyl and propofol during the procedure, ± a propofol infusion at a sedating dose. See *PROPOFOL*.

3 Topically anaesthetise the airway with:

(a) 3 mL of 2% lignocaine nebulised in a salbutamol type nebuliser and inhaled by the patient. Alternatively a Devilvis nebuliser can be used with topical 4% lignocaine.

(b) For nasal intubation, soak four cotton pledgets in 4% cocaine solution. Insert a cotton pledget gently and gradually along the floor of the nose on each side. The nasal mucosa will be anaesthetised as the pledget is advanced. Insert the other pledgets between the inferior and middle turbinates bilaterally to anaesthetise the sphenopalatine ganglion. Alternatively use 2% lignocaine with adrenaline 1:200 000 or cophenylcaine forte on the pledgets.

(c) Gargle 2 mL of 4% lignocaine topical dripped onto the back of the pharynx and larynx with a Cass needle. The patient must resist the urge to swallow the solution for ≈ 1 minute.

(d) Cricothyroid puncture is then performed. See *LARYNX, ANATOMY AND INNERVATION*. To perform this procedure:

(i) Anaesthetise the skin over the cricothyroid membrane with a bleb of LA.

(ii) Attach a 22 G cannula to a 5 mL syringe containing 2 mL of 2% plain lignocaine.

    (iii) Insert the cannula through the cricothyroid membrane and confirm tracheal puncture by aspirating air.

    (iv) Remove the needle stylet and re-attach the syringe to the cannula, then inject lignocaine. Warn the patient that this will cause coughing.

  (e) Consider bilateral superior laryngeal nerve blocks, although these are not usually necessary. See *SUPERIOR LARYNGEAL NERVE BLOCK*.

4   Prepare the fibre-optic bronchoscope (FOB). Ensure the FOB is correctly focused and orientated. Form a cylinder with the fingers of the right hand and inspect this 'tunnel' through the FOB to check orientation and focus. Apply demisting solution to the tip of the instrument.

5   For nasal intubation, soften the endotracheal (ET) tube tip by immersing it in hot water. Load the ET tube onto the FOB (size 7–7.5 for an adult male, size 6.5–7.0 for an adult female), ensuring the tube is well lubricated and the Murphy eye is orientated anteriorly facing the epiglottis. Place the patient in the same position as for conventional intubation and ask the patient to protrude the tongue and/or ask an assistant to gently grasp tongue with gauze and pull it forward. Give supplementary O_2 via a nasal catheter in the contralateral nostril. Consider passing the ET tube through the nose first into the nasopharynx, then passing the tip of the FOB through the ET tube and then into the larynx.

6   For oral intubation use a Burman airway as a guide, placed exactly in the midline.

7   Airway anaesthesia can be supplemented by inserting an epidural catheter down the suction port of the FOB and injecting 4% lignocaine directly onto the site to be anaesthetised. The FOB suction port is of little use for suctioning. It is more effective

to suck out secretions with a Yanker sucker, or suction catheter placed blindly into pharynx.

8   Intubate the larynx and trachea with the FOB and identify the carina. Pass the ET tube over the FOB while the view of the carina is maintained. As the FOB is removed ensure the ET tube tip is well into the trachea but above the carina. For nasal intubations the ET tube should be at about 26–28 cm at the nares in adults.

9   There are many variations and modifications to the above techniques.

Awareness

Awareness is a surprisingly common and potentially devastating complication of anaesthesia. As stated by one patient, '... The pain was so acute I couldn't move a finger. My screams stayed in my head... the pain was overwhelming.'[74]

Incidence

The risk of conscious awareness with explicit recall and severe pain is estimated to be < 1:3000 general anaesthetics.[75] Conscious awareness with explicit recall but without severe pain is estimated to be 3:1000 general anaesthetics.[76]

Implicit memory refers to subconscious processing of information while anaesthetised and can be revealed by hypnosis or behavioural suggestions.

The risk of awareness is highest in patients undergoing cardiac and obstetric anaesthesia, and is usually due to drug error such as failure of delivery of volatile agent.[77]

The incidence of awareness is also increased in patients undergoing opioid-based anaesthetics and anaesthetics utilising total intravenous anaesthesia (TIVA).[76]

Detection of Awareness

Signs suggesting awareness (and light anaesthesia) include:

1 tachycardia and hypertension
2 diaphoresis and lacrimation
3 movement.

These signs are very unreliable and frequently do not occur in patients with awareness.[78]

Fortunately there are now available specific monitors for 'wakefulness', including the BIS monitor and the M-Entropy monitor. See *BISPECTRAL INDEX (BIS) EEG MONITOR* and *TIME FREQUENCY BALANCED SPECTRAL ENTROPY*.

Management of Significant Awareness

1 Treat the patient with appropriate concern and respect. Believe the patient's account.
2 Post-traumatic stress disorder and other physiological conditions may result from awareness under anaesthesia. Every effort must be made to appropriately refer and manage patients who have undergone this complication.
3 Notify your medical defence organisation.

Bb

Bacterial Endocarditis Prophylaxis

The following guidelines are based on recommendations of the American Heart Association, the Victorian Medical Post Graduate Foundation and Prasad and Fraser.[1,2,3]

Topics Covered in this Section
▶ Lesions Predisposing to Subacute Bacterial Endocarditis
▶ Procedures for Which Antibiotic Prophylaxis is Recommended
▶ Procedures for which Antibiotic Prophylaxis is Not Recommended
▶ Antibiotic Prophylaxis Regimens in Adults
▶ Antibiotic Prophylaxis Regimens in Children

Lesions Predisposing to Subacute Bacterial Endocarditis

These lesions can be divided into high, moderate and negligible risk.

▶ *High Risk Lesions*
1 Prosthetic heart valves.
2 Previous endocarditis.
3 Complex cyanotic congenital heart disease.
4 Surgically constructed systemic pulmonary shunts or conduits.

▶ *Moderate Risk Lesions*
1 Acquired valvular dysfunction
2 Uncorrected patent ductus arteriosus or repair within 1 year.
3 Uncorrected ventricular septal defect.

B

4 Uncorrected coarctation of the aorta.
5 Hypertrophic cardiomyopathy.
6 Mitral valve prolapse with valvular regurgitation and/or thickened leaflets.

▶ *Negligible Risk Lesions*
1 Surgically corrected ventricular septal defect, atrial septal defect or patent ductus arteriosis (without residual defect and allowing for a 6 month healing period).
2 Mitral valve prolapse without regurgitation.
3 Innocent heart murmurs.
4 Previous rheumatic fever without valvular damage.
5 Cardiac pacemakers.

Procedures for which Antibiotic Prophylaxis is Recommended:

▶ *Oral and Respiratory Tract*
1 Dental extractions, scaling, root planning, implants, dental procedures associated with bleeding.
2 Tonsillectomy/adenoidectomy, surgical operations on the respiratory mucosa.
3 Rigid bronchoscopy.
4 Nasotracheal intubation.

▶ *Gastrointestinal Tract*
1 Sclerotherapy of oesophageal varices and stricture dilatation.
2 Endoscopic retrograde cholangiography with biliary obstruction.
3 Biliary tract surgery.
4 Operations involving intestinal mucosa.

▶ *Genitourinary Tract*
1 Prostate surgery.
2 Cystoscopy.

3   Urethral dilatation.
4   Lithotripsy.

▶ *Other Procedures*
1   Operations involving infected material. Use antibiotics appropriate to the type of infection.
2   Proctoscopy, sigmoidoscopy or colonoscopy, especially in high risk patients and especially if deep biopsies.
3   Vaginal hysterectomy.
4   Vaginal delivery in high risk patients.
5   Per vaginal procedures involving infected material in high risk patients.
6   Dilatation of cervix and curettage of uterus in high risk patients.
7   Implantation of prosthetic valve or permanent pacemaker.

Procedures for which Antibiotic Prophylaxis is Not Recommended:
1   Flexible bronchoscopy.
2   Orotracheal intubation.
3   Panendoscopy.
4   Endoscopic banding or ligation of varices.
5   Normal vaginal delivery.

Antibiotic Prophylaxis Regimens in Adults
▶ *Dental, Oral, Respiratory Tract or Oesophageal Procedures*
Amoxycillin 2 g PO or ampicillin 2 g IV. If allergic to penicillin give clindamycin 600 mg PO or IV or cephalexin 2 g PO or cefazolin 1 g IV. If the patient has had a penicillin type antibiotic more than once in the previous month, use clindamycin (instead of ampicillin or a cephalosporin). Give oral therapy 2 h before procedure and IV/IM therapy within 30 min of procedure.

▶ *Genitourinary/Gastrointestinal Procedures*

Ampicillin and gentamicin 1.5 mg/kg up to 120 mg. Give amoxy-cillin 1 g PO or ampicillin 1 g IV or IM 6 h after procedure. If aller-gic to penicillin or recent exposure to penicillin, give vancomycin 1 g IV over 1–2 h plus gentamicin as above.

Antibiotic Prophylaxis Regimens in Children

The same regimen as above is used. Doses are:

- amoxycillin 50 mg/kg PO
- ampicillin 50 mg/kg IM or IV, second dose 25 mg/kg IM or IV
- clindamycin 20 mg/kg PO, 20 mg/kg IV
- cephalexin 50 mg/kg PO, cephazolin 25 mg/kg IV or IM
- gentamicin 1.5 mg/kg IV
- vancomycin 20 mg/kg IV

Total children's dose should not exceed the adult dose.

Bier Block

IV regional anaesthetic technique that can be used for surgery of the upper or lower limb.

Technique for Upper Limb Anaesthesia

1. Insert an IV cannula in each arm. Place the cannula distally in the limb to be anaesthetised.
2. Apply a single cuffed surgical tourniquet to the arm to be blocked. Prior to inflation, drain blood from the venous system by either of the following:
   (a) Apply Esmach bandage from distal to proximal.
   (b) Occlude the brachial artery at the elbow and elevate the limb for 1 min.
3. Inflate the tourniquet to 100 mmHg above the measured systolic blood pressure or a maximum of 300 mmHg.
4. Inject LA solution over at least 90 s. Use lignocaine 0.5% 3 mg/kg.

Do not use adrenaline-containing solutions. For a 70 kg person use ≈ 40 mL of LA solution. Onset of block takes ≈ 5–10 min.

5   *Deflation of tourniquet*: Do not release the tourniquet if less than 20 min has elapsed. If 45 min has elapsed, the tourniquet can be released as a one-step procedure.[4] Between 20 and 45 min, release the tourniquet cuff pressure for 10 s then reinflate cuff for 1 min before final release.

Biphasic Defibrillators

See *DEFIBRILLATORS*.

Bispectral Index (BIS) EEG Monitor

This monitor is a continuous highly processed electroencephalograph that measures changes in interfrequency coupling. BIS is used to provide a measure of hypnosis during anaesthesia and thus diminish the risk of awareness.

Underlying Principles of BIS

Part of the cortical EEG is influenced by neuronal activity of subcortical structures, and this interaction is reflected in harmonic and phase relationships in the EEG signal called 'biocoherence'.[5] Broadly speaking, EEG measurements change from low amplitude, high frequency signals while awake to large amplitude, low frequency signals while anaesthetised. Biocoherence patterns also change with increasing concentrations of hypnotic drugs. The BIS monitor analyses these EEG pattern changes using measurement algorithms which were derived empirically. This involved applying a stepwise regression analysis to EEGs from over 2000 subjects in various phases of anaesthesia, sedation and wakefulness. The regression equation obtained combines several features such as burst suppression and β wave activation. This regression equation is converted to a 1–100 scale where:[6,7,8]

100...........awake
70.............light hypnosis/sedation
60.............moderate hypnosis (aim for a BIS level of < 60 to prevent
                awareness).
40.............deep hypnosis (excessive hypnosis for routine anaesthe-
                sia).
0...............isoelectric EEG

Advantages of BIS

1 By using BIS monitoring there is the potential to safely minimise
   anaesthetic dosage, resulting in fewer unwanted anaesthetic
   drug side-effects, faster wake up time and earlier discharge.[9]
2 BIS monitoring may enable a reduced possibility of patient
   awareness under anaesthesia. The B-Aware trial concluded that
   BIS monitoring reduced the risk of awareness in high risk
   patients by 82%.[10] High risk patients were defined as patients
   having general anaesthesia with muscle relaxation and another
   risk factor such as Caesarean section surgery or coronary artery
   bypass surgery. See *AWARENESS*.

Disadvantages of BIS

1 BIS monitoring can be affected by brain ischaemia or hypoxia
   and hypothermia. BIS is also affected by forehead muscle activity, which must be considered in evaluating the non-paralysed
   patient.[11] See *TIME FREQUENCY BALANCED SPECTRAL ENTROPY*.
2 BIS values must be interpreted in the light of other patient monitors and clinical evaluation of the patient.
3 The equipment, including electrode costs, is expensive.[11]

Practical Aspects of Using BIS

A typical device is the Aspect A-1000 EEG monitor. To use this device:
1 Attach four Zipprep or other suitable electrodes to the head. Two
   of these are positioned over both temporal bones, laterally from
   the eyes. A reference electrode is placed on the centre of the fore-

head between the eyebrows. A fourth ground electrode is placed on the forehead.

2   BIS values are calculated by the Aspect monitor and displayed.

3   BIS values between 40 and 60 are recommended as optimal to prevent awareness while avoiding excessive anaesthesia.[10]

Bleomycin (BLM)

Anthracycline antibiotic type anticancer drug used for the treatment of malignancies such as testicular cancer and Hodgkin's disease. BLM can cause pulmonary toxicity and possibly acute severe lung toxicity in the presence of hyperoxia.[12]

Pre-operative Evaluation

1   Assess the patient for evidence of pulmonary and/or renal toxicity (which can result in delayed clearance of BLM).

2   Possibly increased risk if:
    (a) exposure to BLM within 1–2 months[12]
    (b) > 450 mg total dose received.

3   Consider corticosteroid pretreatment.[12]

Intra-operative Management

Avoid an inspired O_2 concentration > 30%. Use the minimum inspired O_2 concentration required to maintain an O_2 saturation > 90%.

Blind Nasal Intubation

1   If patient is to be awake, anaesthetise the airway and provide sedation. See AWAKE FIBRE-OPTIC INTUBATION.

2   If the patient is undergoing GA, maintain spontaneous ventilation.

3   Use a mucosal vasoconstrictor in nose, e.g. cocaine, oxymetazoline or cophenylcaine.

4   Place the patient in the usual intubation position.

B

5   Soften the endotracheal (ET) tube tip in hot water prior to use.

6   Gently introduce well-lubricated ET tube (7–7.5 for male, 6.5–7 for female) into the nose with its concave side facing the feet. If the patient is breathing spontaneously, occlude the other nostril to increase the volume of breath sounds audible through the ET tube. Listen for breath sounds and monitor capnography as the tube is advanced.

7   If breath sounds disappear, look for a visible bulge in the neck which may indicate in which direction to manipulate the tube. Advance the tube during inspiration or coughing.

8   Methods to increase likelihood of successful placement include:

   (a) Inflate the ET tube cuff in the oropharynx. Advance tube until slight resistance is felt, at which point the cuff may be against the vocal cords. Deflate the cuff and advance the ET tube into the trachea.[13]

   (b) If the oesophagus is intubated, reattempt intubation with increased neck flexion.

   (c) Rotation of the ET tube and manipulation of the larynx may also be helpful.

Blood Loss Assessment and Initial Management

Topics Covered in this Section

▶ Grading Blood Loss

▶ Initial Management of Severe Blood Loss

▶ Anaesthesia in the Presence of Severe Blood Loss

Grading Blood Loss

Blood loss is graded into four classes, based on blood loss as a percentage of total blood volume (TBV).[14] Figures quoted for blood loss assume a TBV of 5 L.

- *Class 1* (up to 15% TBV) (≈ 800 mL). Associated with minimal clinical symptoms/signs.
- *Class 2* (15–30% TBV) (≈ 800–1500 mL). Clinically see tachycardia, tachypnoea and narrowing of the pulse pressure with increased diastolic blood pressure. The patient is usually anxious/agitated. Urine output is reasonably well maintained.
- *Class 3* (30–40% TBV) (≈ 1500–2000 mL). Clinically see marked tachycardia and tachypnoea, a fall in systolic blood pressure and the patient may become confused. Urine output is reduced.
- *Class 4* (> 40% TBV) (> 2000 mL). A marked tachycardia occurs with a very depressed systolic blood pressure and narrow pulse pressure. There is little or no urine output. The patient's skin is pale and cool, with decreased capillary return. There is also marked depression of the central nervous system with loss of consciousness if > 50% of TBV is lost.

Initial Management of Severe Blood Loss

1 Secure the airway and ensure adequate ventilation. Give high concentration O_2.
2 Control haemorrhage, e.g. direct pressure to the wound site, suturing of skin bleeders. Elevate the site of bleeding if possible. The patient may require immediate surgical intervention.
3 Secure large bore IV access, i.e. insert a 'Rapid Infusion Device'. See *RAPID INFUSION CATHETER EXCHANGER SET*. Insert a second large bore IV cannula. A pulmonary artery (PA) catheter introducer sheath can also be used. A new device for large bore central venous access is the Arrow MAC (see *ARROW MAC 2 LUMEN CENTRAL VENOUS ACCESS DEVICE*).
4 Send blood specimens off for urgent full blood count, coagulation studies and cross-match.
5 Give IV fluids rapidly.

In adults: Give 1–2 L of colloid (e.g. gelofusine) rapidly and assess response. If the patient is still cardiovascularly unstable, he or she will probably need blood urgently ± urgent surgery.

In children: Give 20 mL/kg of Hartmann's solution. If the patient is still cardiovascularly unstable give a second bolus of crystalloid 20 mL/kg.[15] If there are persistent signs of shock, give 10 mL/kg of type specific or O -ve blood (packed cells).

6 Establish intra-arterial blood pressure monitoring and central venous pressure monitoring.

7 For ongoing management see *BLOOD TRANSFUSION, Massive Blood Transfusion Management.*

Anaesthesia in the Presence of Severe Blood Loss

The general principles are:

1 Ensure adequate airway and ventilation.

2 Establish large bore IV access as described above. Resuscitate the patient with intravenous crystalloid, colloid, blood as required.

3 Insert an arterial line to measure blood pressure accurately and enable frequent blood sampling.

4 Prep and drape the surgical area prior to the induction of anaesthesia if possible. This is because anaesthesia may cause:

   (a) a reduction in sympatho-adrenal stimulation[16]

   (b) loss of the tamponading effect of abdominal musculature that may occur in the awake patient.[16]

5 Perform a rapid sequence induction but induce anaesthesia cautiously. For example use:

   (a) fentanyl 100–200 μg plus thiopentone in a reduced dose (e.g. 50–100 mg depending on the severity of haemorrhagic shock) or

   (b) ketamine 1.5–2.5 mg/kg[17] or

   (c) etomidate 0.3 mg/kg plus

   (d) a rapidly acting muscle relaxant such as suxamethonium or rocuronium.

6 Maintain anaesthesia with O_2 ± a low concentration of isoflurane or sevoflurane as tolerated by the patient.

7 As soon as practically possible organise:
   (a) two or more blood warmers and/or a rapid warmed fluid delivery system such as the 'Level One'
   (b) urinary catheter insertion
   (c) patient-warming devices such as a Bair Hugger
   (d) nasopharyngeal temperature probe
   (e) blood scavenging device such as a cell saver.

7 Insert a CVP line to aid in the estimation of intravascular filling.

8 It is essential to prevent or minimise hypothermia and prevent the deleterious effects of hypothermia on coagulation.[18]

9 Ensure there are adequate numbers of trained theatre staff in attendance. Call more staff in if required.

10 Communicate with blood bank and haematologist early regarding:
   (a) number of units required and urgency of request
   (b) need for other blood products such as fresh frozen plasma (FFP) and platelets.

See also *BLOOD TRANSFUSION, Massive Blood Transfusion Management.*

Blood Loss Prevention

Pre-operative Measures

1 Identify/investigate patients with possible bleeding tendencies.

2 Cease drugs which may cause increased bleeding prior to surgery or reverse their effects. These include the following:
   (a) Aspirin. Aspirin irreversibly inhibits platelet function (for the life-time of the platelet ≈ 7–10 days) by inhibiting cyclo-oxygenase 1 (COX1) enzyme. Cease 1 week before surgery. If aspirin is ingested within 5 days of surgery, and surgery is

urgent and likely to be associated with severe blood loss, consider the use of desmopressin (DDAVP) and/or platelet transfusion. See *DESMOPRESSIN (DDAVP)*.

(b) *Heparin, low molecular weght heparin and warfarin.* See *ANTI-COAGULATION THERAPY AND SURGERY*.

(c) *Non-steroidal anti-inflammatory drugs* (other than aspirin). NSAIDs are of two types: non-selective (inhibiting both COX1 and COX2 enzymes) and selective (COX2) inhibitors. The non-selective NSAID drugs reversibly inhibit platelet aggregation only while effective plasma concentration is maintained. Cease the drug 3 days before surgery if the intra-operative bleeding risk is of particular concern.

(d) *New antiplatelet drugs.* These include platelet glycoprotein IIb/IIIa receptor antagonists (such as abciximab, tirofiban and eptifibatide) and platelet adenosine diphosphate (ADP) receptor antagonists (e.g. ticlopidine and clopidogrel). These drugs cause profound platelet inhibition making surgery hazardous. See *PLATELET GLYCOPROTEIN IIb/IIIa RECEPTOR ANTAGONISTS* and *PLATELET ADENOSINE DIPHOSPHATE (ADP) RECEPTOR ANTAGONISTS* for specific recommendations.

Intra-operative Measures

1 Meticulous surgical technique.
2 Modest hypotension and avoidance of hypertension.
3 Maintainance of normal body temperature to prevent the adverse effects of hypothermia on coagulation.[18]
4 Use of a tourniquet during limb surgery.
5 Positioning of surgical site uppermost.
6 Use of regional anaesthesia.[19]
7 Use of pharmacological agents such as:
   (a) aprotinin (see entry)

(b) DDAVP (see *DESMOPRESSIN*)

(c) antifibrinolytic agents such as epsilon aminocaproic acid or tranexamic acid. See *TRANEXAMIC ACID*.

Blood Patching

See *EPIDURAL ANAESTHESIA*.

Blood Transfusion

Topics Covered in this Section

▶ Strategies to Avoid Allogenic Blood Transfusion

▶ Haemoglobin Level as a Transfusion 'Trigger'

▶ Decision to Transfuse Based on Volume of Blood Loss

▶ Massive Blood Transfusion Management

Strategies to Avoid Allogenic Blood Transfusion

1 Pre-operative autologous blood donation. This technique is associated with poor cost effectiveness and high wastage rates.[20]

2 Pre-operative use of iron therapy and/or erythropoietin to increase haemoglobin levels. This treatment can be combined with pre-operative autologous blood donation.[21]

3 Acute normovolaemic haemodilution.

4 Intra-operative blood salvage through such devices as a cell saver.

5 Intra-operative blood loss prevention strategies (see above).

6 Postoperative blood recovery, e.g. from surgical drains.

7 Blood substitutes. These include O_2 carrying perfluorochemicals (e.g. Fluosol DA) and cell free haemoglobin based substances.

Haemoglobin Level as a Transfusion 'Trigger'

There is little evidence-based medicine support for deciding to transfuse a patient solely on a haemoglobin (Hb) level.[22] Blood transfusion is rarely indicated if the Hb levels are > 10 g/100 mL and almost always indicated if Hb < 6 g/100 mL.[22]

Transfusing 1 unit of blood will increase the Hb level by ≈ 1 g/100 mL.

The following guidelines are suggested transfusion 'triggers' based on measured Hb levels and assuming that intravascular volume is maintained.

▶ *Healthy Young Patients*

Tolerate Hb levels of ≥ 7–8 g/100 mL provided that intravascular volume is well maintained.[23] Transfusion is probably indicated if Hb level falls below 7–8 g/100 mL in these patients.[24] Jehovah's Witnesses do not usually die from anaemia alone if the Hb level is > 3 g/100 mL.[21]

▶ *Patients Requiring a Minimum Hb Level of 10 g/100 mL*

- Patients older than 60 years[23]
- Significant systemic disease.
- Known or possible coronary artery disease.
- Cerebrovascular disease or severe lung disease.

Decision to Transfuse Based on Volume of Blood Loss

1   *Loss of up to 15% Total Blood Volume (TBV)* (≈ 700 mL in a 70 kg patient). In young healthy patients, this amount of loss is usually well tolerated with little or no haemodynamic effects.

2   *Loss of 15–30% TBV* (≈ 800–1500 mL). Blood transfusion is likely to be required in an unfit or elderly patient but can be tolerated by a young fit patient as long as intravascular volume is maintained.

3   *Loss of 30–40% TBV* (≈ 1500–2000 mL). In a young fit patient, can be treated adequately with crystalloid therapy.[22] Blood

transfusion will almost certainly be required in all other patients.

4   *Loss of > 40% TBV (> 2000 mL)*. Severe life-threatening haemorrhage requiring blood transfusion in almost all circumstances.

Massive Blood Transfusion Management
See *BLOOD LOSS ASSESSMENT AND INITIAL MANAGEMENT*.

Massive blood transfusion is defined as acute administration of greater than 1 total blood volume within a 24 h period.[25] In a 70 kg patient this equates to about 12 units of blood.[25] Ongoing severe haemorrhage treated with transfusion of packed cells will lead to coagulopathy and thrombocytopenia. However, these clotting deficits are multifactorial in origin and are not due just to the amount of blood lost and replaced. Other factors such as hypothermia and prolonged periods of hypotension are also important.[23]

1   Obtain fully cross-matched blood as soon as possible in adequate quantities. Fully cross-matched blood requires $\approx$ 20–30 min to process. Saline compatible group specific blood requires $\approx$ 5–10 min. If blood is required before a cross-match is available give Group O Rh -ve blood. If the O -ve blood supply is exhausted and patient's life is threatened give O Rh +ve blood (but O Rh -ve blood is preferable particularly in women of childbearing age or younger).[26] If O Rh +ve blood or platelets are given to an O Rh –ve female with childbearing potential give anti-D if the patient does not already have an anti-D antibody detected.

2   Give fresh frozen plasma (FFP) when coagulation studies (PT/APTT) are $> 1.5 \times$ normal.[22] Expect dilution of coagulation factors sufficient to cause coagulopathy after transfusion of $1–1.5 \times$ TBV or about 12–18 units of packed cells in a 70 kg patient.[22,25] Give 4–8 units of FFP.[23]

3   Give platelets if platelet count drops below 50 000/mm³ (50 $\times$ 10⁹/L) or on clinical grounds if the wound looks 'oozy'.

B

Significant thrombocytopenia is expected after transfusion of 1.5–2 × TBV or 18–24 units of packed cells in a 70 kg patient.[23,25] See also *PLATELET THERAPY*.

4   Other clotting factor products to consider include cryoprecipitate, prothrombinex-HT, Factor VIII, Factor IX and recombinant activated Factor VII. See *CRYOPRECIPITATE (AND CRYO-DEPLETED PLASMA)* and *RECOMBINANT ACTIVATED FACTOR VII*. Cryoprecipitate is indicated if fibrinogen concentrations fall below 80–100 mg/100 mL.[22] Consult a haematologist early in resuscitation for advice on type and quantity of clotting factors to give.

5   Prevent or reverse hypothermia which inhibits platelet function and increases bleeding times.

▶ *Problems Associated with Massive Blood Transfusion*

1   Anticipate/treat 'citrate toxicity' due to citrate binding to calcium in the serum, leading to low levels of ionised calcium. See *CALCIUM*. This occurs when blood is being given so rapidly that the liver has insufficient time to metabolise the citrate, i.e. > 1 unit of blood per 5 min. Effects of citrate-induced ionised hypocalcaemia include hypotension, decreased cardiac output, electromechanical dissociation and prolongation of the QT interval. To prevent/treat citrate toxicity give 1 g calcium gluconate IV 10% solution (10 mL) for every 5 units of blood. Give the same amount of calcium gluconate if FFP given at 5 units per min or faster. Patients with liver disease have an increased susceptibility to citrate toxicity.

2   Anticipate/treat hyperkalaemia due to high potassium content of stored blood (e.g. 40 mmol/L at 4 weeks).[27] Monitor the ECG closely for evidence of hyperkalaemia. For a description of the ECG changes seen with hyperkalaemia see *ELECTROCAR-DIOGRAPHY*.

Blood Volume

See Tables B1 and B2.

Table B1 Total blood volume in mL/kg at various ages	
Age	Blood volume
Premature infant	100 mL/kg
Term infant	90 mL/kg
6–8 years	Adult levels
Adult male	70 mL/kg
Adult female	60 mL/kg

Table B2 Distribution of 5 L of blood in a 70 kg patient	
Volume	Site
1000 mL	Heart, arterial circulation and capillaries
1000 mL	Pulmonary circulation
3000 mL	Venous circulation

Blunt Airway Trauma

Assessment of Injury

1 Classic symptoms/signs are:
   (a) pain, dysphagia and stridor
   (b) haemoptysis
   (c) surgical emphysema
2 Identify/exclude other injuries such as fractured base of skull
   and cervical spine injury.

3 If patient's condition permits obtain an urgent ENT surgical opinion ± indirect laryngoscopy/fibre-optic laryngoscopy. Obtain a lateral airway X-ray if the patient's condition permits.

4 If the patient is able to maintain their own airway but intubation is required consider the following options:

(a) awake tracheostomy under LA.

(b) awake fibre-optic bronchoscopy and inspection of the trachea for disruption, prior to placement of endotracheal (ET) tube.

(c) direct laryngoscopy with the patient awake. Anaesthetise back of tongue and larynx with 10% lignocaine spray prior to laryngoscopy.

(d) inhalational induction. The risk of aspiration must be weighed against risk of 'losing the airway' if the patient is paralysed.

(e) a retrograde intubation technique. See *DIFFICULT AIRWAY MANAGEMENT*.

5 If neither the patient nor the anaesthetist is able to maintain the patient's airway the options to be considered are:

(a) rapid sequence induction with thiopentone and suxamethonium

(b) immediate surgical airway with LA. See *CRICOTHYROID PUNCTURE AND CRICOTHYROTOMY*.

Body Mass Index (BMI) and Obesity

$$BMI = \frac{weight\ (kg)}{height\ (m)^2}$$

Ideal body weight in kg ≈ for men height in cm – 100, and for women height in cm – 105.

Normal BMI 23–26.

See Table B3.

Table B3 Obesity classification and BMI	
Weight description	BMI
Overweight	27–29
Obese	30–35
Morbidly obese	> 35

Obesity can be defined as a body weight more than 20% greater than ideal body weight (IBW).

Morbid obesity is a body weight > 2 × IBW or a BMI > 35.[28]

Bone Cement Implantation Syndrome

See *FAT EMBOLISM SYNDROME AND BONE CEMENT IMPLANTATION SYNDROME*.

Brachial Plexus Block

Topics Covered in this Section

▶ Introductory Comments
▶ Anatomy of the Brachial Plexus
▶ Interscalene Approach
▶ Supraclavicular Approach
▶ Axillary Approach
▶ Intersternocleidomastoid Brachial Plexus Block
▶ Infraclavicular Brachial Plexus Block
▶ Infraclavicular Brachial Plexus Block, Coracoid Technique
▶ Continuous Brachial Plexus Infusions

Introductory Comments

Interscalene block is recommended for surgery on the upper arm and shoulder. The block is most dense in the C4–C7 root distribution. Interscalene blocks tend to be of shorter duration than axillary or supraclavicular blocks due to increased LA absorption in this area.[29]

Supraclavicular block can be used for surgery on the forearm and upper arm.

Infraclavicular block is useful for surgery on the elbow, forearm, wrist and hand but not the shoulder. *Axillary block* is suitable for surgery on the wrist and hand. As a rough guide lignocaine with adrenaline will provide reasonable anaesthesia for up to 3 h and analgesia for up to 6 h. Ropivacaine will provide anaesthesia for 6–8 h and analgesia for 9–16 h.[29] With all the blocks described, when the tip of the block needle is in position near the plexus always aspirate first for blood (or CSF), then give a test dose of 2 mL. If the needle tip is intraneural this may produce pain and the needle tip should be withdrawn slightly. Give the rest of the dose of LA in 5 mL increments, observing the patiently closely for any side-effects.

Anatomy of the Brachial Plexus

The brachial plexus is formed from the anterior rami of C5–T1 nerve roots. It is the main sensory, motor and sympathetic innervation of the upper limb. Some of the important anatomical features of the brachial plexus are discussed in the descriptions of the various types of brachial plexus blocks. See Figure B1.

Interscalene Approach

The five roots of the brachial plexus form three trunks (upper, middle and lower). These trunks are sandwiched between *scalenus anterior* and *scalenus medius*. The fasciae of these muscles form a sheath around the plexus.

▶ *Technique*

1 Insert IV cannula in the contralateral arm.

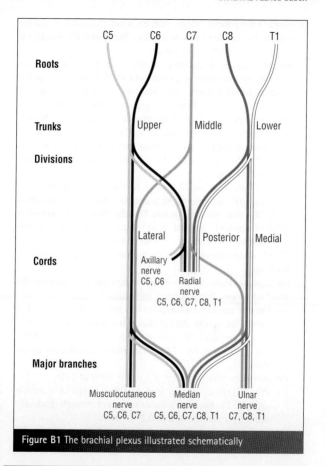

Figure B1 The brachial plexus illustrated schematically

B

2 Position the patient supine, with the head turned away slightly, with a small folded towel as a pillow. The ipsilateral shoulder is depressed by reaching for knee.

3 Identify the cricoid cartilage at the level of C6. At this level identify the interscalene groove behind the lateral edge of the sternomastoid muscle. The external jugular vein almost always crosses the interscalene groove at the level of C6. The transverse process of C6 (Chassaignac's tubercle) may be palpated in the interscalene groove. At the base of the groove the pulsations of the subclavian artery may be palpable. The roots of the brachial plexus lie closer to middle than the anterior scalenus muscle.

4 Insert a short bevelled 22 G block needle into the groove, closer to the scalenus medius, in a direction that is ≈ perpendicular to the skin in every plane. The direction of placement is slightly caudad, medial and posterior angling towards Chassaignac's tubercle. If bone is contacted redirect the needle slightly anteriorly or posteriorly but never cephalad or directly medially.

5 Elicit paraesthesia or use a nerve stimulator to identify the brachial plexus. To use a nerve stimulator:[30]

(a) Use an insulated short bevelled block needle such as a Stimuplex needle. Attach this to a suitable nerve stimulator via the black electrode (negative electrode). Attach the red electrode to an ECG dot positioned on the ipsilateral shoulder.

(b) Stimulate with a current of 2 mA initially at 1 Hz.

(c) When contractions are seen in either biceps or a muscle group in the forearm, reduce the current strength gradually, aiming for contractions at 0.2–0.4 mA.

6 Once paraesthesia or satisfactory nerve stimulation is obtained, inject a 2 mL test dose of LA. If pain occurs with injection of the

test dose withdraw the needle slightly (to avoid intraneural injection) and repeat the test dose injection.

7   Use a LA volume of ≈ 30 mL in a 70 kg patient. Suitable anaesthetic agents include lignocaine 1.5% with adrenaline 1:200 000 or lignocaine 2% with adrenaline mixed with an equal volume of bupivacaine 0.5% with adrenaline. Alternatively 30–40 mL of ropivacaine 5 mg/mL can be used. Inject the LA cautiously in 5 mL increments. Aspirate for blood or cerebrospinal fluid before each injection.

▶ *Complications of Interscalene Block*

1   Block of the phrenic nerve is almost unavoidable.[29,31]

2   Inadvertent epidural or subarachnoid injection can occur. See *BRAINSTEM ANAESTHESIA*.

3   Vertebral artery injection. Seizures are likely with this complication. The incidence of vertebral artery injection was 0.3% in one series.[29]

4   Nerve damage, particularly associated with sharp needles and repeated stabs.

5   Horner's syndrome, which has an incidence of about 60%.[32]

6   Hoarse voice.

7   Bronchospasm.

8   CVS instability, including hypotension, bradycardia and asystole. The mechanism of these episodes may be due to the Bezold-Jarisch reflex and may be resistant to atropine. Ephedrine appears to be an effective treatment.

Supraclavicular Approach

The three trunks emerge from between the scalenus anterior and medius and pass in a closely grouped cluster downwards and laterally across the base of the posterior triangle of the neck and across the first rib. See Figure B2.

B

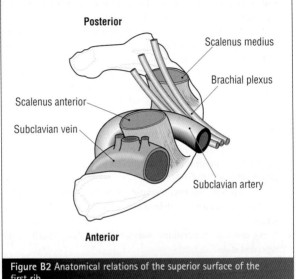

Posterior

Scalenus medius

Brachial plexus

Scalenus anterior

Subclavian vein

Subclavian artery

Anterior

Figure B2 Anatomical relations of the superior surface of the first rib

▶ *Technique*

1 Position the patient supine, with the head turned slightly to the opposite side.

2 Identify the lateral edge of the sternomastoid muscle, then the interscalene groove behind this muscle. Palpate groove as caudally as possible. Attempt to palpate the subclavian artery overlying the first rib.

3 From behind the top of the patient's head insert a 22 G short bevelled needle in a caudad direction parallel to the floor and

just behind the subclavian artery. Insert the needle closer to the edge of the scalenus medius than scalenus anterior. Obtain paraesthesia or use a nerve stimulator (see above). Inject a test dose, then the full dose of LA as described for interscalene block.

▶ *Complications of Supraclavicular Block*
1 Pneumothorax may occur. A pneumothorax rate of 2–5% is quoted.[29]
2 Phrenic nerve block occurs in a majority of patients.[29]
3 Nerve damage.
4 Intravascular injection.

Axillary Approach

After crossing the first rib, the trunks divide into six divisions. These divisions stream into the axilla and then rejoin to form three cords (medial, lateral and posterior). The cords then divide into five terminal branches. The fascial layers from the scalene muscles that envelop the brachial plexus extend into the axilla to form a tubular sheath that includes the axillary artery. A multiple injection technique may improve success rate up to 97%.[29] See Figure B3.

▶ *Technique*
1 Position patient supine with forearm pronated, shoulder abducted to 90° and elbow flexed to 90°.
2 Palpate the axillary artery as proximally as possible.
3 The *musculocutaneous nerve* is sought first. Insert the block needle, aiming to position the tip just above and deep to the axillary artery. Stimulation of the musculocutaneous nerve causes arm flexion. Use a current of 2 mA initially, reducing the current to 0.3–0.5 mA with ongoing arm flexion confirming good position. Inject 5 mL of LA if aspiration is negative.
4 The needle is then repositioned so that the tip lies just superior and anterior to the axillary artery, aiming for the *ulnar and*

median nerves indicated by wrist and finger flexion. Again 2 mA is used initially, reducing to 0.3–0.5 mA. Inject 15 mL of LA incrementally (after -ve aspiration).

5   For the third injection the needle point is redirected to just inferior to the axillary artery, aiming for the radial nerve. With stimulation using the same pattern as above, extension of fingers and thumb is seen. Inject 10 mL of LA after -ve aspiration.

6   Onset of block with lignocaine will take 10–20 min.[29]

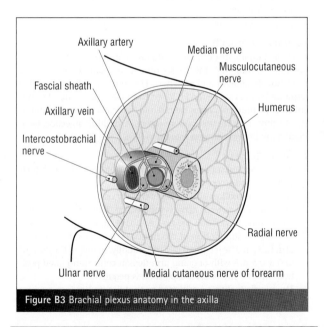

Figure B3 Brachial plexus anatomy in the axilla

▶ *Complications of Axillary Block*

There is less risk of major complications than with the other techniques.[32]

1 May get nerve damage.
2 Risk of intravascular injection and haematoma if the artery is punctured.

▶ *Continuous Axillary Blockade (Adults)*

This can be achieved by passing a catheter into the brachial plexus sheath. The steps in placement of the catheter are the same as for axillary brachial plexus block, except that a catheter through needle technique is used. Kits are available for this technique such as the Contiplex Katheterset. Insert the catheter 1–3 cm beyond the needle tip, then remove the needle.

Give a standard bolus dose as described above. Wait 1 h, then run an infusion of *Bupivacaine* 0.25% at 10 mL/h. This rate of infusion does not result in accumulation of Bupivacaine.[33]

Intersternocleidomastoid Brachial Plexus Block

Pham-Dang et al. describe a novel approach to supraclavicular brachial plexus block.[34] This technique involves the following steps:

1 Position the patient supine with the head turned away from the side to be blocked.
2 Identify the triangle formed by the heads of the sternocleidomastoid muscle (SCM) at the base of the neck. Also identify and mark the midpoint of the clavicle.
3 Aseptically insert the stimulating block needle at the medial border of the sternal head of SCM 3 cm above the sternal notch.
3 The needle is angulated caudal, dorsal-posteriorly and laterally towards the midpoint of the clavicle. The needle is passed behind the clavicular head of SCM at a 40–50° angle to the bed.
4 Use the nerve stimulator to identify the position of the brachial plexus.

The authors claim the risk of pneumothorax is minimal with this technique.

B

Infraclavicular Brachial Plexus Block

The steps in this technique are:

1 Position the patient supine with the arm to be blocked flexed at the elbow 90° and abducted at the shoulder 90°. Stand on the side of the patient opposite to the arm to be blocked.

2 Identify the midpoint of the clavicle (halfway between the sternal notch and the shoulder tip). The midpoint of the clavicle can also be identified above the clavicle by locating the pulsation of the subclavian artery.

3 Identify the axillary artery pulsation in the axilla as proximally as possible.

4 Using sterile technique as described above, insert a stimuplex needle 2.5 cm below the midpoint of the clavicle, at a 45° angle, towards the pulsations of the axillary artery. Use a nerve stimulator starting with a stimulating current of 1.5–2 mA.

5 The needle will pass through the pectoralis group of muscles, causing twitches. Reduce the stimulating current and continue to insert the needle. The pectoralis contractions should cease. The current can again be increased to 1.5–2 mA.

6 As the needle is passed still further, contractions of the muscles of the arm and/or hand should be observed, and the current should be reduced. Twitches with a current of 0.2–0.3 mA indicate that the tip of the needle is near the brachial plexus.

7 Inject 2 mL of LA (which should *not* cause pain) and the twitches should cease. Then inject the rest of the solution.

Infraclavicular Brachial Plexus Block, Coracoid Technique

This is another infraclavicular approach using the coracoid process as the major landmark. A technique using a nerve stimulator and insulated Stimuplex needle is described.[35] It involves the following steps:

1 Identify the coracoid process. The injection site is 2 cm medial and 2 cm caudad to the tip of this process.
2 The Stimuplex needle is passed in a 'plumb bomb' (directly posterior) parasagittal direction until nerve stimulation is achieved, usually at a depth of 4–4.25 cm.[35] Start with a stimulation current of 1 mA, looking for movement in the forearm, wrist and/or hand. Reduce the stimulation current to 0.4 mA to ensure close proximity to the plexus. Do not insert the needle medially and not beyond a depth of 6 cm.

▶ Complications
1 Pneumothorax is described, but uncommon.
2 Vascular puncture occurs reasonably frequently.[36]

Continuous Brachial Plexus Infusions
Catheter through needle kits are available for continuous brachial plexus infusions. A suggested regimen is 0.2% ropivacaine 10–15 mL/h. If pain occurs give a bolus of 10 mL and increase infusion rate by 3 mL/h to a maximum of 15 mL/h.[37]

Bradycardia

Defined as a pulse rate < 60 beats/min. Bradycardia requires treatment if it is associated with inadequate cardiac output. Management includes the following:
1 Ensure adequate airway, ventilation, and palpable pulse. Check blood pressure.
2 Identify/treat cause. See *COVER ABCD CRISIS MANAGEMENT ALGORITHM*. Common causes include:
   (a) *physiological derangements*, e.g. hypoxia
   (b) *pharmacological causes*, e.g. suxamethonium
   (c) *surgical causes*, e.g. traction on the eye muscles
   (d) *pathological causes*, e.g. heart disease.

3 Diagnose type of bradycardia, e.g. sinus bradycardia, heart block. If sinus bradycardia give atropine up to 20 µg/kg IV. The maximum IV dose for the adult is 3 mg.

4 If significant symptoms or signs consider:
   (a) Pacing either transvenous, oesophageal or transcutaneous approach. See *PACEMAKERS*.
   (b) Isoprenaline (see entry). Give a bolus dose of 1–10 µg, then infusion of 1–8 µg/min. Adrenaline can also be used. See *ADRENALINE*.
   (c) If severe symptoms/signs treat as for cardiac arrest (see *CARDIAC ARREST*).

Brainstem Anaesthesia

Aetiology

Brainstem anaesthesia is due to accidental intrathecal injection or intrathecal spread of a local anaesthetic drug to the region of the brainstem. This condition has been associated with various types of regional anaesthesic blocks performed around the head and neck including:[38]

1 deep cervical plexus block
2 stellate ganglion block
3 interscalene brachial plexus block
4 retrobulbar block with accidental subarachnoid injection.

Diagnosis

This syndrome is characterised by the rapid (over 2–10 min)[38] appearance of:

1 restlessness, drowsiness and confusion
2 vomiting
3 cardiac depression
4 respiratory arrest
5 absence of brainstem reflexes on laryngoscopy.

Treatment

Supportive measures are required until the local anaesthetic effect wears off. These include:

1 intubation of the airway and ventilation
2 circulatory support with IV fluids and vasopressor agents.

Breastfeeding and Anaesthesia

Patients who require anaesthesia while breastfeeding should be advised as follows:

1 Continue breastfeeding up until the time of anaesthesia.
2 When the next feed is due postoperatively, express and discard the first breast milk that has accumulated and provide formula feed for the infant.
3 Resume breastfeeding at the usual intervals.

Broad Complex Tachycardia

Diagnosis

Differential diagnosis is between ventricular tachycardia (VT) and supraventricular tachycardia (SVT) with left bundle branch block (LBBB). Diagnostic features on the ECG to differentiate between these two dysrhythmias include:

1 *P Waves.* If P waves are present before each QRS, this favours SVT whereas atrioventricular (AV) dissociation favours VT.
2 *QRS axis.* A bizarre axis or a change in axis from the patient's usual ECG favours VT.
3 *QRS duration.* A QRS duration < 0.14 s favours SVT, whereas a duration $\geq$ 0.14 s favours VT.
4 *Lead V1.* A monophasic positive QRS in V1 favours VT, but a right bundle branch block (RBBB) pattern in V1 favours SVT. If QRS in V1 is biphasic and the first R wave is taller than the second r wave, this favours VT. See Figure B4.

B

This pattern in V1 favours VT.

This pattern in V1 favours SVT with LBBB.

Figure B4 Lead V1 QRS morphology in the differentiation of broad complex tachycardia

This pattern in lead V6 favours SVT.

Figure B5 Lead V6 QRS morphology in the differentiation of broad complex tachycardia

5 *Lead V6.* A deep S in V6 strongly favours VT. A positive QRS in V6 favours SVT especially if the QRS is double peaked and the R (first) peak is smaller than the r (second) peak. See Figure B5.
6 *Concordance* favours VT (all the QRS complexes look similar in shape).
7 *Fusion beats* favour VT (QRS complexes that look halfway between a normal QRS and the broadened QRS complexes).
8 *Capture beats* also favour VT (a normal looking QRS between two broad QRS complexes).
9 Always consider the clinical picture. An elderly patient with ischaemic heart disease is much more likely to have VT than SVT. Young patients without heart disease are more likely to have SVT.
10 *Cannon waves* visible in the jugular venous pulse wave indicate AV dissociation. These waves support the diagnosis of VT.

Management of Broad Complex Tachycardia

1 If unstable cardiovascularly, DC cardioversion.
2 If stable, it is much safer to treat as VT than SVT. If a patient with VT is treated with verapamil on the assumption that the patient has SVT with LBBB, the result could be fatal. If there is a strong suspicion of SVT with LBBB the safest course of action is to treat with adenosine. See *ADENOSINE, SUPRAVENTRICULAR TACHYCARDIA* and *VENTRICULAR TACHYCARDIA*. Adenosine may revert SVT but will have little effect on VT and has a high safety profile.
3 If the origin of the hemodynamically stable broad complex tachycardia remains obscure, treat with amiodarone, procainamide or sotalol.

B

Bronchial Tree Anatomy and Bronchoscopy

Bronchial Tree Anatomy and Bronchoscopy

The trachea is ≈ 15 cm long in the adult. See Figure B6.

Right Lung

The right main bronchus is wider and more vertical than the left, and gives off the right upper lobe bronchus after ≈ 2.5 cm. It is then called the lower part of the right main bronchus, which is ≈ 3 cm long. In the right upper lobe bronchus, three openings come into view, for the *anterior*, *posterior* and *apical* bronchi. Continuing down the lower part of the right main bronchus, the opening of the *middle lobe bronchus* is seen anteriorly. Just below this and posteriorly, the opening to the *apical bronchus* of the lower lobe is noted. Travelling past this opening further into the lower lobe bronchus, the *medial (cardiac) basal bronchus* is identified on the medial wall. Finally three openings are observed: the *anterior basal*, *lateral basal* and *posterior basal bronchi*.

Left Lung

Advancing into the left main bronchus which is ≈ 5 cm long, the first orifice seen is the *left upper lobe bronchus* on the lateral wall.

The lingual orifice can only be seen with a retrograde telescope attachment. Advancing into the lower lobe bronchus the next orifice observed is the *apical bronchus* on the posterior aspect. Beyond this orifice three openings come into view: the *anterior*, *lateral* and *posterior basal bronchi*.

Bronchopleural Fistula (BPF)

This condition can result from a wide variety of causes including:

1   post-thoracic surgery with breakdown of a suture line
2   ruptured lung abscess, bulla or cyst

1 Right main bronchus

Right upper lobe
2 Apical
3 Posterior
4 Anterior

Right middle lobe
5 Lateral
6 Medial

Right lower lobe
7 Apical
8 Anterior basal
9 Lateral basal
10 Posterior basal
11 Medial basal (cardiac)

12 Left main bronchus

Left upper lobe
13 Apical
14 Posterior
15 Anterior

Lingular
16 Superior lingular
17 Inferior lingular

Left lower lobe
18 Apical
19 Anterior
20 Lateral basal
21 Posterior basal

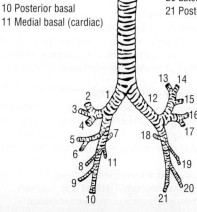

Figure B6 Bronchial tree anatomy

3   erosion by malignancy
4   barotrauma.

Diagnosis

The lesion may be small, chronic and have little clinical impact. Clinical symptoms and signs for acute large bronchopleural fistulas include:

1   sudden dyspnoea, cyanosis, respiratory distress
2   subcutaneous emphysema
3   deviation of the trachea
4   tension pneumothorax
5   failure of a chest tube to drain a pneumothorax, often with a massive air-leak.[39]

Treatment

1   *Airway.* Optimise airway.
2   *Breathing.* Ensure adequate ventilation.
3   *Circulation.* Ensure adequate pulse and blood pressure. Tension pneumothorax can cause pulseless electrical activity. See *CARDIAC ARREST.* If tension pneumothorax is suspected insert a chest tube.
4   Provide adequate IV fluid resuscitation.
5   Establish the usual non-invasive monitoring plus consider insertion of an arterial line to detect early pericardial compression.
6   Pre-anaesthetic bronchoscopy should be performed if possible and may provide information regarding the site and extent of the BPF.
7   Options for induction of anaesthesia include:
    (a) rapid sequence induction if patient is in extremus
    (b) awake fibre-optic bronchoscopy and intubation.
    (c) inhalational induction
8   A double lumen tube is usually required to isolate the lung with the BPF.

Bronchospasm

Topics Covered in this Section
▶ Prevention
▶ Treatment
▶ Ventilation Strategies for Patients with Severe Bronchospasm
▶ Dosages in Children

Prevention
See *ASTHMA*.

Treatment
1 Identify the cause (see *COVER ABCD CRISIS MANAGEMENT ALGORITHM*). Always consider asthma, anaphylaxis and pneumothorax as possible causes.
2 Assess airway, breathing and circulation.
3 Increase FiO_2 to 100% if oxygen saturation is reduced.
4 Remove any airway irritation, e.g. secretions, endotracheal tube tip touching carina. Suck out the endotracheal tube and consider withdrawing it slightly.
5 Cease surgical stimulation and deepen anaesthesia if it is suspected that the patient is 'too light'.
6 Give salbutamol aerosolised down the endotracheal tube via a 'spacer' device attached between the endotracheal tube and the breathing system.
7 Give salbutamol 200–300 µg IV over 5 min, then infusion run at 2–20 µg/min. Mix 15 mg salbutamol in 250 mL N/S, run at 2–20 mL/h.
8 Give adrenaline if bronchospasm is severe and not responding to the above measures. The dose depends on the urgency of the situation. In general, give between 50–100 µg and 0.5 mg IV

(the higher dose for imminent cardiorespiratory arrest). Follow up with an infusion of adrenaline. Mix 6 mg in 100 mL N/S and titrate to effect starting with 5 mL/h. If IV access is not available, give 0.3 mg subcut 20 min repeat × 2.[40]

9   Aminophylline may also be useful. Give a loading dose of 5 mg/kg over 15–30 min (unless the patient is on oral theophylline, in which case a loading dose is contraindicated). Then give an aminophylline infusion of 0.5 mg/kg/h.

10 Give hydrocortisone 200 mg IV.

11 Be aware of the constant risk of tension pneumothorax, which may be bilateral and may result in cardiac arrest.

▶ Other Treatments of Bronchospasm to Consider

1   Give ipratropium bromide (inhaled anticholinergic drug), which can be used in combination with nebulised salbutamol. *Dose in adult*: 2 mL of 0.025% solution 2 h initially, then 4–6 h.

2   Consider ketamine. For non-intubated patients, give 0.1–0.2 mg/kg followed by an infusion of 0.5 mg/kg/h.[40] Atropine 0.1 mg or more should be given with ketamine to prevent excessive oral secretions. For intubated, ventilated patients a ketamine infusion of 1–5 mg/kg/h can be used.[41]

3   A lignocaine infusion can be tried, run at 1–3 mg/kg/h.[42]

4   Give magnesium sulphate IV 2–3 g IV over 3 minutes.[40]

5   Sevoflurane has significant bronchodilating effects, and is superior to halothane in this regard.[43]

6   Give sodium bicarbonate in ventilated patients to normalise pH. Acidosis is thought to oppose the bronchodilator effects of sympathomimetic drugs.

7   Do external chest compression to assist expiration. At the end of inflation firmly squeeze the lower chest wall bilaterally until the next inflation.

8   Intratracheal injection of recombinant human deoxyribonuclease,

which acts as a mucolytic agent, has produced dramatic improvement in some cases.[44]

9   Heliox (helium/oxygen) mixture reduces airflow resistance and decreases the work of breathing. A 60:40 mixture of helium and O_2 is commonly used and may be of some benefit with severe bronchospasm.[45]

10 Cardiopulmonary bypass.

Ventilation Strategies for Patients with Severe Bronchospasm

The overall principles are small tidal volumes, slow respiratory rate and a long expiratory time.

1   Aim for adequate oxygenation at acceptable airway pressures. Allow permissive hypercapnoea up to 80 mmHg if necessary.[40]

2   Aim for a ventilation rate of 8–10 breaths per minute (bpm) and a tidal volume of 5–7 mL/kg.

3   Peak flow should be 60 L/min.

4   If this pattern still results in unacceptably high airway pressures, decrease ventilation rate to 6–8 bpm, reduce tidal volume to 3–5 mL/kg, increase peak flow to 90–120 L/min to further decrease the inspired to expired time ratio. Also ensure that the patient is fully paralysed and adequately sedated.

▶ *Hypotension and/or Desaturation Immediately After Intubation*

Causes to consider include:

1   incorrect ET tube position (bronchial intubation, oesophageal intubation)

2   ET tube obstruction (biting, secretions)

3   tension pneumothorax

4   massive auto-PEEP buildup, which can cause profound hypotension. Treat by disconnecting the patient from the ventilation device for a brief period to allow auto-PEEP to dissipate.

Dosages in Children

1 Salbutamol IV bolus 5–10 µg/kg slowly (max. 250 µg), then infusion 5–7.5 µg/kg/h.
2 Aminophylline 5 mg/kg over 1 h IV, then infusion. No loading dose if on oral theophylline. Rate of infusion depends on age: age 1–9 years 1 mg/kg/h, 10–16 years 0.8 mg/kg/h.
3 Hydrocortisone IV 4 mg/kg 6 h.

Bupivacaine

Amide type local anaesthetic agent. Suitable for all types of local and regional anaesthesia except for intravenous regional blockade (see *BIER BLOCK*) and obstetric paracervical block.

Advantages

1 Longer acting than lignocaine.
2 Due to tissue binding, the addition of adrenaline is not needed to prolong bupivacaine's duration of action.

Disadvantages

1 More cardiotoxic than lignocaine, levobupivacaine or ropivacaine.
2 Cardiovascular collapse due to bupivacaine is much more difficult to treat than CVS collapse due to ropivacaine or lignocaine.[46]
3 May get more motor block with bupivacaine than with ropivacaine.

Maximum Dose

Adult: 2–2.5 mg/kg.
Child: 3 mg/kg. This is equivalent to 0.7–1 mL/kg of the 0.25% solution or 0.35–0.5 mL/kg of the 0.5% solution.

Effects of Accidental IV Injection

As blood bupivacaine levels increase the following effects may be seen:

1 tingling in the lips and tongue, dysphoria, tinnitus
2 loss of consciousness/seizure
3 respiratory arrest
4 hypotension, cardiac dysrhythmia, cardiovascular collapse, cardiac arrest.

Treatment of IV Bupivacaine Toxicity

1 Cease bupivacaine administration.
2 *Airway*: Ensure the patient has a clear and protected airway. Intubate the patient if there is an aspiration risk and consciousness is reduced.
3 *Breathing*: Ensure adequate ventilation. Hyperventilate the patient if possible. Note that acidosis and hypoxia markedly increase the cardiotoxicity of bupivacaine.[46]
4 *Circulation*: Support the patient's cardiovascular system by such measures as these:
   (a) If hypotension occurs increase intravascular volume by elevating the legs, and giving IV fluids and vasopressors (e.g. metaraminol, adrenaline).
   (b) If cardiac arrest occurs see *CARDIAC ARREST*.
   (c) If there is marked bradycardia give atropine 0.6 mg. Ventricular tachycardia/fibrillation may occur, which may be difficult to revert electrically or pharmacologically. Consider using lignocaine. In very resistant cases consider cardiopulmonary bypass as recovery may take hours.
   (d) If seizures occur, treat with diazepam 5–10 mg IV incrementally. If ineffective give thiopentone 50 mg IV incrementally.

B

Burns

Topics Covered in this Section
▶ Initial Management and Assessment in the Emergency Department
▶ Calculating Area of Burns as a Percentage of Body Surface Area
▶ Definition of Major Burns
▶ Fluid Management for Major Burns
▶ Management of Carbon Monoxide (CO) Poisoning
▶ Anaesthetic Considerations for Burns Patients

Initial Management and Assessment in the Emergency Department

1 Obtain a detailed history of the injury, which may provide an indication of additional injuries and the likelihood of airway burns and carbon monoxide poisoning.

2 Ensure the burning process is stopped, e.g. removal of burning clothing.

3 As for any trauma, assess *airway*, ensure patient is *breathing* adequately and assess and optimise patient's *circulation*. Inspect the airway for any evidence of inhalational injury such as pharyngeal burns, sooty sputum, a hoarse voice, and singed nasal hair. Intubate early if the airway is compromised or is likely to become compromised, e.g. in the case of severe neck/facial burns. The options to be considered are:

   (a) Rapid sequence induction. Suxamethonium does not cause a significant hyperkalaemic response in burn patients for at least 24 h, and probably for a few days.[47,48] After this time *suxamethonium is contraindicated* until several months after burns have completely healed.[47]

   (b) Awake fibre-optic intubation.

(c) Inhalational induction and direct laryngoscopy and/or fibre-optic intubation.

4 Establish large bore IV access. Take blood for FBC, electrolytes and creatinine, ABG, blood group and save, coagulation studies and CO levels. Obtain a CXR.

5 The burnt area should be irrigated with tepid H_2O (15°C) for 20–30 min if possible to minimise the eventual depth and area of burn.[49]

6 Exclude/manage associated trauma. Immobolise the cervical spine if neck injury is possible. If the patient is unconscious consider head trauma, drug/alcohol use, carbon monoxide (CO) poisoning and/or smoke inhalation. Always log roll the patient to identify injuries on the back.

7 Provide tetanus prophylaxis.

8 Hypovolaemic shock, if present, will not usually be due to the burn itself in the early stages, but due to other injuries, which must be identified.[49]

9 Give adequate analgesia (usually opioids) only when all other injuries are elucidated.

10 Calculate the percentage of skin area burnt.

11 Early escharotomy may be required for circumferential burns to areas such as the chest. This procedure may be urgent and life-saving.

12 Cling film can be used as an initial dressing.

Calculating Area of Burns as a Percentage of Body Surface Area

The percentage of total body surface area (TBSA) burnt in adults and children can be calculated from Tables B4 and B5. Only areas of skin with partial or full thickness burns should be included.

B

Table B4 Calculating area of burns (Rule of Nines) in the adult	
Region	% of TBSA
Arm	9
Trunk	36
Head	9
Leg	18
Perineum	1

Table B5 Calculating % burns in the child		
	% of TBSA	
Region	0–3 years	>3 years
Head and neck	18	12
Trunk and groin	32	38
Both arms	20	20
Both legs	30	30

Definition of Major Burns

Major burns are defined as:

- *Adult*: > 15% TBSA having partial and full thickness burns or > 10% TBSA full thickness burns.[50]
- *Child*: > 10% TBSA full thickness burn or > 20% partial and/or full thickness burns.[51]

Fluid Management for Major Burns

1 Commence *fluid resuscitation*. Various formulae are used; these in general aim at providing about 2–4 mL/kg per % TBSA burns in the first 24 h post burn. An example is the Parkland formula:[47]

On the first day of therapy, give Hartmann's 4 mL/kg per % TBSA burn over first 24 h (from time of burn). Give half this over the first 8 h. Also add the patient's normal maintenance fluid.

2 Aim for at least 0.5–1 mL/kg/min urine output in adults and at least 1 mL/kg/min in children.[50] If oliguria occurs increase IV fluids by 50%.[49]

Management of Carbon Monoxide (CO) Poisoning

▶ *Clinical Effects of CO Poisoning*

Haemoglobin has 240 × more affinity for CO than O_2. The oxygen–haemoglobin dissociation curve is shifted to the left and the O_2 content of the blood is severely reduced with significant poisoning.

Effects of CO poisoning include confusion, fitting or coma. Cerebral irritability may persist for weeks.[55] Cherry pink skin and mucosa can occur but cyanosis is more common. Basal ganglia damage can occur, and patients may suffer loss of higher mental function and depression.[52] Cardiac dysrhythmias may occur and cardiac output may fall.[53]

▶ *Relevant Investigations*

ECG may show ST segment changes.[54] Pulse oximetry is misleading because only oxyhaemoglobin and deoxyhaemoglobin are detected. In the presence of carboxyhaemoglobin (COHb) a falsely elevated O_2 saturation reading will be obtained.[55] A low co-oximeter O_2 with raised COHb levels is diagnostic.[53]

Table B6 Significance of COHb levels[56,57]

COHb level	Significance
< 2%	Normal
Up to 12%	Heavy smokers
15%	Monitor closely
30%	Life-threatening hypoxia
> 50%	Lethal

▶ *Treatment*

In addition to general supportive measures, treat CO poisoning with 100% O_2. This reduces the half-life of COHb from 240 min to 30–40 min.[49] Hyperbaric O_2 therapy is recommended but its management value is doubted by some researchers.[49]

Table B7 Half-life of CO in blood under various conditions of FiO_2 and pressure[58]

CO Half-life in blood	Pressure and concentration of inhaled O_2 (%)
250 min	21% at 1 atm
50 min	100% at 1 atm
22 min	100% at 2.5 atm

Anaesthetic Considerations for Burns Patients

1   Suxamethonium is *contraindicated* after the first 24–48 h post burn due to the risk of severe hyperkalaemia. Suxamethonium

remains contraindicated until well after the burns have healed, some authorities recommending a period of 2 years after the burn injury.[59] Burns patients are resistant to the effects of non-depolarising neuromuscular blocking drugs.

2 Pay meticulous attention to maintaining the patient's body temperature peri-operatively.

3 Prepare for moderate to severe blood loss during grafting procedures. Try to limit the area excised at each debridement to less than 20% of TBSA and blood loss to < 50% of total blood volume. Encourage the surgeon to use vasoconstrictor infiltration, such as POR 8 diluted to 0.1–0.2 units/mL (use a maximum dose of 0.5 units/kg).[51] Adrenaline can also be used topically on skin donor sites. Use 1:10 000 solution liberally as there is very little systemic absorption.[51]

Cc

Caesarean Section (CS)

Topics Covered in this Section
- Choice of Anaesthetic Technique
- Pre-operative Assessment and Preparation
- General Anaesthesia—Induction and Intubation Phase and Failed Intubation Drill
- Anaesthetic Management after Intubation
- Epidural Anaesthesia
- Subarachnoid Block Anaesthesia

Choice of Anaesthetic Technique

Regional anaesthesia has a lower maternal risk than general anaesthesia.[1] Hawkins et al. calculated that the relative risk of maternal mortality is $16.7 \times$ greater with GA compared with a regional technique.[2]

The risk of failed intubation in the obstetric population is estimated to be about 0.4%.[3] The majority of anaesthesia-related maternal deaths are due to failed intubation and/or aspiration.[4]

General anaesthesia is often still required for failed regional anaesthesia, for patient refusal of regional anaesthesia and for some obstetric emergencies. Although tracheal intubation for CS has long been thought to be the 'gold standard' the laryngeal mask airway has been used successfully in at least one large trial in selected patients.[5]

Pre-operative Assessment and Preparation

In addition to routine history and examination:

1 Carefully assess the airway to identify possibly difficult intubation. Prepare for unanticipated difficult intubation.

2 Acid aspiration prophylaxis:

(a) Ranitidine 150 mg PO the night before and the morning of surgery.

(b) Sodium citrate 0.3 M 30 mL on call to op-suite, or in op-suite.

(c) Metoclopramide. Consider 10 mg IV or IM if the patient has had a recent meal, to increase gastric emptying.

General Anaesthesia—Induction and Intubation Phase and Failed Intubation Drill

1 Position the patient in left lateral tilt with a wedge placed under the right buttock to prevent aortocaval compression. See *SUPINE HYPOTENSIVE SYNDROME*.

2 *Rapid sequence induction*:

(a) Pre-oxygenate patient for 5 min.

(b) Give thiopentone 4–5 mg/kg, followed immediately by suxamethonium 1–1.5 mg/kg (or rocuronium 0.6 mg/kg if suxamethonium is contraindicated).

An assistant must apply cricoid pressure as the patient begins to lose consciousness and does not release cricoid pressure until the trachea is intubated and the anaesthetist requests its release.

For a more detailed discussion of this manoeuvre see *RAPID SEQUENCE INDUCTION*.

3 *Always* be prepared for the possibility of failed intubation and be familiar with an appropriate failed intubation drill.

▶ *Suggested Failed Intubation Drill for CS*

1 Send for help and alert the surgeon. Maintain cricoid pressure.

2 *Oxygenation must be maintained* via mask and bag using an

C

oral and/or nasal airway as required. If unable to maintain oxygenation insert a laryngeal mask airway (LMA) or ProSeal LMA. It may be necessary to release cricoid pressure temporarily while placing the LMA/ProSeal.[6] See *DIFFICULT AIRWAY MANAGEMENT*.

3 If *able to maintain oxygenation* consider re-attempting intubation with whatever aids are available (e.g. teflon introducer, Kessels blade, Belscope, McCoy blade). Do not attempt intubation more than three times in total.

4 If *able to maintain oxygenation* but *unable to intubate*, decide whether CS *must proceed immediately* to save the life of the baby (foetal distress) and/or the mother (e.g. bleeding placenta praevia or ruptured uterus). Morris argues that the decision to continue should be made only if there is serious threat to the life of the mother.[6] Other clinicians feel that if foetal distress is severe and maternal oxygenation is well maintained, then it is reasonable to proceed with CS.[7] Note also that uneventful CS using a LMA is a well documented technique.[5]

5 If CS *must proceed immediately* maintain anaesthesia with bag and mask or LMA/ProSeal, volatile anaesthetic agent and intermediate acting NMBD, e.g. vecuronium or rocuronium, with maintenance of cricoid pressure throughout the procedure.[7] Cricoid pressure must be maintained until the patient is able to protect her own airway.

6 If *able to maintain oxygenation* and CS *not urgent* allow the patient to 'wake up' and use epidural, spinal or awake intubation technique.

7 If *unable to maintain oxygenation* obtain a *surgical airway* via cricothyrotomy or cricothyroid membrane needle puncture. See *CRICOTHYROID PUNCTURE AND CRICOTHYROTOMY*.

Anaesthetic Management After Intubation

1   Maintain anaesthesia with O_2, N_2O and volatile agent.
2   Maintain muscle relaxation with intermediate acting muscle relaxant such as rocuronium.
3   Avoid hypocapnia, which may result in decreased placental perfusion.
4   Give 10 IU syntocinon IV + opioid (e.g. morphine 10 mg) once baby is delivered. The surgeon may request a syntocinon infusion (40 IU in 1000 mL of Hartmann's solution).
5   Extubate the patient in the left lateral position 'awake', i.e. when she is able to protect her own airway. Selecting the optimum time to extubate is a matter of experience but usually a patient can be extubated when she has a vigorous cough and shows evidence of voluntary muscle control, e.g. opening eyes to voice, trying to self-extubate.

Epidural Anaesthesia

Aortocaval compression must be prevented at all times. The epidural anaesthetic dose required is ≈ 20–25 mL of lignocaine 2% with adrenaline 1:200 000 + fentanyl 100 µg epidurally. Preload patient with 500 mL–1 L of IV crystalloid fluid. Do not use 5% glucose. See *EPIDURAL ANAESTHESIA*. The onset time of adequate epidural anaesthesia can be decreased by placing the patient in a modified Trendelenburg position (15° Trendelenberg with 10° of 'head up').[8]

Subarachnoid Block Anaesthesia

Anticipate hypotension, which may be of a more rapid onset than with epidural. Preload patient with 1–1.5 L of crystalloid (not 5% glucose) and consider prophylactic ephedrine 15 mg IV immediately after LA injection. For the subarachnoid block use 'heavy' bupivacaine 0.5% (which contains glucose 80 mg/mL). Use 2.5 mL for the average-sized patient. Opioids can be added to improve the quality of spinal block, e.g. fentanyl 25 µg. Position the patient to

C

avoid aortocaval compression at all times (e.g. left lateral tilt with 10–15° of 'sitting up'). See *SUBARACHNOID BLOCK ANAESTHESIA*.

Calcium

Calcium is an essential electrolyte for body metabolism. It is particularly important for nerve conduction and skeletal, cardiac and smooth muscle contraction and in many enzymatic processes such as coagulation.

NR 2.25–2.6 mmol/L. To correct for the serum albumin level, actual Ca^{2+} level equals measured Ca^{2+} + (40 – measured albumin) × 0.024. It is the ionised calcium level that is clinically significant.

Hypercalcaemia
Severe if Ca > 3.5 mmol/L.

▶ *Clinical Effects*
1 Drowsiness, lethargy, weakness.
2 Nausea and vomiting.
3 Abdominal pain.
4 Pancreatitis.
5 Polydypsia, polyuria and dehydration.
6 Dysrhythmias including bradycardia, tachycardia, heart block.
7 Hypertension.
8 ECG may show shortened a Q-T interval in prolonged PR and QRS intervals, and T wave flattening and widening. AV nodal block progressing to complete heart block may occur.
9 Coma, cardiac arrest.

▶ *Treatment*
1 Rehydrate with N/S.
2 Establish forced saline diuresis with 1000 mL N/S over 4 h, then 1000 mL N/S + 20 mEq KCl + 20 mg frusemide 4 h. Monitor the following:
   (a) Potassium, calcium, and magnesium levels.

C

(b) Intravascular volume status (including use of CVP measurement).

(c) Urine output and urinary sodium. Aim to keep urinary Na^+ greater than 100 mmol/L.

3 If the hypercalcaemia is due to myeloproliferative disorder, give mithramycin (plicamycin) 25 µg/kg by infusion over 3 h. Give one dose only.

4 Calcitonin is effective for hypercalcaemia associated with cancer. Give 3–4 U/kg IV, then 4 U/kg subcutaneously 12–24 h.

5 Hydrocortisone 200–400 mg/day IV.

6 EDTA 15–50 mg/kg.

7 Dialysis.

Hypocalcaemia

▶ Clinical Effects

Clinical manifestations occur when serum $Ca^{2+} < 2$ mmol/L. These include:

- tetany, cramps, carpo-pedal spasm
- positive Chvostek and Trousseau's signs
- mental changes
- reduced cardiac output, hypotension
- perioral and peripheral paraesthesia
- ECG may show a prolonged Q-T interval, T wave inversion, heart blocks and ventricular fibrillation.

▶ Treatment

1 Provide adequate airway and ventilation.

2 Provide circulatory support if cardiac output is inadequate.

3 Give IV calcium, either calcium chloride 10% 10 mL (6.8 mmol) or calcium gluconate 20 mL (4.4 mmol). The final dose depends on the degree of deficiency although the maximum daily dose should not exceed 33 mmol (15 g).

Calcium Gluconate

Calcium gluconate is presented in 10 mL ampoules containing 1 g (2.2 mmol) of calcium. Calcium gluconate is useful in the treatment of:

- hypocalcaemia
- hyperkalaemia
- hypermagnasaemia
- calcium channel blocker overdose.

Adult Dose

- *Hyperkalaemia/hypermagnasaemia*: 2.2 mmol by slow IV injection (over 5 min), repeat if required.
- *Hypocalcaemia*: See *CALCIUM* above.
- *Calcium channel blocker poisoning*: 2.2–4.4 mmol by slow IV injection (over 5 min).

Precautions: Do not give in the presence of digoxin toxicity.

Carbon Monoxide Poisoning

See *BURNS, Initial Management and Assessment in the Emergency Department*.

Cardiac Arrest

Topics Covered in this Section

▶ Basic Life Support—Adult
▶ Advanced Life Support—Adult
▶ Basic Life Support—Child
▶ Advanced Life Support—Child
▶ Cardiac Arrest in Pregnancy
▶ Administration of Drugs by the Endotracheal Route

Basic Life Support—Adult

The steps in basic life support (BLS) can be summarised as:

D   Danger
R   Response
A   Airway
B   Breathing
C   Circulation
D   Defibrillation

▶ *Danger*

Ensure the safety of the rescuer, victim and bystanders, e.g. the victim may have been overcome by smoke and needs to be removed from this environment.

▶ *Response*

Establish that the patient is unresponsive to simple commands, e.g. 'open your eyes', and physical stimulation that will not put the patient at risk of further injury, e.g. squeezing the shoulders. If the patient is unresponsive, *call for help/summon the cardiac arrest team.*

▶ *Airway*

Ensure that the unconscious patient has a clear airway. This can be achieved by backward head tilt (extending the head on the neck), jaw thrust, opening the mouth slightly (jaw support) and removal of any obvious loose foreign body in the mouth such as loose dentures. Well fitting dentures should be left in place.[9]

▶ *Breathing*

Look for evidence of breathing by listening for breath sounds and feeling for exhaled gas. If the patient is not breathing commence artificial ventilation. This can be achieved by mouth-to-mouth, mouth-to-mask or bag–mask ventilation. Give 5 fast deep breaths within 10 seconds. Provide oxygen supplementation if possible, e.g. mouth-to-mask technique with oxygen tubing attached to a suitable port on the mask.

C

▶ *Circulation*

1 Identify whether a palpable pulse is present by feeling the carotid artery. If no pulse is palpable commence external cardiac compression (ECC). ECC is achieved by compressing the lower half of the sternum at a rate of 100/minute. The point of compression is found by identifying the midpoint between the sternal notch and the xiphisternum. The upper edge of the compressing hands are placed against this midpoint and over the lower half of the sternum. The depth of compression should be one-third the anterior-to-posterior diameter of the chest or 5 cm. To coordinate ECC and ventilation use the following ratios:

- one rescuer: 15 ECCs per two chest inflations.
- two rescuers: 15 ECCs per two chest inflations or 5 ECCs per one chest inflation (both ratios are acceptable).[10]

2 Give ECC at a rate of 100 per minute with a compression-to-relaxation ratio (or 'duty cycle') of 1:1.

3 Check for the return of spontaneous circulation after 1 minute, then after every 2 minutes. With properly performed ECC, cardiac output is 25–35% of normal.[11] Although systolic blood pressures of 40–80 mmHg can be achieved, diastolic blood pressure is very low.

▶ *Defibrillation*

1 If a defibrillator is immediately available, defibrillation of VF/pulseless VT takes precedence over the other steps in BLS in the witnessed arrest situation. If an automated external defibrillator (AED) is available, apply this to the patient's chest as quickly as possible. Follow the voice prompts. Do not use an AED to defibrillate patients less than 8 years old, patients less than 25 kg or if the patient is wet.

2 For a witnessed monitored arrest due to ventricular fibrillation (VF) or pulseless ventricular tachycardia (VT), or a witnessed cardiac arrest due to electrocution, where a defibrillator is not

immediately available, give a precordial thump. This manoeuvre consists of a blow to the mid-sternum with the ulnar surface of the clenched fist. This may revert these dysrhythmias.[12]

Advanced Life Support—Adult

Subsequent management of cardiac arrest after BLS depends on diagnosing the underlying cardiac rhythm. The three common types of cardiac arrest are:

1 *ventricular fibrillation or pulseless ventricular tachycardia*. About 85% of cardiac arrests are associated with these rhythms, at least initially.[13]
2 *asystole*
3 *pulseless electrical activity (electromechanical dissociation).*

▶ Ventricular Fibrillation (VF) or Pulseless Ventricular Tachycardia (VT)

1 Early defibrillation is the most important aspect of management. If a monophasic defibrillator is used, defibrillate with 200 J, 200–300 J, then 360 J. Do not remove the paddles from the chest between shocks. Deliver these as rapidly as possible, recharging immediately after each shock is delivered. Continue ECC between shocks only if recharging time is > 20 s. If a biphasic defibrillator is available, defibrillate with three shocks of 150 J.[13]
2 If the initial three shocks are unsuccessful continue ECC, establish IV access, and intubate the patient. Ventilate with 100% O_2 and give adrenaline 1 mg IV flushed through with 20 mL of N/S (as with all other drugs given IV). *Give adrenaline 1 mg IV every 5 minutes of arrest time.* Alternatively, vasopressin 40 IU can be given (1 dose lasts ≈ 20 min).[14] If no venous access is available give adrenaline 2 mg diluted in 10 mL of N/S down the endotracheal tube.[15] See p. 112, *Administration of Drugs by the Endotracheal Route*. Continue cardiac massage for

C

  1 min, then repeat defibrillation: monophasic defibrillator 360
  J × 3, biphasic defibrillator 150 J.

3 If the patient is still in VF/pulseless VT give an anti-arrhythmic
  drug, one of:

  (a) amiodarone 300 mg IV or 5 mg/kg. Give the drug in 20 mL
    5% glucose IV bolus over 1–2 min. Two recent studies have
    supported the efficacy of amiodarone in shock-resistant VF
    compared to placebo[16] and lignocaine.[17] *or*

  (b) sotalol 1 mg/kg IV *or*

  (c) lignocaine 1 mg/kg IV.

  Continue ECC for 1 min, then repeat defibrillation, three shocks
  as described above.

4 If still VF/pulseless VT give a second dose of the chosen anti-
  arrhythmic drug using half the initial dose:

  (a) amiodarone 150 mg IV

  (b) sotalol 0.5 mg/kg

  (c) lignocaine 0.5 mg/kg.

  Continue ECC for 1 min, then repeat defibrillation three shocks
  as described above.

5 If still VF/pulseless VT give a second antidysrhythmic drug (e.g.
  lignocaine if *sotalol* given initially).

6 Consider *magnesium sulphate* IV, which is particularly useful in torsade de pointes, and dysrhythmias associated with digoxin toxicity and documented hypokalaemia. See *TORSADE DE POINTES*
  and *MAGNESIUM SULPHATE*. Give 5 mmol as a bolus IV which
  may be repeated once, then an infusion of 20 mmol over 4 h.

7 Consider sodium bicarbonate IV 1 mmol/kg. Sodium bicarbonate may be beneficial in the following circumstances:

  (a) documented metabolic acidosis prior to arrest

  (b) hyperkalaemia

  (c) arrest time > 15 min

  (d) tricyclic antidepressant overdose-induced dysrhythmia.

8 *Potassium* may be indicated in the following situations:
   (a) persistent VF in a patient on a potassium wasting diuretic without K$^+$ supplement
   (b) documented hypokalaemia.
   Give potassium chloride 2–5 mmol IV.
9 Attempt to diagnose the cause of the arrest, in particular confirm/exclude:
   (a) hyper- or hypokalaemia
   (b) hypothermia
   (c) hypoxia
   (d) digoxin toxicity.

▶ Asystole

Asystolic cardiac arrest is associated with a very poor prognosis and low survival (< 2%).[18]

1 *Adrenaline* 1 mg IV, repeated every 3–5 min of arrest time.
2 *Atropine* 1 mg IV up to a maximum dose of 0.04 mg/kg (3 mg in a 70 kg adult).
3 *Pacing.* There are reports of efficacy[19] in special circumstances but pacing is usually ineffective in asystole. If pacing is used in asystole it should be initiated as early as possible. Pacing is strongly indicated for complete heart block and severe bradycardia. See *PACEMAKERS*.
4 Consider sodium bicarbonate. See above.

▶ Pulseless Electrical Activity (PEA) (Electromechanical Dissociation)

This is defined as organised cardiac electrical activity (other than VF/VT) without a palpable pulse. Cardiac output may or may not be present. In addition to the non-specific treatments outlined below, the most important management strategy is to identify and treat the cause of PEA. The common causes are summarised as the 5 Hs and 5 Ts.

C

5Hs	5Ts
Hypovolaemia	Tablets (e.g. drug overdose)
Hypoxia	Tamponade, cardiac
Hydrogen ion (acidosis)	Tension pneumothorax
Hyper/hypokalaemia	Thrombosis, coronary
Hypothermia	Thrombosis, pulmonary

Another approach is to consider five groups of causes:
1 inadequate circulating volume (haemorrhage, anaphylaxis)
2 something in the cardiac chambers other than liquid blood—gas, fat, clot, bone cement or amniotic fluid embolus filling the heart and pulmonary vasculature
3 impaired cardiac muscle function—inadequate myocardial pumping ability due to hypothermia, hypoxia, ischaemia, drugs or metabolic disturbances
4 compression of the heart muscle—tension pneumothorax, cardiac tamponade.

Non-specific treatment measures include:
1 adrenaline 1 mg IV repeat every 3–5 min of arrest time.
2 aggressive IV fluid loading to increase intravascular volume. This will improve cardiac output with many of the causes of PEA, such as hypovolaemia, pulmonary embolus and cardiac tamponade.
3 transcutaneous pacing. This will be of benefit if the PEA is due to disrupted cardiac conduction with otherwise adequate myocardial muscle function.

Basic Life Support—Child
Most cardiac arrests in children result primarily from respiratory insufficiency, trauma, drowning, and sudden infant death

syndrome. Airway and ventilatory management and early intubation are of the highest priority in the child, unlike in the adult, in whom defibrillation takes priority.

▶ *Basic Life Support—Older Child (9–14 Years)*

The approach to BLS in the adult applies also to the older child but with the following qualifications:

1   Compress the chest approximately one-third the antero-posterior (AP) diameter of the chest.
2   The rate of compression is 100 per minute.
3   The ratio of ECC to ventilation is the same as for the adult.

▶ *Basic Life Support—Younger Child (1–8 Years)*

The approach to BLS in the adult applies also to the younger child but with the following qualifications:

1   ECC is performed with the heel of one hand placed over the sternum one finger's breadth above the xiphisternum.
2   Compress the chest approximately one-third the depth of the chest.
3   The rate of compression is 100 per minute.

▶ *Basic Life Support—Infant (1 Month–1 Year Old)*

The approach to BLS in the adult applies also to the infant but with the following qualifications:

1   Head tilt should not be used to optimise the airway.[20]
2   The brachial pulse is easier to feel and locate than the carotid pulse, in the infant.[21]
3   In the infant, compress the chest by placing two fingers one finger's breadth beneath a line joining the nipples. Compress the chest approximately one-third the AP diameter of the chest.
4   The rate of compression is 100 per minute.
5   The ratio of ECC to ventilation is 5:1 for one or two rescuers.

▶ *Basic Life Support—Neonate*
See *NEONATAL RESUSCITATION*.

Advanced Life Support—Child
▶ *Asystole or Severe Bradycardia*
1 Adrenaline 10 μg/kg IV (0.1 mL/kg of 1:10 000 solution). If unable to obtain IV access give 100 μg/kg (i.e. 10 × the IV dose) via the endotracheal (ET) tube. If the child is less than 6 years and IV access cannot be obtained use the interosseous (IO) route. See *INTEROSSEOUS PUNCTURE*. If asystole or severe bradycardia persists give adrenaline 100 μg/kg via the IV, ET tube or IO route. Repeat this dose every 3–5 min of resuscitation.
2 If still unsuccessful give sodium bicarbonate 1 mmol/kg IV. Do not give sodium bicarbonate via the ET tube or IO route.
3 Atropine 20 μg/kg IV, IO or ET tube.
4 Attempt pacing (oesophageal, transcutaneous or transvenous).
5 If hypovolaemia is suspected give crystalloid 20 mL/kg and repeat this dose until hypovolaemia is reversed.

▶ *Ventricular Fibrillation/Pulseless Ventricular Tachycardia*
1 DC cardioversion (monophasic defibrillator) 2 J/kg, then 2–4 J/kg, then 4 J/kg.
2 If no response give adrenaline 10 μg/kg IV or IO or 100 μg/kg via the ET tube. Give adrenaline 100 μg/kg for every 3–5 min of arrest time.
3 Repeat DC shock 4 J/kg × 3.
4 If still unsuccessful give an anti-arrythmic drug, either:
   (a) lignocaine 1–1.5 mg/kg IV, IO or ET tube *or*
   (b) amiodarone 5 mg/kg IV or IO.
5 Repeat DC shock 4 J/kg × 3.
6 If still unsuccessful try an alternative anti-arrhythmic, e.g. amiodarone if lignocaine was used first.
7 Consider sodium bicarbonate 1 mmol/kg IV.

▶ *Pulseless Electrical Activity (Electromechanical Dissociation)*

1 As in the adult identify/treat the cause.
2 Adrenaline 10 µg/kg IV or IO or give 100 µg/kg via ET tube. If a second dose of adrenaline is required give 100 µg/kg via any of the above routes.
3 IV fluid bolus 20 mL/kg (colloid or crystalloid).
4 Consider sodium bicarbonate 1 mmol/kg.

▶ *Supraventricular Tachycardia*

1 If there is severe hypotension or no palpable pulse administer a DC shock 0.5–1 J/kg.
2 If the patient's circulation is adequate treat with pharmacotherapy. Adenosine is the drug of choice (see entry). *Do not use verapamil or other Ca^{2+} channel blocker to treat SVT in the infant.* Other options to consider are:
   (a) carotid sinus massage (never perform bilaterally at the same time)
   (b) Valsalva during ventilation using an ET tube
   (c) ice pack applied to face
   (d) overdrive pacing.

▶ *Defibrillation in Children*

Small paddles, with a cross sectional area of 12–20 cm^2, are used.

Cardiac Arrest in Pregnancy

1 The patient who is in the second or third trimester must be placed in the left lateral tilt position in the arrest situation to prevent aorto-caval compression by the gravid uterus. See *SUPINE HYPOTENSIVE SYNDROME*. If this position cannot be achieved it may be necessary for a rescuer to hold the uterus towards the victim's left side manually.
2 ECC should be performed slightly higher on the sternum e.g. mid-sternum compared with the non-pregnant adult.[22]

C

3 Failure to achieve successful resuscitation within 5 min is an indication for immediate Caesarean section in the best interests of the mother and foetus.

Administration of Drugs by the Endotracheal Route

The endotracheal route can be used for the administration of adrenaline, lignocaine and atropine. These should be given at 2–2.5 × the recommended IV dose and diluted in 10 mL of N/S. A catheter should be passed beyond the tip of the ET tube, and chest compression is stopped as the drug solution is sprayed quickly through the catheter. Give two or three quick insufflations to aerosolise the medication and hasten absorption.[15]

Cardiac Arrest in the Newborn

See *NEONATAL RESUSCITATION*.

Cardiac Failure

See *CONGESTIVE CARDIAC FAILURE*.

Cardiac Investigations

Can be divided into non-invasive and invasive tests.

Non-invasive Tests

1 *Electrocardiograph (ECG)*. The resting ECG is normal in 25–50% of patients with coronary artery disease.[23] Patients with a previous Q wave myocardial infarct (MI) may be at less anaesthetic risk than patients with a previous non-Q wave MI.[24]
2 *Chest X-ray*.
3 *Exercise stress test*. A positive stress test is indicative of an increased anaesthetic risk but a negative stress test may not exclude increased risk.[24]
4 *Echocardiography*. This is able to show wall motion, chamber size and valvular function. This test also gives a semi-quantitative

estimate of left ventricular ejection fraction (LVEF). The two types are *transthoracic* and *transoesophageal* (see below).

5   *Ambulatory ST segment analysis.*

6   *Dobutamine stress and exercise stress echocardiography.* This may help estimate dynamic cardiac reserve. An exercise-induced reduction in ejection fraction may be highly indicative of increased risk.[24]

7   *Dipyridamole and exercise thallium isotope scan (nuclear stress test).* Thallium 201 is a potassium analogue that penetrates into the myocardium. Exercise (or dipyridamole if patient unable to exercise) causes coronary vasodilatation. Dobutamine can also be used to increase myocardial O_2 demand. Ischaemic myocardium takes up little thallium and appears as a cold spot on gamma imaging. A second scan is performed after 3–4 h and may show delayed uptake, indicating ischaemic myocardium (thallium redistribution). Failure to take up thallium suggests an area of infarction. The sensitivity and specificity of this procedure as a screening test have been challenged recently.[23]

8   *Sesta-MIBI scan.* Similar principle to above.

9   *Metabolic cart.*[25] Also called cardiopulmonary exercise testing. The basis of this test is the premise that the metabolic stress of major surgery is comparable to the metabolic stress of exercise. With exercise, CO_2 production and O_2 consumption increase in a linear fashion. A point is reached where O_2 delivery (by heart and lungs) is unable to keep up with O_2 demand and anaerobic metabolism must supplement aerobic metabolism. This causes an inflection point in the CO_2 production graph called the *anaerobic threshold* (AT). This AT occurs at $\approx 40\%$ of the maximum O_2 consumption, and the test is considered to be inherently safe. The level of exercise at which the AT occurs allows a measure of the patient's cardiorespiratory reserve.

C

Postoperative cardiovascular mortality is much more likely in patients with an AT < 11 mL/min/kg O_2 uptake.

▶ *Invasive Tests*

1 *Transoesophageal echocardiography* is more sensitive than transthoracic echocardiography for the detection of prosthetic valve dysfunction, atrial thrombus, atrial septal defect, aortic dissection and infective endocarditis.

2 *Coronary angiography* is the 'gold standard' for elucidating coronary vascular disease. It also enables study of ventricular contraction and pressure measurements in chambers and across valves. This test has a mortality of < 0.1% and a coronary dissection or embolism rate of 0.2%.[26]

▶ *Notes on Ventricular Ejection Fraction*

This can be measured by echocardiography, gated blood pool scan, radionucleotide angiocardiography and cardiac catheterisation. This measurement gives an indication of the effectiveness of myocardial contraction. Normal left ventricular ejection fraction is 50–75%. A left ventricular ejection fraction of < 40% indicates significant left ventricular impairment.

Cardiac Ischaemia

See *MYOCARDIAL ISCHAEMIA*.

Cardiac Risk Factors

See *CARDIOVASCULAR PERI-OPERATIVE RISK PREDICTION FOR NON-CARDIAC SURGERY*.

Cardiac Tamponade

General Measures

1   Ensure the airway is patent and that ventilation is optimal.

2 Give IV fluid loading to optimise ventricular diastolic filling and improve cardiac output.

3 Inotropic support may be required.

4 Maintain systemic vascular resistance to support coronary perfusion.

5 Maintain a heart rate of 90–140 bpm.

6 Perform emergency pericardiocentesis if pericardial fluid results in a life-threatening reduction in cardiac output. Opening of the chest by a trained cardiothoracic surgeon may be required for patients who have had recent heart surgery.

Technique for Pericardiocentesis

1 Position patient sitting at 45° in bed.

2 Connect the limb leads of the ECG monitor to patient's limbs and a chest lead to a 16 FG aspiration needle (or other suitable needle such as a 18 G spinal needle).

3 Insert the needle between the xiphisternum and the seventh costal cartilage on the left side, at an angle of ≈ 35° to the midline and ≈ 45° to the skin.[27] Aim for the left shoulder. Aspirate constantly with a syringe while inserting the needle.

4 Elevation of the ST segments or ectopic beats suggests the needle is entering the myocardium and that it needs to be pulled back.

5 Drain fluid using a three-way tap. If possible consider leaving a plastic cannula in place for continuous or repeated pericardial sac drainage. This can be done by a Seldinger technique utilising a guide wire passed through the drainage needle.

Cardiogenic Shock

See *CONGESTIVE CARDIAC FAILURE.*

Cardiomyopathy of Pregnancy

See *PERIPARTUM CARDIOMYOPATHY.*

Cardiovascular Peri-operative Risk Prediction for Non-cardiac Surgery

Topics Covered in this Section

▸ Clinical Predictors of Cardiac Risk Factors in Patients Having Non-cardiac Surgery

▸ Surgery-specific Cardiac Risk Factors

▸ MET Concept as a Measure of Functional Capacity

▸ Specific Issues in Cardiovascular Peri-operative Risk Prediction

Clinical Predictors of Cardiac Risk Factors in Patients Having Non-cardiac Surgery

The following information is based on recommendations from the American College of Cardiology and the American Heart Association (ACC/AHA guidelines).[28]

▸ *Major Clinical Predictors*

1 Unstable coronary syndromes, e.g. recent myocardial infarct (< 1 month), unstable or severe angina.

2 Decompensated congestive cardiac failure (CCF).

3 Significant arrhythmias such as high grade atrioventricular block.

4 Severe valvular disease.

▸ *Intermediate Predictors*

1 Mild angina.

2 Prior myocardial infarct.

3 Compensated or prior CCF.

4 Diabetes mellitus.

5 Renal insufficiency.

▶ *Minor Predictors*
1. Advanced age.
2. Abnormal ECG/rhythm rather than sinus.
3. Low functional capacity.
4. History of cerebrovascular accident.
5. Uncontrolled systemic hypertension.

Surgery–specific Cardiac Risk Factors[29]

▶ *High Risk Surgery*
(> 5% peri-operative risk of a cardiac event such as MI)
1. Major emergency surgery, especially in the elderly.
2. Aortic surgery.
3. Surgery associated with large fluid shifts or blood loss.

▶ *Intermediate Risk*
(1–5% peri-operative risk of a cardiac event)
1. Carotid surgery.
2. Head and neck procedures.
3. Prostate surgery.
4. Intrathoracic and intraperitoneal surgery.
5. Orthopaedic surgery.

▶ *Low Risk*
1. Breast surgery and superficial procedures.
2. Endoscopic procedures.
3. Cataract surgery.

MET Concept as a Measure of Functional Capacity

MET stands for 'metabolic equivalent', and 1 MET = the O_2 consumption of a resting adult (3.5 mL/kg/min).

Myocardial ischaemia induced at an exercise level of < 5 MET or at a heart rate < 100 indicates a high risk group.[29]

Achievement of exercise > 7 MET or a heart rate of > 130 indicates a low risk group.[29] A patient who is unable to climb two flights of stairs is considered to have poor functional capacity.

Table C1 MET exercise equivalents[29]	
1–4 MET	Walk around house Walk on flat 200 m
5–9 MET	Climb 1 flight of stairs Walk > 6 km Run short distances
> 10 MET	Strenuous sport (swimming, bicycle riding)

Specific Issues in Cardiovascular Peri-operative Risk Prediction

1 Coronary artery bypass graft (CABG) surgery has an overall peri-operative mortality of ≈ 3%.[30] For patients with vascular disease the mortality for CABG increases to 6.5%.[29] The combination of risk of cardiac revascularisation surgery and non-cardiac major surgery will often be higher than the risk of performing major non-cardiac surgery alone in stable patients. The American College of Physicians concludes that coronary revascularisation is not likely to improve peri-operative short-term outcome if only done specifically to reduce the risk for non-cardiac surgery.[30]

2 Percutaneous transluminal coronary angioplasty and coronary artery stenting carry less risk than CABG (≈ 0.5% mortality at 30 days).[30] However, these less invasive procedures have, as yet, an uncertain effect on peri-operative morbidity and mortality for

major non-cardiac surgery. Note that discontinuing antiplatelet therapy within 2 weeks of stenting or angioplasty carries a high mortality (32% in one study).[31] Surgery within 14 days of stent placement is associated with significantly increased mortality and should only be undertaken in an emergency.[29] Surgery should be delayed for at least 3 months post stenting if possible.[29]

3 Patients who have had a MI are at maximal risk for the first 6 weeks and at intermediate risk until 3 months post infarct.[29]

4 *Peri-operative β receptor blockade appears to significantly reduce morbidity and mortality (> 50%) in at risk patients undergoing non-cardiac surgery.*[32] Relative contraindications to β receptor blockade therapy include:
   (a) asthma
   (b) CCF
   (c) symptomatic bradycardia or heart block
   (d) allergy to β receptor blockers.

▶ Which Patients Require a Cardiologist Consultation Pre-operatively?

1 For patients who require elective non-cardiac surgery, cardiologist consultation may be indicated if:[33]
   (a) the patient has an intermediate clinical predictor and poor functional status and there is an intermediate risk surgical procedure being undertaken
   (b) the patient has an intermediate clinical predictor or poor functional status and surgery is high risk
   (c) the patient has one or more of the major clinical predictors of cardiac risk outlined above.

2 In general, patients who have had coronary revascularisation within 5 years or cardiac evaluation within 2 years, with stable symptomatology, do not require cardiology review prior to non-cardiac surgery.[33]

C

3   Algorithms are available based on complex guidelines from the ACC/AHA to aid decision making but are beyond the scope of this manual.[28]

Cardioversion

Adult-sized cardioversion paddles have an area of 50–80 cm^2 (14 cm diameter) whereas the paediatric type have an area of 12–20 cm^2 (5–8 cm diameter).

Paddle or Electrode Pad Positions
Increasingly, paddles are being superseded by gel electrode pads.
1   Right paddle or electrode placed to the right of the sternum below the clavicle over the second intercostal space.
2   Left paddle or electrode placed laterally to the left nipple and centred over the mid-axillary line and the sixth intercostal space.

Alternative Paddle or Electrode Pad Position
1   Anterior paddle or electrode placed over the left precordium.
2   Posterior paddle or electrode placed behind the heart below the scapula.[11]

Table C2 DC monophasic cardioversion electrical energy for the various dysrhythmias

Dysrhythmia	Suggested initial electrical energy for cardioversion
Atrial fibrillation	Adult: 100, 200 J
Atrial flutter	Adult: 50, 100 J
Supraventricular tachycardia (with pulse)	Adult: 30, 50 J Child: 0.5–1 J/kg

Supraventricular tachycardia (pulseless)	Adult: 100, 200, 360 J Child: 0.5–1, 2, 4 J/kg
Ventricular tachycardia	
Monomorphic	Adult: 100 J
Polymorphic	Adult: 200 J
Ventricular fibrillation	Adult: 200, 360 J Child: 2–4 J/kg

Table C3 DC biphasic cardioversion electrical energy for the various dysrhythmias

Dysrhythmia	Suggested initial electrical energy for cardioversion
Atrial fibrillation	Adult: 100 J
Atrial flutter	Adult: 50 J
Supraventricular tachycardia	Adult: 25, 50 J
Ventricular tachycardia	Adult: 100 J
Ventricular fibrillation	Adult: 150 J

Points to Note

1 Defibrillate during expiration to minimise impedence.
2 Synchronise shock with the R wave when cardioverting a supraventricular dysrhythmia (SVT, AF or atrial flutter) or ventricular tachycardia with a palpable pulse. Do not synchronise the shock if pulseless VT or VF is present.
3 Do not defibrillate over ECG electrodes or nitrate patches, or over implanted devices such as pacemakers, and ensure the patient is not in contact with metal.

C

4   Use conductive gel pads and ensure these are not touching each other.

5   Digoxin toxicity reduces the threshold for inducing ventricular arrythmias with cardioversion shocks.

6   Provide adequate sedation/anaesthesia.

Carotid Endarterectomy (CEA)

Pre-operative Evaluation and Assessment

1   CEA patients have a high incidence of ischaemic heart disease. See *CARDIAC INVESTIGATIONS* and *CARDIOVASCULAR PERI-OPERATIVE RISK PREDICTION FOR NON-CARDIAC SURGERY*. CEA surgery is considered to be an intermediate risk operation for myocardial infarction. However, there is little evidence that CABG surgery performed either before or in combination with CEA lowers the overall risk of stroke and MI.[34]

2   Patients requiring both CEA and CABG are usually operated on sequentially with the most urgent surgery performed first.[35]

3   Hypertension is common and should be controlled between reasonable limits. Aim for a pre-operative blood pressure less than 180 mmHg systolic.[36]

4   Document pre-existing neurological deficits.

5   Assess the patient's respiratory function carefully, especially if cervical plexus block is planned as this will affect phrenic nerve function.

6   Commence the patient on β blocker therapy pre-operatively if there are no contraindications to reduce the incidence of tachycardia and myocardial ischaemia and improve long-term prognosis.[32]

7   The debate about whether regional anaesthesia is preferable to general anaesthesia is unresolved and either technique can be combined with meticulous surgical technique to provide a good outcome.[37]

Anaesthesia Aims

1 Ensure peri-operative cardiovascular stability. Maintain high normal (for the patient) blood pressure throughout the procedure. Use light anaesthesia rather than vasoconstrictors to achieve this, as the use of sympathomimetics such as metaraminol is associated with an increased risk of myocardial ischaemia and infarction.[38]

2 Prevent/identify/treat cerebral and/or myocardial ischaemia.

3 Aim for prompt awakening at the end of surgery if GA is used.

4 *Hyperglycaemia* must be avoided as it can increase the incidence of cerebral cellular damage.[38] Similarly, glucose-containing solutions should be avoided.

5 Consider pre-operative evaluation of vocal cord function if the patient has had previous contralateral carotid surgery, to detect recurrent laryngeal nerve injury. Bilateral nerve injury may cause acute airway compromise.[38]

General Anaesthesia Technique

▶ *Pre-induction Phase*

1 In addition to routine monitoring use a 5 lead ECG system displaying leads II and V. See *ST SEGMENT ANALYSIS*. Invasive arterial blood pressure measurement, initiated before induction, is also required.

2 Monitoring of cerebral function and perfusion must be undertaken. Techniques include:

(a) *internal carotid artery stump pressure*. The artery is temporarily occluded and the back pressure in the artery downstream from the clamp is measured. A mean arterial stump pressure of > 50–60 mmHg is generally accepted (by surgeons who measure stump pressure) as indicative of adequate perfusion.[38] Stump pressures do not correlate

C

consistently with other measures of cerebral perfusion, such as assessment of the awake patient.[39]

(b) *EEG monitoring.* Variations of EEG techniques include compressed spectral array and density spectral array.

(c) *somatosensory evoked potentials.*

(d) *regional cerebral blood flow studies.* Utilise a radioactive tracer such as xenon[133] or krypton[85] and an external array of scintillation monitors.

(e) *transcranial Doppler ultrasonography.* Measure middle cerebral artery blood flow.

(f) *near infrared spectroscopy.* This technique provides a measure of neuronal cellular oxygenation.

(g) *jugular venous oximetry.*

(h) *direct neurological assessment* of the awake patient.

▶ *Induction and Maintenance Phase*

1 Aim for cardiovascular stability on induction and throughout the peri-operative period. Appropriate drugs to use include:

(a) midazolam 3 mg

(b) fentanyl 100–250 µg

(c) thiopentone or propofol

(d) rocuronium 0.6 mg/kg

Consider lignocaine 1.5 mg/kg IV 1 minute prior to intubation to blunt the haemodynamic response to intubation. See *HYPERTENSIVE RESPONSE TO INTUBATION (ATTENUATION OF).*

2 Maintain anaesthesia with oxygen, N_2O and isoflurane.

3 Consider a cervical plexus block prior to incision to reduce intra-operative nociceptive stimulation and postoperative pain.[38] See *CERVICAL PLEXUS (CP) BLOCK.*

4 Stretching of the carotid baroreceptor can result in severe bradycardia and hypotension. This can be avoided by the

surgeon infiltrating around the carotid bifurcation with 1% lignocaine. However, this technique has been associated with postoperative hypertension and is not recommended routinely.[40]

5 Prior to clamping of the common carotid artery, give heparin ($\approx$ 100 U/kg). The surgeon may choose to insert a shunt between the common carotid artery and the internal carotid artery downstream from the clamp.

6 Some centres use EEG monitoring and barbiturate cerebral protection. Thiopentone reduces cerebral metabolic rate of O_2 consumption, decreases intracranial pressure and reduces cerebral oedema.[41] Immediately before clamping a slow bolus of thiopentone 9 mg/kg is given and isoflurane and N_2O are ceased. About 125–250 mg of thiopentone is given every 3–10 min during clamp time to maintain burst suppression. The total average dose given is $\approx$ 19 mg/kg.

7 Adjust ventilation to ensure normocarbia.[38] Both hypocarbia (causing cerebral vasoconstriction) and hypercarbia (causing cerebral vasodilation and a potential steal' phenomenon) are undesirable.[38]

8 Consider the use of mild hypothermia ($\approx$ 35°C) up until the point of completion of the carotid endarterectomy which may reduce ischaemic brain injury.[38] Begin active rewarming after the clamp is removed.

9 If severe hypertension occurs with carotid clamping notify the surgeon immediately. This may indicate cerebral ischaemia and the need for clamp release and shunt insertion.

10 The surgeon may request a dose of protamine to reverse the effects of heparin.

▶ Emergence and Immediate Postoperative Phase

1 Aim for smooth emergence with minimal CVS disturbance. Consider using a drug to reduce the hypotensive response to

C

extubation, such as IV lignocaine 1.5 mg/kg 1–2 min, before extubation or esmolol 2–3 mg/kg IV.

2   Aggressively treat postoperative hyper/hypotension, tachycardia or bradycardia. Aim for values within the patient's usual pre-operative range for pulse rate and blood pressure.

Regional Anaesthesia Technique

This technique is used in many centres.

1   Perform a deep and superficial cervical plexus block. See *CERVICAL PLEXUS (CP) BLOCK*.

2   Monitoring is identical to that used for GA except that patient assessment is used for neurological evaluation.

3   Give O_2 by facemask throughout the procedure.

4   Sedation can be provided with midazolam. Fentanyl can be added if midazolam is inadequate.[36] However, the sedation must not impair patient cooperation.

5   An inadequate cervical plexus block can be supplemented by LA infiltration by the surgeon.

6   Phrenic nerve block occurs commonly with cervical plexus block. It is well tolerated in patients with normal respiratory function but may cause severe respiratory compromise in patients with underlying respiratory disease.[42]

7   Conversion rate to general anaesthesia is normally very low, of the order of 1–3%.[42]

Postoperative Complications

1   Airway compromise can occur due to oedema, haemorrhage, recurrent laryngeal nerve palsy (if previous contralateral recurrent laryngeal nerve injury). See *NECK HAEMATOMA* for management of airway compromise due to haemorrhage.

2   *Postoperative neurological deterioration* is a surgical emergency and the surgeon must be notified immediately. In addition to thromboembolic phenomena the hyperperfusion syndrome can also

cause neurological dysfunction. This syndrome is usually associated with surgery on severely stenotic lesions and may cause headache, seizures and/or intracranial haemorrhage.[42]

3　Aggressively treat any cardiovascular instability. Hypertension is the most common abnormality and can be treated with esmolol, hydralazine and/or glyceryl trinitrate, depending on its severity.

4　Bilateral carotid body dysfunction can result if surgery on both sides of the neck has occurred, leading to a decreased ventilatory response to hypoxia.[38]

Caudal Anaesthesia

Useful for analgesia during and after surgery to areas supplied by the sacral segments. Appropriate operations include haemorrhoidectomy and circumcision.

Anatomy

The dural sac terminates at S2 and the extradural space terminates at the sacral hiatus. This triangular hiatus is formed by the unfused lamina of S5 and lies at the posterior aspect of the lower end of sacrum. The sacral cornua are part of the S5 lamina remnants. It is roofed by the sacrococcygeal ligament, which is equivalent to the ligamentum flavum. This site thus provides an access point to the epidural space.

Technique

1　Establish IV access.

2　Position the patient laterally with the legs drawn up towards the chest. Palpate the posterior superior iliac spines (PSISs). An imaginary line drawn between the PSISs forms the base of an inverted equilateral triangle. At the caudal apex of this triangle is the sacral hiatus at the lower end of the sacrum. As stated above the triangular shaped sacral hiatus is formed by the

C

deficient laminae of S5, which bears the sacral cornua and the spinous process of S4 or S3 above.

3 Using aseptic technique and a suitable needle such as a 22 G short bevelled needle, penetrate the skin and subcutaneous tissue at an angle of about 45° to the skin.

4 Next, penetrate the posterior sacrococcygeal ligament and then flatten the needle to insert the tip 2–3 mm into the sacral canal. Use a syringe and extension tubing to aspirate on the needle to check for CSF or blood. If no fluid is aspirated inject 0.5 mL of air. There should be no resistance to injection. By placing a stethoscope over the sacrum, injected air can be heard entering the epidural space in the sacral canal (called the 'whoosh' test).[43]

Dose of LA

▶ *Adults*

For surgery such as circumcision, inject bupivacaine 0.5% with adrenaline 1:200 000 10 mL + 5 mL N/S.

▶ *Child*

For surgery such as circumcision, inject bupivacaine 0.25% (with adrenaline) 0.5 mL/kg up to 20 mL. To cover upper lumbar and lower thoracic segments, e.g. for hip surgery, inject 0.75 mL/kg of bupivacaine 0.25% with adrenaline. Do not exceed 3 mg/kg of bupivacaine in the child.

Complications

1 Dural puncture with total spinal anaesthesia.

2 Intravascular or interosseous injection of LA and adrenaline with dysrhythmias and cardiac arrest has been reported.[44] The risk of this complication may be reduced by the 'whoosh' test described above, plus careful aspiration.

3   In pregnant patients, injection into the foetal scalp, with fatal results, has been described.[45]

4   Periosteal injection or haematoma with postoperative pain that may last weeks.

5   Urinary retention.

6   Infection.

7   Neurological injury.

Celecoxib

Cyclo-oxygenase 2 (COX2) inhibitor non-steroidal anti-inflammatory analgesic drug without COX1 effects at clinical doses. Useful for the treatment of osteo- and rheumatoid arthritis.

Dose
Adult: 100 mg–200 mg 12 h.

Note
Celecoxib is contraindicated in patients who have a history of sulfonamide allergy. See *NON-STEROIDAL ANTI-INFLAMMATORY DRUGS*.

Cell Saver

These devices consist of suction tubing, filter, reservoir, and a washing bowl that is centrifuge-driven. Heparinised saline (30 000 units of heparin per litre of N/S) is added to blood sucked from the surgical site to prevent clotting. The heparinised blood is washed in saline and the final product consists of RBCs suspended in saline (without heparin), which is retransfused back into the patient. The haematocrit of the recollected blood is 50–60%. About 75% of shed blood can be collected and retransfused,[46] provided that blood loss does not exceed the rate at which it can be sucked up. Suction pressure should be < 150 mmHg.

Problems with this Technique
Most of the platelets and clotting factors are lost in this process.

Contraindications to Cell Saver Use
1 *Infected material* at operative site, e.g. bowel contents.
2 *Malignancy.* Tumour cells may not be removed by standard washing techniques, but limited studies do not suggest a reduced patient survival rate.[47] This may therefore be a relative contraindication. A leucocyte filter[48] and gamma irradiation[49] can be used to remove malignant cells. Irradiation of the salvaged blood takes 1–2 h.
3 *Amniotic fluid.* This should be sucked away before blood is sucked into the cell saver.

Cement Implantation Syndrome

See *FAT EMBOLISM SYNDROME AND BONE CEMENT IMPLANTATION SYNDROME.*

Central Anticholinergic Syndrome

This is a confusional state due to the effects of anticholinergic drugs, such as atropine and scopolamine, on the brain.

Treatment
Adult: Give physostigmine 1 mg IV.

Prevention
Avoid anticholinergics that cross the blood–brain barrier (scopolamine, atropine) especially in patients over 60 years. Use glycopyrronium as an alternative drug (see *GLYCOPYRRONIUM*).

Cerebral Aneurysm Surgery

C

Topics Covered in this Section

▶ Cerebral Aneurysm Rupture and Subarachnoid Haemorrhage (SAH)

▶ Grading the Severity of SAH

▶ Pre-anaesthetic Considerations for Cerebral Aneurysm Repair

▶ Anaesthetic Management up to Aneurysmal Clipping

▶ Aneurysmal Clipping

▶ Postclipping Considerations

▶ Intra-operative Aneurysmal Rupture

▶ Cerebral Vasospasm

Cerebral Aneurysm Rupture and Subarachnoid Haemorrhage (SAH)

About 50% of cases of subarachnoid haemorrhage are due to cerebral aneurysm rupture.[50] The other causes are arteriovenous malformations, extension of an intracerebral haemorrhage and haemorrhage into an infarct or tumour.

Clinical symptoms and signs include:
1 sudden severe headache
2 loss of consciousness, which may be transient or prolonged.
3 neck stiffness
4 hypertension
5 seizures
6 focal neurological signs.

Grading the Severity of SAH

See Tables C4 and C5.

C

Table C4 Classification of SAH: Hunt and Hess modified clinical grades[51]

Clinical presentation	Grade
Unruptured aneurysm	0
Asymptomatic or minimal headache	1
Moderate/severe headache, nuchal rigidity ± cranial nerve palsy	2
Drowsy, confused ± mild focal deficit	3
Stupor, mild or severe hemiparesis, early decerebrate rigidity	4
Deep coma, moribund	5

Table C5 Severity scale for subarachnoid haemorrhage, World Federation of Neurosurgeons grade[52]

World Federation of Neurosurgeons grade	Glasgow coma score	Motor deficit
0 (unruptured aneurysm)	15	Nil
I	15	Nil
II	13–14	Nil
III	13–14	Present
IV	7–12	Present or absent
V	3–6	Present or absent

Pre-anaesthetic Considerations for Cerebral Aneurysm Repair

1   About 50% of patients die within 4 weeks of cerebral aneurysm rupture, and only 30% will have a good neurological outcome.[53]

2   Current management guidelines recommend four-vessel cerebral angiography as soon as practical after presentation, in order to plan ongoing treatment.[53]

3   Patients may be hypertensive due to autonomic hyperactivity secondary to cerebral ischaemia. Increased noradrenaline release from the adrenal medulla and cardiac efferents may result in myocardial ischaemia, ventricular dysfunction and dysrhythmias.[53] ST segment and T wave changes are common and are thought to indicate myocardial dysfunction rather than injury.[52] However, minor or major myocardial damage and left ventricular dysfunction or failure may occur.[54]

4   Cerebral ischaemia and infarction due to vasospasm is common both before and after clipping of the aneurysm.[55] Nimodipine is currently the drug of choice for the prevention of vasospasm and cerebral infarction. It may also be effective in treating established vasospasm.[51] See *NIMODIPINE*. Induced hypertension may be required with refractory cerebral vasospasm.

5   Acute and/or subacute raised intracranial pressure may occur, with impaired level of consciousness, cerebral ischaemia, brain herniation and death.

6   There is a 30% risk of rebleeding in the first 28 days after a subarachnoid haemorrhage due to a cerebral aneurysm. About 70% of these patients will die from the second bleed.[52]

7   Other potential problems include neurogenic pulmonary oedema and hyponatraemia.

C

8 Ensure patients are well hydrated and normovolaemic prior to induction of anaesthesia.[52] Serum osmolarity and electrolytes should also be normalised.

9 Both hyperglycaemia and hypoglycaemia are deleterious and must be prevented or corrected.[56]

Anaesthetic Management up to Aneurysmal Clipping

The anaesthetic aims are to maintain a stable haemodynamic profile, an optimal physiological environment for the brain and favourable operating conditions for the surgeon.

1 In addition to routine monitoring, establish invasive blood pressure monitoring via arterial cannulation. Measure the arterial pressure at the level of the brain. Establish central venous access, although this can be done after induction. Consider use of EEG monitoring. Ensure that the patient's bladder is catheterised after induction. Have a sodium nitroprusside infusion readily available. See *SODIUM NITROPRUSSIDE*.

2 Continue or commence a nimodipine infusion. See *NIMODIPINE*.

3 It is essential to attenuate the sympathetic response to laryngoscopy and intubation. Induce anaesthesia with fentanyl 2–5 µg/kg IV followed by thiopentone 3–5 mg/kg. Give lignocaine 1.5 mg/kg IV 2–3 min before laryngoscopy. Spray the vocal cords with 3 mL of 4% lignocaine topical prior to intubation. An esmolol 0.5 mg/kg IV bolus can also be used. See *HYPERTENSIVE RESPONSE TO INTUBATION (ATTENUATION OF)*. Give a suitable dose of muscle relaxant, e.g. rocuronium 0.6 mg/kg. Do not intubate until a nerve stimulator indicates adequate paralysis. Use of a rapid sequence induction is controversial because the risk of aneurysmal rupture (if the sympathetic responses to laryngoscopy and intubation are inadequately controlled) may exceed the risk of aspiration.[53] Give repeated boluses of thiopentone if hypertension occurs with laryngoscopy or intubation.

4 Application of the head-pin holder can be associated with marked hypertension. This can be attenuated by LA injection at the pin sites prior to their insertion.

5 Maintenance of anaesthesia can be achieved with a combination of O_2, N_2O and isoflurane or sevoflurane. Alternatively, a combination of O_2, air and a propofol infusion ± a remifentanil infusion can be used. A combination of intravenous propofol and volatile anaesthetic agent is also satisfactory.

6 The use of desflurane is not recommended because this agent may impair autoregulation at concentrations greater than 0.5 MAC and is a less suitable agent for patients with raised ICP than sevoflurane or isoflurane.[57] See *DESFLURANE*.

7 The neurosurgeon may request *mannitol, dexamethasone* and/or *phenytoin*. See *NEUROANAESTHESIA*. If mannitol is given, begin the mannitol infusion after the dura is opened. This is to avoid over-aggressive reduction of ICP prior to opening of the dura, as this can result in increased transmural pressure and aneurysmal rupture.[53]

8 Discuss arterial blood pressure requirements with the neurosurgeon. The use of deliberate hypotension has declined but may still be requested by some neurosurgeons.[56] In general, aim to maintain a normal MAP.[52]

9 In some institutions and situations intracranial pressure (ICP) may be reduced through the use of a lumbar drain or a ventricular drain. Cerebrospinal fluid must not be drained before removal of the cranial flap.[52] Drainage of CSF should be limited to a rate not exceeding 5 mL/min.[52]

10 Modest intra-operative hypothermia (35°C) may be beneficial, with active rewarming of the patient undertaken during wound closure.[56]

11 Maintain adequate cerebral perfusion pressure and circulating

C

volume as guided by central venous pressure, urine output and mean arterial pressure (MAP). Use N/S as replacement fluid.

Aneurysmal Clipping

1 The neurosurgeon may temporarily occlude the aneurysm's parent blood vessel to lower pressure stress within the aneurysm. Consider increasing MAP by 10–15% to improve collateral blood flow.[56]

2 Some neurosurgeons may request a bolus of thiopentone sufficient to provide deep burst suppression on the EEG or an isoelectric pattern on the EEG.[56]

Post-clipping Considerations

1 After the cerebral aneurysm is clipped consider increasing MAP to the high normal range, moderate hypervolaemia, and haemodilution (i.e. Hb ≈ 10 g/dL to reduce viscosity). This is referred to as 'Triple H Therapy'. These measures are intended to decrease the incidence of cerebral artery vasospasm.[56]

2 During emergence, aim to avoid coughing, straining, hypercarbia and hyper- and hypotension. Give 1.5 mg/kg lignocaine ≈ 2 min prior to planned extubation. Attempt to extubate the patient 'deep', i.e. as soon as the patient is breathing effectively. Patients with a Hunt and Hess Grade IV and V SAH usually require postoperative ventilation.[58]

Intra-operative Aneurysmal Rupture

Sudden sustained hypertension, massive brain swelling, and bradycardia or other arrhythmias are suggestive of intra-operative aneurysmal rupture. This is an *anaesthetic and surgical emergency* with a mortality approaching 75%.[58] The risk of aneurysm rupture on induction is 1–2% and has the higher mortality than rupture during surgical dissection.[58] Treatment includes the following:

1 Correct all factors that may increase ICP (see *RAISED INTRACRANIAL PRESSURE*).

2 Give boluses of thiopentone to correct hypertension to baseline levels.

3 Give immediate mannitol and frusemide.[59]

4 Once the dura is open and the surgeon has commenced dissection, use a sodium nitroprusside infusion to lower mean arterial pressure to 50 mmHg until the aneurysm is clipped.[59] This will help to decrease bleeding and facilitate surgical exposure.

5 Consider cerebral protection with thiopentone (see above).[56]

6 Cut down onto the ipsilateral cervical internal carotid artery and occlude or externally compress the ipsilateral common carotid artery if required.[56]

Cerebral Vasospasm

Cerebral vasospasm may occur with deterioration in the patient's mental status ± focal neurological deficit.

Treatment includes:

1 hypertension, hypervolaemia and haemodilution ('triple H therapy')

2 nimodipine infusion.

Balloon angioplasty and superselective intra-arterial papaverine may be of benefit.[56]

Cerebral Blood Flow

50 mL/100 g/min	normal cerebral blood flow.
25 mL/100 g/min	the threshold for cerebral ischaemia and neuronal impairment.
20 mL/100 g/min	EEG becomes isoelectric.
15 mL/100 g/min	below this level evoked potentials become unrecordable.
10 mL/100 g/min	neuronal death will occur if flow is maintained at this level or less.

C

Cerebral Oedema

See *RAISED INTRACRANIAL PRESSURE.*

Cerebral Perfusion Pressure

Cerebral perfusion pressure (CPP) is the difference between mean arterial pressure and jugular venous pressure or intracranial pressure, whichever is the greater.

CPP = MAP – (CVP or ICP)

Aim for a CPP of at least 70 mmHg.

Cerebrospinal Fluid

Normal Values

pH	7.32
Glucose	2.8–4.4 mmol/L
Protein	0.45 g/L
PCO_2	50 mmHg
Sodium	144–152 mmol/L
Potassium	2–3 mmol/L
Bicarbonate	24–32 mmol/L
Normal CSF pressure	10–13 cmH$_2$O or 10 mmHg

Cervical Plexus (CP) Block

Anatomy

The cervical plexus (CP) is made up of the anterior rami of C1–C4 and supplies sensory and motor innervation to the neck and posterior scalp. The CP can be divided into superficial cutaneous branches and deep motor branches, the most important of which is the *phrenic nerve* (C3, C4, C5). The superficial cutaneous branches are:

1 lesser occipital nerve (C2)
2 greater occipital nerve (C2, C3)

3   anterior cutaneous nerve of the neck (C2, C3)
4   supraclavicular nerve (C3, C4).

▶ Superficial CP Block

May provide analgesia for surgery such as thyroidectomy, tracheostomy, cervical lymph node biopsy and carotid endarterectomy.

▶ Superficial and Deep CP Block

May be used as the sole anaesthetic technique for carotid artery surgery.

▶ Technique for Superficial CP Block

1   Establish IV access. Identify the midpoint of the posterior border of the sternocleidomastoid muscle (SCM). This point corresponds to the junction of the external jugular vein and the posterior border of the SCM.
2   Insert a 4 cm 22 G needle just behind and deep to the SCM muscle.
3   Inject 10–15 mL of local anaesthetic solution, e.g. ropivacaine 1%. The injection is made in a fan-like pattern along the posterior border of the SCM 4 cm caudally and 4 cm cranially from the entry point.

▶ Technique for Deep CP Block

1   The patient lies supine with the face turned to the contralateral side. Palpate the mastoid process and the transverse process of C6 vertebrae (tubercle of Chassaignac) which lies at the level of the cricoid cartilage. Draw a line between these two landmarks.
2   Identify the transverse process of C2 which will lie 1.5 cm (≈ one finger's breadth) caudal to the mastoid process and 0.5–0.75 cm dorsal to this line. Mark this point.
3   Identify C3 transverse process, which will lie 1.5 cm more caudal to C2. Identify C4 transverse process, which lies another

C

1.5 cm more caudal to C3. The C4 transverse process underlies the point where the external jugular vein crosses the posterior border of the SCM. Clearly mark all three injection points.

4   Using a 4 cm 22 G needle, penetrate the skin over each point, directing the needle in a slightly caudad direction to contact each transverse process. Confirm the position by 'walking' the needle off the tip of the transverse process caudally and/or cranially.

5   Ensure that neither blood nor CSF can be aspirated.

6   Cautiously inject 3–5 mL of LA solution adjacent to the transverse processes of C2, C3 and C4.

7   Anticipate phrenic nerve block on the side of the injections. The incidence of phrenic nerve block is 50–60%.[60]

▶ *Complications of Deep Cervical Plexus Block*

1   Recurrent laryngeal nerve blockade causing hoarseness, paroxysmal coughing, impaired cough reflex.

2   Anxiety.

3   Dyspnoea due to phrenic nerve anaesthesia.

4   Airway obstruction.

5   Seizures and tachycardia from intravascular injection.

6   Hoarseness (due to recurrent laryngeal nerve blockade).

7   Dysphagia.

8   Stellate ganglion block.

9   Horner's syndrome.

10 Brainstem anaesthesia (due to intrathecal injection or spread). See *BRAINSTEM ANAESTHESIA*.

Chest Drain

Site of Insertion

Insert in the 'triangle of safety' (the area bounded by the anterior axillary line, midaxillary line and a line passing dorsally at the level of the nipple). The catheter should be inserted in the fifth or sixth intercostal space.

Alternatively, insert catheter in the second intercostal space in the midclavicular line.

Table C6 Suggested chest drain sizes[61]

Patient	Size
Adult	
Pneumothorax	26–28 FG
Pleural effusion or haemothorax	36–40 FG
Child	
Small child	6–10 FG
Child up to 30 kg	14–20 FG
Adolescent > 30 kg	20–28 FG

Technique

1 Insert IV cannula and sit patient up 30°. Sterilise site of insertion and infiltrate with a 'generous' amount of 1% lignocaine.
2 With a scalpel make an incision long enough to just allow passage of the appropriate size chest drain.
3 Blunt dissect with heavy forceps through the subcutaneous tissues and intercostal muscles to the pleura, ensuring that the route taken is over the top of the rib below and *not* under the rib above.
4 Break through the pleura with a finger, then introduce the chest tube with the trocar removed and the tip held with forceps. Clamp the tube unless air is under pressure in the pleural space, in which case allow the air to escape before clamping.

5   Direct the tube posteriorly and basally if fluid is to be drained, and apically if air is to be drained.

6   Suture the wound with 3.0 silk so that it is closed snugly around the tube and tie the tube securely.

7   Place a separate suture, which is to be tied when the chest tube is removed.

8   Connect the tube to an underwater sealed drain with 2 cm of water above the distal end of the drainage tube.[61]

9   Consider application of low suction (15–20 cmH$_2$O of negative pressure).[61]

For Tension Pneumothorax

If tension pneumothorax is causing respiratory or cardiovascular embarrassment it can be relieved rapidly by inserting a 14 G cannula into one of the sites described above and releasing the air. Then insert a chest tube as described above.

Cholinergic Receptors

These are acetylcholine receptors, classified into nicotinic and muscarinic receptors which are subdivided into the following subtypes:

- *N1* is a receptor in autonomic ganglia, adrenal medulla and also in the central nervous system. Stimulation causes activation of autonomic ganglia (parasympathetic and sympathetic), and has diverse effects such as vasoconstriction.

- *N2* receptors are present at the neuromuscular junction, and are blocked by the neuromuscular blocking drugs. Stimulation of these receptors causes skeletal muscle contraction.

- *M1* receptors are also present in autonomic ganglia and the central nervous system, and in gastric parietal cells. Stimulation of these receptors causes increased gastric acid secretion. These receptors are inhibited by *pirenzepine*.

- *M2* receptors are present mainly in the heart and salivary glands. Stimulation causes bradycardia, increased salivation and pupillary constriction.

Cinchocaine

See *SUBARACHNOID BLOCK*.

Cisatracurium

Non-depolarising neuromuscular blocking drug. Cisatracurium is one of the ten isomers of atracurium. It is $3 \times$ more potent than atracurium and is broken down almost entirely by Hofmann elimination.[62]

Advantages

1 It can thus be used in patients with liver and/or renal failure.
2 Unlike atracurium, cisatracurium does not cause significant histamine release.

Disadvantages

1 As for atracurium, cisatracrium metabolism results in the production of laudanosine, which can cause excitement and seizure activity. However, levels of laudanosine produced are less with cisatracurium than atracurium.[63]
2 Cisatracurium should be refrigerated during storage. Once removed from refrigeration it should be discarded after 30 days.
3 It has a relatively slow onset.

Dose

0.15 mg/kg. Its onset of action is slightly slower than atracurium. Effects last $\approx$ 45 min.

Repeat Bolus Injections

Give 0.03 mg/kg, lasts $\approx$ 20–25 min.

C

Continuous IV Infusion

Mean infusion rate to maintain steady state block is 1.4 µg/kg/min (0.084 mg/kg/h).[64]

Citrate Toxicity

See *BLOOD TRANSFUSION, Massive Blood Transfusion Management.*

Clonidine

A selective α2 presynaptic adreno-receptor agonist (selectivity for α2:α1 ratio 200:1). Stimulation of these receptors results in decreased noradrenaline release from sympathetic nerve endings and a decreased sympathetic outflow via a central action.

Uses

1 Treatment of hypertension.
2 Analgesia when used epidurally or intrathecally.
3 Sedative/anaesthetic sparing properties.

Dose For Hypertension
▶ *IV dose in adult*

150–300 µg, the maximum dose is 750 µg/24 h. May get transient increase in blood pressure prior to the hypotensive effect, which takes about 10 min to come on.

▶ *IV dose in child*

5 µg/kg

Epidural Dose for Analgesia
▶ *Adult*

150 µg. Clonidine enhances both sensory and motor blockade produced by local anaesthetic agents and has sedating effects. Although clonidine does not enhance the hypotensive effects of LA agents, it greatly prolongs the duration of analgesia.[65]

▶ *Child*

2 µg/kg

Premedication Dose

5 µg/kg PO provides effective sedation and reduces intra-operative anaesthetic requirements.[66]

Points to Note

1 Rapid withdrawal of clonidine in patients on long-term clonidine therapy may result in severe rebound hypertension.
2 Clonidine has a long duration of action with a half-life of 6–10 h.

Clopidogrel

Potent antiplatelet drug with significant anaesthetic and surgical implications. See *PLATELET ADENOSINE DIPHOSPHATE RECEPTOR ANTAGONISTS*

CM5 ECG Monitoring

See *ELECTROCARDIOGRAPHY*.

Cocaine

Amino-ester type local anaesthetic and vasoconstricting agent, used for these purposes in nasal surgery and for awake nasal intubation. Presented as pastes and solutions in concentrations of 1–10%.

Maximum Topical Dose To Mucosa

3 mg/kg. Effects last 20–30 min.

Codeine Phosphate

Methylated morphine derivative analgesic drug suitable for mild to moderate pain. Codeine acts primarily by conversion to morphine.

Indications

Codeine is used for:

1 analgesic for pain of mild to moderate severity
2 constipating and antitussive agent.

Use in Neurosurgery

Codeine is traditionally recommended for patients requiring neurological assessment due to a reputedly lower incidence of opioid side effects compared with more potent opioids such as morphine. This lower incidence of side effects is most likely due to codeine's lower potency as an opioid (about 10% as potent as morphine). It has variable efficacy and is ineffective in about 20% of patients following neurosurgery.[52] Morphine is a superior analgesic drug for neurosurgical patients and does not cause confusion between neurological deterioration and opioid side effects.[67] Hirsch argues that the use of codeine in neurosurgical patients should be abandoned.[68]

Use in Paediatrics

Codeine is frequently used in paediatrics due to a perceived low incidence of side effects. As for its use in neurosurgery, this low incidence of side effects is at the cost of poor and variable effectiveness.

Dose

▶ *Adult Oral/IM*

30–60 mg 4–6 h

▶ *Child Oral*

0.5–1 mg/kg 4–6 h

▶ *Subcutaneously*

1 mg/kg up to 4 hourly. Maximum paediatric dose 3 mg/kg/day.[69]

Advantages

Relatively low incidence of opioid-related side-effects unless used in high doses.[69]

Disadvantages

1 Codeine has a relatively low analgesic potency and its effectiveness is variable and unpredictable.[69]

2 IV codeine is not recommended due to the risk of hypotension, probably related to histamine release.[69]

Combined Spinal/Epidural Technique

See *SUBARACHNOID BLOCK*.

Combitube

This device is a plastic double lumen tube. The tubes are joined together for most of their length, except for the proximal portion. One tube has eight openings in the supraglottic region and is occluded at its tip. This is termed the 'oesophageal channel'. The second tube is a simple tube open at each end and is termed the 'tracheal channel'. There are two cuffs: a larger one to occlude the oropharynx and a smaller one to occlude the oesophagus or trachea. The patient's head and neck can be in the neutral position for insertion. The device comes in two sizes: 37F for a small adult and 41F for an adult.

Technique for Insertion of Combitube[70]

1 Insert the device gently into the mouth. Placement is almost always into the oesophagus. Insert to the depth indicated on the device.

2 Inflate the oropharyngeal balloon with 100 mL of air using the enclosed large syringe. This cuff presses against the base of the tongue and the soft palate, thus sealing the hypopharynx from the oral and nasal cavities. Then inflate the distal cuff with 10–15 mL of air. This cuff seals the oesophagus.

3 Attempt ventilation via the 'oesophageal' lumen (which has the supraglottic openings). If successful the 'tracheal'

C

channel can be used for gastric fluid aspiration.

4 If attempted ventilation via the 'oesophageal' lumen is unsuccessful, attempt ventilation via the 'tracheal' lumen as the Combitube may be in the trachea.

5 If still unable to ventilate the patient's lungs, consider pulling the device back slightly as the oropharyngeal balloon may be obstructing the larynx.

Common Peroneal Nerve Block

See *POPLITEAL FOSSA BLOCK*.

Confusion, Decreased Level Of Consciousness, Postanaesthetic

There are numerous causes of postanaesthetic confusion/decreased level of consciousness. These can be divided into:

1 *pharmacological causes.* All drugs given to the patient should be considered as a possible cause, particularly opioid, benzodiazepines, atropine/scopolamine (see *CENTRAL ANTICHOLINERGIC SYNDROME*), ketamine, and droperidol. Also consider drugs the patient may be taking, such as alcohol, amphetamines. Other causes to consider are toxins and poisons such as carbon monoxide.

2 *metabolic/physiological causes.* These include hypoxia, hypercarbia, hypotension, and electrolyte disorders such as hyponatraemia and hypoglycaemia. Also consider severe pain, bladder distension and hypothermia as possible causes.

3 *pathological causes.* These include cerebral injury due to CVA, embolism or tumour, and encephalopathy due to such causes as liver failure. Look for systemic causes such as overwhelming sepsis, malignant hyperthermia, haemorrhage

and endocrinopathies such as thyrotoxicosis. Consider an acute exacerbation of dementia in the elderly patient.

4 *psychiatric causes.* Only consider psychiatric causes when organic causes have been excluded.

Management of Postoperative Confusion

1 Check the patient's response to verbal and tactile stimulation.
2 The combative or aggressive patient must be restrained to prevent self-injury and injury to staff.
3 Ensure the patient's airway is patent and that ventilation is adequate. Exclude hypoxia and check patient's pulse oximetry.
4 Check the patient's pulse and blood pressure. Exclude a significant dysrhythmia, hypotension or hypertension.
5 Examine the patient carefully for causes of postoperative confusion, looking in particular for any neurological signs, bladder distension, or evidence of haemorrhage.
6 Check patient's temperature, looking for hypothermia or hyperthermia (sepsis, MH).
7 Review the patient's history and pre-anaesthetic state.
8 Review all drugs given to the patient and dosages, and consider the possibility of a drug error. Consider antagonists such as naloxone, flumazenil. Consider central anticholinergic syndrome.
9 Inform the surgeon of the patient's condition.
10 Check arterial blood gas (hypoxia/hypercarbia/acidosis), electrolytes and blood sugar level. Exclude hypoglycaemia. Check FBC for anaemia and raised WCC (sepsis). Consider blood and urine screen for illicit drugs.
11 Consider cerebral CT/MRI scan, neurological/geriatric consultation and ICU transfer.
12 If significant correctable causes are ruled out or unlikely, consider small doses of opioid (if pain suspected) and/or midazolam. Consider haloperidol for ongoing severe agitation. Keep

the patient warm. Attempt to verbally calm and reassure the patient and keep him or her orientated.

Congestive Cardiac Failure

(See also *PULMONARY OEDEMA*.) Congestive cardiac failure (CCF) is usually secondary to ischaemic heart disease. Other causes include cardiomyopathy, and hypertensive and valvular heart disease. Ejection fraction (EF) is an important prognostic indicator; an EF < 40% is indicative of significant cardiac impairment.

Treatment of Mild to Moderate CCF

1 *Dietary modification*, including salt and water restriction and correction of excess weight.
2 *Diuretic therapy*. This results in a loss of sodium and water from the body, decreasing preload and thus ventricular volume overload.
3 *ACE inhibitors*. These are beneficial by decreasing systemic vascular resistance and ventricular filling.
4 *Digoxin*. Marginally improves EF ($\approx$ 4–5%) and is the only oral positive inotropic agent available.
5 β *blockers*. These improve survival in patients with CCF after myocardial infarction.[71]

Severe CCF/Cardiogenic Shock

Treat the cause of cardiogenic shock (e.g. myocardial ischaemia, hypertensive heart failure, dysrhythmias) if possible. Invasive monitoring with a pulmonary artery catheter and arterial line will usually be required. In addition to general supportive measures such as O_2 therapy and sitting the patient up, the basic principles of management are to optimise preload, contractility and afterload:

1 *Preload optimisation*. A PCWP of 15–18 mmHg is usually optimal. If the initial PCWP is < 18 mmHg provide plasma volume expansion incrementally.[72] If PCWP > 18 mmHg preload needs

to be reduced. Reducing excessive preload decreases left ventricular wall stress and O_2 consumption and enables resolution of pulmonary congestion through reduced right atrial pressure. Reduced preload also enables more effective ventricular contraction, lessens physiological mitral regurgitation and improves myocardial perfusion during diastole. Preload can be reduced by:

(a) *loop diuretic*, e.g. frusemide 40–120 mg IV

(b) *vasodilators* such as glyceryl trinitrate (GTN) or sodium nitroprusside (see below). Nitroglycerine is predominantly a venodilator at lower dosages and decreases ventricular filling pressure and ventricular dilatation. As many patients with ventricular overload have functional mitral + tricuspid regurgitation, reduced ventricular volume decreases the regurgitant fraction and improves forward cardiac output.[73] Nitrates can be given sublingually for a more immediate effect while a GTN infusion is prepared.

2 *Inotropes and other drugs to improve contractility*

(a) *Dobutamine* acts on β1 adreno-receptors, leading to increased contractility and heart rate. In addition dobutamine stimulates β2 adreno-receptors, leading to decreased systemic vascular resistance. Its use is most appropriate when there is mild to moderate hypotension and severe congestive heart failure.[74] Dobutamine is not the inotrope of choice if there is profound hypotension/shock as it lacks significant α effects.[72,74] See *DOBUTAMINE*.

(b) *Dopamine* is used for its ability to increase coronary blood flow, and for its positive inotropic effects with a slight decrease in systemic vascular resistance at a dose of < 15 μg/kg/min. At doses > 15 μg/kg/min α adreno-receptor effects predominate. See *DOPAMINE*.

(c) *Adrenaline*.

(d) *Phosphodiesterase inhibitors*. See *AMRINONE* and *MILRINONE*. Milrinone may be preferable to inotropic drugs in patients with critical coronary artery disease[74] due to its ability to increase cardiac output without increasing myocardial O_2 demand.

(e) *Levosimendan* is a new drug that increases contractility by enhancing the sensivity of myocardial cells to calcium. See *LEVOSIMENDAN*.

3   *Afterload reduction* with an arterial vasodilator such as sodium nitroprusside or a phosphodiesterase inhibitor such as milrinone can be obtained. These drugs may be particularly effective in patients with heart failure due to hypertensive disease.

4   *Ventilation strategies* such as positive pressure ventilation with positive end-expiratory pressure (PEEP) can be used. This can result in decreased work of breathing and improved ventilation:perfusion matching. PEEP may also reduce left ventricular preload beneficially.

5   *Mechanical assist devices* such as an intra-aortic balloon pump may be of benefit by reducing left ventricular work and increasing cardiac output.

6   *Angiographic/surgical intervention*, including cardiac transplant, angioplasty and urgent coronary artery bypass grafts, can be considered.

COVER ABCD Crisis Management Algorithm[75]

(Summarised with the permission of the Australian Safety Foundation.) This algorithm is an easy reference summary for the rapid identification of the aetiology of a crisis during anaesthesia. It is both systematic and comprehensive.

   'COVER ABCD' applies to patients with a tracheal tube. 'AB COVER ABCD' refers to patients receiving mask anaesthesia.

COVER ABCD covers 95% of incidents, of which 3% are cardiac arrests. The percentages quoted below in brackets are the percentage of incidents caused by or related to the corresponding letter of the algorithm.

C1 Circulation
Feel pulse (rate, rhythm and character of pulse). If pulseless (3%) start CPR, get help and complete the core algorithm as soon as possible. See *CARDIAC ARREST*.

C2 Colour
Note saturation (cyanosis?). Test pulse oximetry probe on your own finger if necessary, while proceeding with O1 and O2.

O1 Oxygen
Check rotameter settings (hypoxic mixture?). Increase FiO_2 to 1.0 and check that only the O_2 flowmeter is operating. (2%)

O2 Oxygen Analyser
Check that the oxygen analyser shows a rising O_2 concentration distal to the common gas outlet. (0.2%)

V1 Ventilation
Ventilate the lungs by hand and assess breathing circuit integrity, airway patency (is patient biting the tube?), chest compliance and air entry. Observe chest movement and auscultate the chest. Also inspect the capnography trace. (20%)

V2 Vaporiser
Note settings and level of contents in the vaporiser and check for leaks. Consider the possibility of the wrong agent being in vaporiser. (4%)

E1 Endotracheal Tube
Check the endotracheal tube for patency, kinks and any possible obstruction. Check the capnography trace to confirm tracheal

intubation. Consider the possibility of endobronchial tube place-ment. If necessary adjust, deflate cuff, pass a catheter through the ET tube, or remove and replace the ET tube. (14%)

E2 Elimination

Eliminate the anaesthetic machine and ventilate with a self-inflat-ing bag using 100% O_2 (from an alternative source if necessary). Retain the gas monitor sampling tubing, but be aware of the possibility of gas sampling/monitoring problems. (15%)

R1 Review Monitors

Review all monitors in use. They should all be correctly sited, checked and calibrated. (4%)

R2 Review Equipment

Review all other equipment in contact with or relevant to the patient, e.g. diathermy, humidifiers, heating blankets, endoscopes, probes, prostheses, retractors and other appliances. (2%)

A Airway

Check patency of the unintubated airway. Consider laryngospasm (6%) or the presence of a foreign body in airway (1%), or aspira-tion/regurgitation (5%). (Total 12%)

B Breathing

Assess pattern, adequacy and distribution of ventilation. Exclude hypoventilation (2%), bronchospasm (2%), pulmonary oedema, lobar collapse and pneumo/haemothorax. (1%)

C Circulation

Evaluate peripheral perfusion, pulse, blood pressure, ECG. Exclude obstruction to venous return (e.g. supine hypotensive syndrome of pregnancy), raised intra-thoracic pressure (e.g. inadvertent PEEP) or direct interference to, or tamponade of, the heart. Note any trends on records, e.g. bradycardia/bradyarrhythmia (5%), tachycardia/tachyarrhythmia (2%), hypotension (5%), hypertension (1%) or ischaemia (1%). (Total 14%)

D Drugs

Review intended and unintended drug or substance administration (e.g. bone cement). Consider failure of drug to reach patient, e.g. kinked cannula. (Total 3%)

A SWIFT CHECK

A SWIFT CHECK is a second crisis algorithm to be applied when the cause of an emergency is not revealed by the COVER algorithm. A covers 4% and SWIFT CHECK 1% of anaesthetic emergencies.

▶ *A Air Embolus, Anaphylaxis, Air in Pleura Awareness*

▶ *S1 Surgeon/situation*

Vagal stimulation, caval compression, bleeding, direct myocardial stimulation.

▶ *S2 Sepsis*

Hypotension, desaturation, acidosis, hyperdynamic circulation.

▶ *W1 Wound*

Trauma, bleeding, tamponade, pneumothorax, problems due to retractors.

▶ *W2 Water Intoxication*

Electrolyte disturbance, fluid overload.

▶ *I1 Infarct*

Myocardial conduction, ST or rhythm problem, hypotension or poor cardiac output.

▶ *I2 Insufflation*

Vagal tone, reduced venous return, pulmonary or paradoxical arterial gas embolism.

C

▶ *F1 'Fat Syndrome'*

Desaturation ± hypotension, especially after induction and in lithotomy position (with obese or distended abdomen), profuse bronchial secretions.

▶ *F2 Full Bladder*

May cause marked haemodynamic changes ± sympathetic stimulation.

▶ *T1 Trauma*

Consider spinal injury, undiagnosed sub- or extra-dural haematoma, bronchial or diaphragmatic injury, ruptured viscus, concealed haemorrhage, myocardial contusion.

▶ *T2 Tourniquet Down*

LA toxicity, unseen bleeding, failed block.

▶ *C Catheter/IV Cannula, Chest Drain Problems, Cement*

▶ *H Hyper-/hypothermia, Hypoglycaemia*

▶ *E1 Embolus*

Fat, thrombus, amniotic fluid.

▶ *E2 Endocrine*

Hyper- or hypothyroid/adrenal medulla or cortex/pituitary/diabetes/5-HT.

▶ *C Check*

Check right patient, right operation, right body part, correct side. Check case notes, old notes for pre-operative status, diseases, drugs.

▶ *K1 K^+*

Exclude potassium (and any other) electrolyte abnormality.

▶ *K2 Keep*

Unless surgery can be ceased immediately, keep the patient asleep until a new anaesthetic machine can be obtained.

99.9% of incidents should have been identified by now. If the problem has not been solved, direct available resources to its solution. Get experienced help. Work from first principles. Think laterally.

COX2 Inhibitors

See *NON-STEROIDAL ANTI-INFLAMMATORY DRUGS*.

Creutzfeldt–Jacob Disease (CJD)

Also called subacute spongiform encephalopathy, this illness is an infectious fatal neurological disorder. It is caused by prions, which are extremely resistant to destruction by routine sterilisation and decontamination measures.

Operating Theatre Guidelines when CJD is Suspected

1 Schedule the case as last for the day.
2 Remove all unneccesary staff, equipment and supplies from the operating theatre and cover all essential exposed surfaces with plastic or impervious disposable drapes.
3 Minimise traffic through the theatre.
4 Use disposible anaesthetic and surgical equipment.
5 Air powered surgical equipment should not be used.
6 All operating theatre staff must wear appropriate disposable protective clothing and eye protection.
7 All relevant staff (such as domestic services, pathology staff) must be notified of CJD risk. All CJD material must be clearly labelled.
8 After the procedure, surfaces are cleaned with 1–2 M sodium hydroxide.

Cricoid Pressure

See *RAPID SEQUENCE INDUCTION*.

Cricothyroid Puncture and Cricothyrotomy

Anatomy

The cricothyroid ligament or membrane connects the cricoid cartilage to the base of the thyroid cartilage. The thyroid cartilage can be identified by feeling for the subcutaneous thyroid notch at the top of the laryngeal prominence (Adam's apple). Run your finger caudally down the laryngeal prominence until a gap is felt. This is the cricothyroid ligament or membrane. The next structure felt moving caudally is the cricoid cartilage, which feels like a prominent hard ring. The cricoid cartilage lies at the level of C6 in the adult. See *LARYNX, ANATOMY AND INNERVATION*.

Technique for Cricothyroid Membrane Puncture and Conversion of a TUTA IV Solution 'Pump Set' into a Ventilation Device

1   Identify the cricothyroid membrane between the cricoid and thyroid cartilages.

2   Insert a 14 G cannula in the midline through this membrane and into the trachea. Remove the stylet.

3   Attach the cannula to the distal luer lock end of a 'pump set'. Cut the hand pump section obliquely and fit this over the common gas outlet. Then use the O_2 flush button to 'jet' O_2 into the trachea. A patent larynx must be present for exhalation to occur or exhalation can occur through the venous access port on the pump set with the bung removed. Occlude the venous access port for each inflation.

4   Alternatively, transtracheal jet ventilation can be provided

through the cannula using a device such as a Sanders injector. See *TRANSTRACHEAL JET VENTILATION*

Cricothyrotomy

1   Identify cricothyroid membrane and make a transverse incision through the skin and membrane with a scalpel.
2   With the handle of the scalpel, widen this incision sufficiently to enable passage of an endotracheal tube. Insert the tube through the incision into the trachea.
3   Inflate the cuff of the ET tube and ventilate.

See *DIFFICULT AIRWAY MANAGEMENT*.

Cryoprecipitate (and Cryodepleted Plasma)

Cryoprecipitate

Cryoprecipitate is formed when fresh frozen plasma from a single unit of whole blood is thawed between 1 and 6°C and the precipitate is recovered. The precipitate is then refrozen. It is rich in Factor VIII (100 units) and fibrinogen (250 mg).[76,77] It also contains Factor IX, Factor VIIa, Factor XIII, fibronectin and von Willebrand's Factor in a total volume of 15 mL. It is stored at –30°C, and is stable for 6 months.[32] 1 unit of cryoprecipitate should increase fibrinogen levels by 5–10 mg/100 mL in the adult.[78] Once thawed cryoprecipitate should be used within 6 h (or within 4 h if the unit has been opened).

Indications for Cryoprecipitate[76,78]

Cryoprecipitate is indicated for the treatment of fibrinogen deficiency or dysfibrinogenaemia associated with blood loss or potential blood loss. The half-life of fibrinogen is 3–5 days. Cryoprecipitate can be used for the following conditions but only if specific therapies are not available:

*   haemophilia A (Factor VIII) deficiency—aim to increase Factor VIII to > 30% of normal

C

- von Willebrand's disease
- Factor XIII deficiency
- fibrinonectin deficiency.

Cryo-depleted Plasma (CDP)

This is the plasma remaining after cryoprecipitate has been removed. CDP can be used:

- for plasma exchange in ITP
- as an alternative to FFP in the treatment of warfarin overdose or reversal
- for coagulopathy with bleeding not requiring those factors in croprecipitate.

Cyanide Poisoning—Treatment

See *SODIUM NITROPRUSSIDE*.

Dd

Dalteparin (Fragmin)

A type of low molecular weight heparin. See *HEPARIN, UNFRAC-TIONATED AND LOW MOLECULAR WEIGHT HEPARINS* and *DEEP VENOUS THROMBOSIS (DVT) PROPHYLAXIS*.

Dantrolene

See *MALIGNANT HYPERTHERMIA*.

D–dimer Test

This test detects elevated levels of fragments of fibrin and is a specific measure of fibrin degradation. See *FIBRIN DEGRADATION PRODUCTS (FDPs)*. Elevated D-dimers occur with disseminated intravascular coagulation (DIC) and the D-dimer test is the most reliable lab test for DIC. See *DISSEMINATED INTRAVASCULAR COAGULATION (DIC)*.

The normal level of D-dimer is < 500 ng/mL.[1]

Decreased Level Of Consciousness Postanaesthetic

See *CONFUSION, DECREASED LEVEL OF CONSCIOUSNESS, POSTANAESTHETIC*.

Deep Venous Thrombosis (DVT) Prophylaxis

Topics Covered in this Section

▶ Risk of DVT

▶ Categories of DVT Risk

▶ Points to Note Regarding DVT Prophylaxis

▶ Strategies for DVT Prophylaxis

▶ Treatment of DVT

The following guidelines are based mainly on recommendations from the National Working Party on the Management and Prevention of Venous Thromboembolism (for Australia and New Zealand).[2]

Risk of DVT

The importance of DVT prophylaxis is indicated by the very high risk of DVT associated with many conditions and procedures. For example the risk of DVT for elective hip replacement without DVT prophylaxis is over 50%.[2] Patients can be divided into low, medium and high risk groups for DVT.[2,3] Major surgery is defined as intra-abdominal surgery and other operations lasting more than 45 min.[2] Risk factors for DVT include increasing age, obesity, cancer, previous DVT or PE, smoking, varicose veins, pregnancy, immobility, dehydration, sepsis, thrombophilia and HRT or OCP therapy. Thrombophilia can be due to congenital or acquired causes. Congenital causes include activated protein C resistance (Factor V Leiden), protein C deficiency and protein S deficiency. Aquired causes include lupus anticoagulant, antiphospholipid antibodies and myeloproliferative disease. Thrombophilia should be suspected in patients with:

1   family history of DVT/PE

2 recurrent DVT

3 unexplained DVT or PE before the age of 40.

Categories of DVT Risk

▶ *Low Risk (Risk of DVT < 10%, risk of pulmonary embolus (PE) 0.01%)*

- Minor surgery lasting < 30 min in patients < 60 years.
- Major surgery in a patient < 40 years with no other risk factors.

▶ *Moderate Risk (Risk of DVT 10–40%, risk of PE 0.1–1%)*

- Major surgery in patient 40–60 years without other risk factors.
- Minor surgery in patients aged between 40 and 60 years with other risk factors.
- Minor surgery in patient aged greater than 60 years.

▶ *High Risk (Risk of DVT 40–80%, risk of PE 1–10%)*

Patients at high risk include:

- major surgery in patients > 60 years old
- major orthopaedic surgery (e.g. hip fracture, hip replacement) or fracture of pelvis, hip or knee
- multitrauma
- abdominal or pelvic surgery for cancer
- major surgery in patients aged 40–60 years with other risk factors
- lower limb paralysis or amputation
- thrombophilia.

Points to Note Regarding DVT Prophylaxis

1 Consider stopping hormone replacement therapy (HRT) or the oral contraceptive pill (OCP) in patients in the high and moderate risk categories.[2] Cease HRT 6 weeks before surgery. The OCP should be stopped the cycle before planned surgery.

2 Start subcutaneous heparin 2 h before surgery and continue heparin therapy until the patient is ambulant.

3   Spinal or extradural anaesthesia reduces the incidence of DVT and PE.

4   Despite the high incidence of DVT in neurosurgery the risk of intracranial or intraspinal haemorrhage is also high with anticoagulation. Recommendations for patients having neuro-surgery are:

   (a) Mechanical methods of prophylaxis should be used in the peri-operative period. Mechanical methods include intra-operative and postoperative pneumatic compression stockings and graduated compression stockings.

   (b) Five days should elapse after surgery before anticoagulant drugs are commenced.

Strategies for DVT Prophylaxis[4]

▶ Low Risk Group

Use intra-operative pneumatic compression stockings plus gradu-ated compression stockings. Aim for early mobilisation post opera-tively.

▶ Medium Risk Group

Use either fractionated or unfractionated heparin in the following dose:

- *heparin* 5000 units subcutaneously 8 h or 12 h
- *dalteparin* (Fragmin) 2500 units subcutaneously as a single dose per 24 h
- *enoxaparin* (Clexane) 20 mg subcutaneously as a single dose per 24 h
- *nadroparin calcium* (Fraxiparine) 0.3 mL (2850 IU) subcuta-neously as a single dose per 24 h.

Continue preferred drug for 7 days or until patient is mobile. Use compression stockings on the ward plus intra-operative pneumatic compression stockings.

▶ *High Risk Group*

Use one of the following recommended regimes. If the risk of perioperative bleeding is high consider withholding the pre-operative dose and give the first postoperative dose 24 h or more after surgery:

- *dalteparin* (Fragmin) 5000 U subcutaneously on the evening before surgery and then every evening after surgery until at least 10 days postoperatively. Reduce dose to 2500 U/24 h if the patient is < 50 kg or > 80 years old.
- *enoxaparin* (Clexane) 40 mg subcutaneously on the evening before surgery and then every evening after surgery until at least 10 days postoperatively. Reduce the dose to 20 mg if the patient is < 50 kg or > 80 years old.

Consider extending the duration of prophylactic drug use for 2–6 weeks, depending on the degree of risk. Use compression stockings on the ward plus intra-operative pneumatic compression stockings.

Treatment of DVT

See *HEPARIN, UNFRACTIONATED AND LOW MOLECULAR WEIGHT.*

Defibrillation

See *CARDIOVERSION.*

Defibrillators

Four different types of defibrillators are discussed:

1 manual monophasic
2 manual biphasic
3 automated external defibrillators (AEDs)—these are all biphasic
4 implantable (all biphasic).

Monophasic Defibrillators

These defibrillators deliver the shock (current) in a single direction from one electrode to the other. This is the 'traditional' type of manual defibrillator.

Biphasic Defibrillators

These deliver a shock in two directions, from one paddle to the other, then the current reverses direction. Biphasic waveforms decrease the threshold for successful defibrillations. This means biphasic defibrillators are more effective than monophasic defibrillators and use less electrical energy to defibrillate or cardiovert (around half the energy of monophasic defibrillators).[5] Using less electrical energy results in less postshock myocardial dysfunction and a lower risk of skin burns.[6]

Automated External Defibrillators (AEDs)

Also called semi-automatic defibrillators, these devices are intended for use by rescuers with any level of CPR training from doctors to lay people. For example, emergency out-of-hospital defibrillation by security guards at casinos has resulted in a survival rate to hospital discharge of 74% (compared to 15% with in-hospital cardiac arrests).[7]

AEDs are indicated for use with patients who have collapsed and are apnoeic and pulseless. Lay people are not expected to feel for a pulse.[8] The steps to use these devices are:

1 Turn the machine 'on'. With some devices this will be achieved by opening the lid.
2 Voice prompts instruct the user to attach defibrillation electrode pads to the chest wall in the positions illustrated on the electrode packet.
3 The voice prompt then requests that the patient not be touched and advises that the patient's rhythm is being analysed.
4 If VF or rapid VT is diagnosed the device will verbally advise that

a shock be given and a button will 'light-up'. The machine will advise to stand clear and for the operator to push the button.

5   If 'no shock advised' the machine will recommend BLS measures.

Points to Note with AEDs

1   Do not use these devices in children under 8 years unless recommended by the manufacturer.[9]

2   Do not use them on wet patients. The patient must be dried off.

3   The distribution of AEDs in the community is increasing constantly. For example, almost all long-haul passenger aircraft carry an AED.

Dermatomes

See Table D1 and Figure D1.

Table D1 Key dermatome landmarks	
Dermatome	Anatomical site
C5–T1	Upper limb
C7	Middle finger
T3	Apex of axilla
T5	Nipple
T7	Tip of xiphoid
T10	Umbilicus
T12–L1	Inguinal ligament
L3	Front of knee
L4	Medial side of calf
L5	Outer calf
S1	Outer border of foot
S2	Back of knee

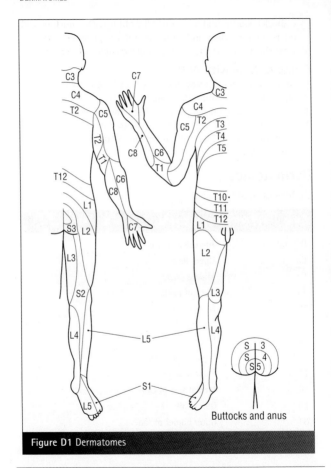

Figure D1 Dermatomes

Desflurane

Methyl ethyl ether inhalational anaesthetic agent, very similar in structure to isoflurane.

Physical Properties and MAC

Blood:gas solubility coefficient	0.42
Oil:gas solubility coefficient	18.7
Saturated vapour pressure (20°C)	664 mmHg (88.5 kPa)
Boiling point	22.8°C
MAC	6.0

Comments and Dosing Guide (based on Dosing Guidelines from Baxter)

1 MAC varies with age. For children aged 1–12 years 8.1–9.1% is suggested. For elderly patients 5.2% is suggested.

2 Following IV induction of anaesthesia, a reasonable initial vaporiser setting is 4–6% with a fresh gas flow (FGF) of 3–5 L/min.

3 Gradually increase the delivered desflurane concentration by increments of 1% or less every few breaths with a FGF of 4–6 L/min, until the desired anaesthetic depth is reached. Do not attempt to increase anaesthetic depth quickly by rapidly increasing the inhaled desflurane concentration.

4 Once an adequate anaesthetic depth has been attained FGF rates can be reduced to a low flow, e.g. 1 L/min.

5 Use of desflurane is associated with rapid emergence. Therefore, ensure that surgery is complete and that the timing of emergence is appropriate (e.g. turning patient from the prone position) prior to ceasing desflurane. Also ensure that muscle relaxation is reversed and the patient is adequately analgesed prior to ceasing desflurane.

6 Coughing on emergence can be attenuated with a small dose of opioid, propofol or lignocaine.

Advantages

1 Rapid onset and offset of effects due to low blood gas solubility. Desflurane has the lowest blood gas solubility of the potent inhalational anaesthetic agents.

2 Metabolised to a very small extent (0.02%). This is less than isoflurane.

3 Pharmacodynamic effects are similar to isoflurane.

Disadvantages

1 Requires a unique and complex vaporiser, which is electrically heated and thermostatically controlled. Output from the vaporiser is determined by an electronically controlled pressure-regulating valve.

2 It has a low potency and is the least potent of the modern anaesthetic agents.

3 Its severe pungency makes it unsuitable for inhalational induction. Irritation of the airways by desflurane may be of particular concern in patients with bronchospastic disease.[10] Desflurane can cause bronchoconstriction, particularly in smokers.[11]

4 Rapidly increasing the inhaled concentration of desflurane or exceeding 1.25 MAC can result in significant sympathetic nervous system stimulation with tachycardia and hypertension.[12]

5 Desflurane impairs cerebral autoregulation at concentrations greater than 0.5 MAC.[12] It may be less suitable for neurosurgery and patients with raised ICP than sevoflurane.[12]

6 Interaction between desflurane and CO_2 absorbers can result in significant carbon monoxide formation. This tends to occur when the absorbent is dried, e.g. by a flow of dry fresh gas over the absorbent for several hours between cases.[13]

7 Desflurane can cause malignant hyperthermia.

Desmopressin (DDAVP)

An analogue of vasopressin, desmopressin may be useful:
1 for treatment of diabetes insipidus
2 to boost Factor VIII concentration in mild to moderate haemophilia A
3 to boost levels of von Willebrand Factor. Although DDAVP is useful for the treatment of Type I von Willebrand's disease, it is contraindicated in Type IIB disease
4 to improve platelet function in illnesses where platelet function may be impaired, e.g. renal disease[14]
5 in situations involving heavy blood loss, e.g. major orthopaedic surgery.[14]

Dose of DDAVP for Bleeding Associated with 2 to 5 Above

0.3 µg/kg/12 h. Give diluted in 50 mL N/S over 30 min. Monitor patient carefully for side-effects such as vasodilatation and hypotension.

Comment

A recent review of desmopressin use to reduce blood loss indicated a small decrease in peri-operative haemorrhage and a 2.4-fold increase in the risk of myocardial infarction.[15]

Dexamethasone

Powerful, long-acting glucocorticoid drug with minimal mineralo-corticoid activity, useful for the treatment of:
- cerebral oedema due to brain tumour
- adrenal insufficiency
- prevention of nausea and vomiting. A dose of 4–10 mg IV is effective in adults.[16,17] A dose of 0.5 mg/kg has been found to be effective in children.[18] The combination of dexamethasone plus

D

a 5-HT$_3$ antagonist such as ondansetron is probably the most effective drug combination to prevent postoperative nausea and vomiting.[19]

Note: If given in the awake patient, dexamethasone can cause brief, unpleasant burning sensations in the lower pelvis, the cure of which is unknown.

Dexmedetomidine

Dexmedetomidine is a potent, highly selective α2 adreno-receptor agonist. The α2 to α1 ratio is 1600:1.

Mechanism of Action

Dexmedetomidine acts by decreasing noradrenaline release centrally and peripherally. This results in decreased sympathetic outflow from the CNS and decreases plasma noradrenaline concentrations.

Clinical Uses

It can be used in ICU by IV infusion to provide satisfactory analgesia and sedation as a single agent.[20]

Dose

Give an IV loading dose of 1 μg/kg over 10 min, then an infusion of 0.2–0.7 μg/kg per h. Do not run infusion for more than 24 h.[21]

Adverse Effects

- Hypotension and bradycardia
- Hypoxia
- Atrial fibrillation[21]
- Sinus bradycardia[22]
- Dizziness[23]

Dextran

Dextran is a polysaccharide derived from sucrose. Dextran 40 (10% solution) and dextran 70 (6% solution) are mixed with either 5%

glucose or N/S. Severe hypersensitivity reactions occur in 1 in 3300 patients.

Dextran 1 (Promit) should be infused (100 mL) just prior to the other dextrans. This decreases the incidence of anaphylactoid reactions by a factor of 15–20.[24]

Dextran 70

Dextran 70 is used for plasma volume expansion via its osmotic effects. It has an intravascular half-life of 6–12 hours.[25]

Dextran 40

Dextran 40 is used for:
- antithrombotic effects by inhibiting platelet adhesiveness and diluting clotting factors[26]
- improving peripheral perfusion by decreasing blood viscosity, thus may be useful for graft and reimplantation procedures.

Dextran 40 is rapidly excreted by the kidney and, if urinary flow is low, a high urinary concentration of dextran 40 can result. This can lead to renal failure.[25] The plasma half-life of dextran 40 is 2–3 hours.[25]

Dextran and Volume Expansion

Titrate the volume infused to the desired clinical response. If more than 20 mL/kg is given within 24 h, increased bleeding may occur due to anticlotting effects. Dextran 40 is less effective than dextran 70 for intravascular volume expansion and the effects are less long lasting. Dextrans are not the solutions of choice for volume expansion.

Dose of Dextran 40 for Thrombosis Prevention and Improving Microcirculation During Low Flow States

Give 500 mL over 4–6 h in the peri-operative period. Repeat the dose in 24 h and, for high risk patients, continue dextran on alternate days for up to 2 weeks.[24]

Diabetes Mellitus, Preparation for Surgery

If possible, schedule the diabetic patient to be first on the morning or afternoon list, to minimise fasting times.

Topics Covered in this Section

▶ Insulin-dependent Diabetics (IDDM or Type I Diabetes)
▶ Preparing and Running an Insulin Glucose Infusion
▶ Non-insulin-dependent Diabetics (NIDDM or Type II Diabetes)
▶ Diet-controlled diabetics

Insulin-dependent Diabetics (IDDM or Type I Diabetes)

▶ *Insulin-dependent Diabetics Unsuitable for Day of Surgery Admission*

1. Poorly controlled or unstable ('brittle') diabetes.
2. Patients requiring prolonged pre-operative fasting, e.g. bowel prep.

▶ *Types of Insulin*

Table D2 Types of insulin and duration of effect[27]

Type of insulin	Duration of effect (h)
Regular (crystalline)	5–8
NPH/Lente/Isophane	18–24
Ultralente	24–36

▶ *Preparation of IDDM for Minor and Major Surgery*
One of several regimes may be used.

Morning Surgery

On the morning of surgery start 5% glucose IV at 80–125 mL/h and give half the patient's usual morning insulin dose subcutaneously. Measure BSL 2 h and give subcutaneous insulin 5 units if BSL > 12 mmol/L.

Afternoon Surgery

If the patient is on unmixed insulin give two-thirds of the usual morning dose of short-acting insulin and omit long-acting insulin prior to a light breakfast. If the patient is on premixed insulin give half the usual insulin dose prior to breakfast. Commence 5% glucose infusion at 1100 hours.

▶ Alternatively

Morning and Afternoon Surgery

On the morning of surgery commence an insulin/glucose infusion. Run 5% glucose at 125 mL/h and insulin at a rate dependent on patient's BSL, i.e. a sliding scale. Any values chosen for the scale need to be revised, depending on the patient's response. Aim to keep BSL at ≈ 5–11 mmol/L. If the patient is on the afternoon list allow an early light breakfast.

▶ Patients with Insulin Pumps

Patients receiving insulin subcutaneously by a pump should have their pump switched off and be commenced on an insulin glucose infusion on the morning of surgery.[27]

Preparing and Running an Insulin Glucose Infusion

Run 5% glucose at 100–125 mL/h.

▶ Insulin Infusion

Load 50 units of soluble insulin, such as actrapid, into a syringe with 50 mL of N/S. Flush the injection tubing with the above solution and discard the flush. This will saturate insulin-binding sites on the plastic tubing. Start the infusion at 1–2 units per h.

Table D3 Example of a sliding scale for an insulin/glucose infusion

BSL (mmol/L)	Units of insulin/h
< 3	0
3–5	0.5
6–7	1
7–10	2
10–15	3
15–20	4

Measure BSL 2 h pre-operatively and 1 h intra- and postoperatively. If hypoglycaemia occurs (BSL < 3 mmol/L) give 25–50 mL of 50% glucose and cease insulin.[28]

Note: The half-life of IV actrapid is only 5 min and with an IV infusion steady state is reached in 25–30 min.[29]

Non-insulin-dependent Diabetics (NIDDM or Type II Diabetes)

▶ *Minor Surgery—Morning or Afternoon Lists*

1 No oral hypoglycaemic drugs on the day of surgery. If taking chlorpropamide cease this for 24 h prior to surgery.

2 Measure BSL pre-surgery, and at 6 h intervals if prolonged fasting. If BSL ≥ 12 mmol/L consider the need for insulin/glucose infusion, depending on such issues as the length of time before surgery and co-morbid conditions. If blood sugars are low (BSL ≤ 5 mmol) commence a glucose infusion.

If the patient is on the afternoon list, give a light breakfast to finish 6 h before the scheduled operation time and clear fluids until 4 h before the operation. The patient should not have his or her usual morning antidiabetic medication and an insulin/glucose infusion commenced if patient becomes hypo-/hyperglycaemic.

3 *Major surgery*:
   (a) Cease oral agents as above.
   (b) Measure BSL pre-operatively. If BSL 6–11 mmol/L no specific preparation is required. If BSL < 6 mmol/L start IV 5% glucose 125 mL/h. If BSL > 11 mmol/L start insulin/glucose infusion as for IDDM (see above).

If an insulin/glucose infusion is not required pre-operatively the anaesthetist may commence one intra-operatively if needed.

Diet-controlled Diabetics

Treat as for non-diabetic patients. As for all diabetics avoid lactate-containing solutions (such as Hartmann's) as lactate is gluconeogenic.

Diamorphine (Heroin, Diacetylmorphine)

Diamorphine is a synthetic diacetylated derivative of morphine with strong analgesic properties. It is 1.5–2 × more potent than morphine. It is a prodrug which acts through its metabolites, 6-monoacetylmorphine and morphine.

Dose in Adults for Analgesia

▶ *IM*

5–10 mg

▶ *IV Boluses*

2.5 mg IV titrated to effect to 10 mg.

▶ *Intrathecal Dose*

0.25–0.375 mg depending on the size and fitness of the patient.[30]

Advantages

Faster onset of action than morphine due to its higher lipid solubility. Possibly less nausea and vomiting than morphine.[31]

Disadvantages

Diamorphine produces marked euphoria and has a high addiction potential. Its medicinal use is banned in the United States but it is a popular analgesic in the United Kingdom.

Diazepam

Benzodiazepine drug useful for sedation, anxiolysis, anterograde amnesia, muscle relaxation and for status epilepticus. Use of the IM route produces a suboptimal effect due to slow and erratic absorption from muscle.

Dose for Status Epilepticus

▸ *Adult*

IV 5–10 mg initially. May require up to 20–30 mg. See *EPILEPSY, STATUS.*

▸ *Child*

0.2 mg/kg/dose IV or 0.5 mg/kg PR.

Note: Diazepam is dissolved in propylene glycol which is very irritating to the veins and can cause pain on injection and thrombophlebitis. Give via a central line if one available. In contrast, diazepam emulsion (diazemuls) is much better tolerated. Midazolam is an appropriate alternative.

Sedation/Anxiolysis

▸ *Adult*

2–60 mg/day in divided doses PO.

▸ *Child*

0.2–0.5 mg/kg/dose 8–12 h PO.

Diazoxide

Benzothiadiazine antihypertensive drug. Acts directly on arteriolar smooth muscle, causing relaxation. Also used to treat intractable hypoglycaemia. Acts by decreasing insulin secretion and inhibiting the peripheral utilisation of glucose.

Dose for Hypertensive Emergencies

▶ *Adult*

Give IV boluses of 30 mg up to a maximum of 150 mg as a single bolus dose. Single bolus doses of 300 mg have been associated with angina and with myocardial and cerebral infarction.[32]

▶ *Child*

1–3 mg/kg IV repeat × 1 prn, then 2–5 mg/kg 6 h.

Diclofenac

Non-steroidal anti-inflammatory drug useful for the treatment of musculoskeletal and postoperative pain. Diclofenac is contraindicated in patients with peptic ulcer disease, gastrointestinal bleeding and hypersensitivity to aspirin. Use with caution or avoid in asthmatic patients. See *NON-STEROIDAL ANTI-INFLAMMATORY DRUGS*.

Dose

▶ *Adult*

25–50 mg PO 8 h with food.

▶ *Child*

1 mg/kg/dose (max. 50 mg) 8 h.

Note: Diclofenac has been associated with hepatic toxicity and, rarely, acute immune haemolytic anaemia.[33] See *NON-STEROIDAL ANTI-INFLAMMATORY DRUGS*.

Difficult Airway Management

Predicting Difficult Intubation

The incidence of difficult intubation is approximately 1–4% and the incidence of impossible intubation is about 0.05–0.35%.[34] Obstetric patients have a higher incidence of failed intubation, about 1 per 250–300. See *CAESAREAN SECTION (CS)*. Up to 16% of difficult intubations cannot be predicted from the risk assessment techniques described below.[35] Predictors of difficult intubation include the following:

1 *Mallampati test* (as modified by Samsoon and Young).[36] The patient is asked to maximally protrude the tongue from the fully open mouth while sitting upright. Visible pharyngeal structures are used to classify the airway as follows.
   * Class 1—soft palate, fauces, uvula and pillars all visible
   * Class 2—as above, but pillars obscured
   * Class 3—only soft palate and base of uvula visible
   * Class 4—hard palate only visible.

The higher the class, the more potentially difficult is the intubation. This test predicts only about 50% of difficult intubations and has a high incidence of false positives.[37]

2 *Thyromental distance.* This is the straight line distance between the thyroid notch and the lower border of the mentum (chin) with the head extended.[38] It is predicted that:
   - > 6.5 cm—easy laryngoscopy
   - 6–6.5 cm—difficult laryngoscopy
   - < 6 cm—very difficult/impossible laryngoscopy[39]

3 *Wilson Risk Sum Score.*[40] Evaluates five factors felt to be correlated with difficult intubation. These are weight, head and neck movement, mouth opening, jaw development (receding or non receding) and prominence of upper incisors. Each factor has three possible scores (0, 1 or 2) and the range of scores is 0–10. A score of 2 predicts 75% of difficult intubations.[37] This scoring system has a sensitivity of ≈ 40–75%,[40,41] a specificity of ≈ 90% and a positive predictive value of ≈ 9%.[41]

Management of Recognised Difficult Airway

The following options are to be considered:

1 Evaluate the suitability of local or regional anaesthesia for the surgery planned.

2 If local or regional anaesthesia not a viable option (e.g. patient refusal) the next best option is to *secure the airway awake. Intubation awake will almost always be the safest option.* Options for securing the airway awake, after adequate airway anaesthesia, include:
   (a) direct laryngoscopy with suitable aides (see *Management of Unrecognised Difficult Airway* below)
   (b) awake fibre-optic intubation (see *AWAKE FIBRE-OPTIC INTUBATION*)
   (c) use of the LMA or Fastrach (see *LARYNGEAL MASK AIRWAY (INCLUDING PROSEAL AND FASTRACH)*)
   (d) blind nasal intubation (see *BLIND NASAL INTUBATION*)
   (e) retrograde intubation techniques (see *RETROGRADE INTU-BATION*)

D

(f) use of the lightwand in the awake patient (see *LIGHTWAND INTUBATION*)

(g) surgical airway under LA (see *CRICOTHYROID PUNCTURE AND CRICOTHYROTOMY*).

3   The next and more hazardous option is to *secure the airway with the patient anaesthetised* via a gaseous and/or a slowly titrated intravenous infusion induction. This technique is especially indicated in patients who refuse awake techniques, or who are unable to cooperate due to such factors as age, mental state or decreased level of consciousness. Once the patient is sufficiently 'deep', attempt direct laryngoscopy or use one or more of the techniques listed above. If using direct laryngoscopy see *Optimising Intubating Conditions* below.

If the patient is an aspiration risk consider applying cricoid pressure when the patient becomes anaesthetised.

The aims of this technique are to maintain oxygenation and to maintain spontaneous breathing. Giving muscle relaxants in this situation may result in loss of airway control and patient asphyxia.

4   If unable to secure the airway with patient anaesthetised, allow the patient to wake up and then plan a different approach. Options are:

(a) further counselling of the patient to accept regional anaesthesia or an awake technique

(b) obtaining more appropriate equipment

(c) obtaining personnel with better skills.

5   If unable to maintain oxygenation insert a ProSeal or LMA. If this is successful and surgery is urgent consider proceeding. If intubation is felt to be mandatory consider a surgical airway or intubating through such techniques as FOB or use of the Fastrach. If surgery is not urgent allow the patient to wake up.

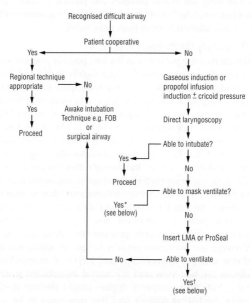

*If able to mask ventilate, decide whether surgery must proceed immediately. If no, wake patient up. If yes, decide whether surgery can be done under mask anaesthesia. If no to mask anaesthesia, insert LMA or ProSeal or intubate using Fastrach, FOB or other technique to obtain a surgical airway.

†If able to ventilate via LMA or Proseal, decide whether surgery must proceed immediately. If no, wake patient up. If yes, decide whether surgery can be done using the LMA or ProSeal. If yes, proceed. If no, intubate using Fastrach, FOB or other technique or obtain surgical airway.

Figure D2 Management of the recognised difficult intubation

D

Management of Unrecognised Difficult Airway

The following discussion assumes the patient is under general anaesthesia and the first attempt at intubation was unsuccessful. Do not attempt intubation more than three times.

▶ Optimising Intubating Conditions

1   Ensure that the patient is in the best possible position for intubation. This means with the neck slightly flexed and the head extended on the neck at the atlanto-occipital joint aligning the oral, pharyngeal and laryngeal axes into a straight line. In the obese it may be necessary to place pillows and/or blankets behind the back shoulders and head to obtain the best 'sniff' position. Placing the patient slightly sitting up by breaking the middle of the bed may help obstacles like large pendulous breasts 'flow away' from the airway rather than towards it.

2   The person attempting the intubation for the second time should be the most 'experienced' anaesthetist immediately available.

3   Optimal external laryngeal manipulation should be undertaken to improve the laryngeal view. This may be backwards, upwards and rightwards pressure—the BURP manouevre.[42] Consider the two-anaesthetist technique in which one anaesthetist uses the laryngoscope and laryngeal manipulation to obtain the best view and the second anaesthetist inserts the tube. Note that inexpertly applied cricoid pressure itself may make intubation difficult and this may need to be relaxed briefly to allow intubation.

4   Mandibular advancement (an assistant pulls the jaw forward) may improve the laryngeal view.[43]

5   Use a specialised laryngoscope. The McCoy laryngoscope, with its hinged distal tip activated by a lever on the handle, is particularly useful in this situation. Other types of laryngoscope to consider are the straight Miller blade, the Kessel blade or the Belscope.

6   Consider using a teflon bougie if there is any view of the epiglottis. In this technique the distal 1 cm of the bougie is formed into a slight hook shape. While an assistant gently steadies the distal end, the proximal end is positioned by the anaesthetist to scrape along the posterior surface of the epiglottis towards the larynx exactly in the midline. The distal tip of the bougie may thus enter the trachea blindly and this can be confirmed by feeling a bumping sensation on the tracheal rings. The ET tube is then railroaded over the teflon bougie.

▶ Unable to Intubate—Steps in Management

The priority at this stage is to maintain oxygenation and ventilation with mask ventilation. To optimise mask ventilation:

1   Optimise the airway by providing maximal jaw thrust, adequate head tilt and use of jaw support (opening the mouth slightly).
2   Use a two-handed grip on the mask, while an assistant squeezes the reservoir bag (two-anaesthetist ventilation technique).
3   Insert an oral (Guedel) and/or nasal airway.
4   If able to mask-ventilate and surgery is not immediately urgent, allow the patient to wake up and formulate a new plan.
5   If surgery is immediately urgent options are:
    (a) surgery under mask anaesthesia
    (b) surgery using a ProSeal or LMA
    (c) intubation using techniques such as the Fastrach or FOB. See *LARYNGEAL MASK AIRWAY (INCLUDING PROSEAL AND FASTRACH), RETROGRADE INTUBATION* and *LIGHTWAND INTUBATION*.
    (d) obtaining a surgical airway.

▶ Unable to Intubate, Unable to Ventilate

This is a *crisis situation*.

1   Summon urgent skilled assistance and notify the surgeon.

2   Insert a LMA, ProSeal or Fastrach. It may be necessary to partly or fully release cricoid pressure to enable correct placement of the laryngeal mask or ProSeal.[44] A new technique of ProSeal insertion has recently been described by Brimacombe[45] and may be ideally suited to this situation. In this technique:

    (a) The ProSeal is deflated and shaped in the usual way in preparation for insertion. See *LARYNGEAL MASK AIRWAY (INCLUDING PROSEAL AND FASTRACH)*.

    (b) A well-lubricated gum elastic bougie (GEB) is passed through the drain tube of the ProSeal.

    (c) A laryngoscope is used to visualise the oesophagus and the GEB is deliberately inserted into the oesophagus.

    (d) The ProSeal is then railroaded over the GEB into place over the larynx. This appears to be the most efficient method yet discovered for insertion of the ProSeal.

3   If an LMA is inserted and ventilation is adequate, this device can be used to enable intubation if this is felt to be necessary. In this technique the LMA cuff is placed over the larynx in the usual way. An ET tube is then inserted through the LMA and into the trachea.

Table D4 Maximum sized ET tube that can be passed through the various LMA sizes[44]

LMA size	Maximum size ET tube that will pass through
1	3.5
2	4.5
2.5	5.0
3	6.0 cuffed
4	6.0 cuffed
5	7.0 cuffed

Use of an extra long size 6.0 ET tube (such as a Mallinckrodt microlaryngoscopy tube) will enable deeper insertion of the tip of the ET tube into the trachea. The LMA is left in position until extubation. In a variation of this technique a Teflon introducer can be passed through the LMA and into the trachea. The tube is then railroaded over the introducer either with or without the LMA left in position. The success rate of this technique is said to be between 19% and 93%.[46,47] Another variation involves passing a fibre-optic bronchoscope (FOB) through the LMA and into the trachea with the tube preloaded on the FOB.

4   If still unable to ventilate the patient and maintain oxygenation then a surgical airway must be obtained. Options are cricothyroid puncture, cricothyrotomy or tracheostomy. See *CRICOTHYROID PUNCTURE AND CRICOTHYROTOMY*.

See Figure D3 overleaf.

Digital Nerve Block

Anatomy
The fingers/toes are supplied by four nerve branches of the digital nerve, two palmar/plantar and two dorsal.

Technique for Finger Block
1   Place the hand palm down on a flat surface.
2   Insert a 25 G needle on one side of the base of the proximal phalanx, aiming to almost transfix the finger as close to the proximal phalanx as possible. Inject a total of 2 mL of 2% lignocaine on each side.

Do not use adrenaline-containing solutions.

Digoxin

Cardiac glycoside. Acts by inhibiting Na^+/K^+-ATP-ase leading to decreased Na^+/K^+ pump function. This results in increased

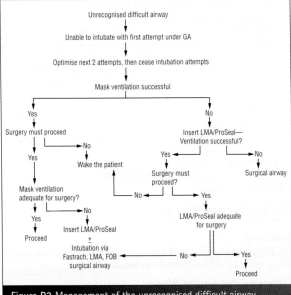

Figure D3 Management of the unrecognised difficult airway

intracellular Na⁺, which in turn causes increased intracellular Ca^{2+}, resulting in a positive inotropic effect on cardiac myocytes. Digoxin also decreases intracellular K⁺, leading to a slowing of atrioventricular conduction and of depolarisation of pacemaker cells. In addition, digoxin increases vagal activity.

Digoxin is useful for the treatment of:
1 atrial fibrillation and flutter
2 congestive cardiac failure.

Dose

See *ATRIAL FIBRILLATION, CHRONIC*.

TR of digoxin is 1–2 ng/mL.

Disseminated Intravascular Coagulation (DIC)

Pathophysiology

DIC is a syndrome characterised by inappropriate, excessive and uncontrolled activation of haemostatic processes. Both thrombin and plasmin may be produced in excess quantities, causing clotting and fibrinolysis in small vessels. The above process results in:

1 haemorrhage due to consumption of platelets and clotting factors and the anticoagulant effect of fibrin degradation products (FDPs). See *FIBRIN DEGRADATION PRODUCTS (FDPs)*

2 microvascular obstruction due to clot and fibrin deposition, leading to end organ damage

3 possible intravascular haemolysis.

Aetiology

DIC can be triggered by any condition that produces damage to vascular endothelium, or that releases damaged or necrotic tissue into the bloodstream. Such precipitating events include:

- obstetric complications. These include haemorrhagic shock, infection, placental abruption, pre-eclampsia/eclampsia, amniotic fluid embolus and foetal death in utero.
- sepsis, e.g. meningococcaemia
- trauma (especially brain and crush injuries) and burns
- transfusion reactions
- malignancy.

There are many other causes and the condition can be acute and fulminant, or chronic and subtle.

Clinical Manifestations of Acute DIC

These are highly variable. The effects of microvascular thrombi may predominate initially, then haemorrhagic effects may be more significant. Clinical symptoms and signs include:

- delirium, coma, cerebral infarction
- renal impairment/failure
- skin ulceration, necrosis, gangrene
- cyanosis, hypoxia, dyspnoea, pulmonary infarction
- bruising, petechiae
- severe haemorrhage from lungs, GIT, genitourinary tract and wounds. Intracranial haemorrhage may occur.

Diagnosis

DIC is characterised by:

1 low fibrinogen levels (NR 200–400 mg/100 mL)

2 elevated FDP levels (NR < 10 µg/mL) in almost all cases.[48] In DIC, FDPs may be > 40 µg/mL.

3 D-dimer test confirms fibrin degradation. D-dimer is a measure of fragments of cross-linked fibrin. See *D-DIMER TEST*.

4 reduced platelet count and reduced levels of antithrombin III and Factors V and VIII

5 abnormal clotting studies. Total clotting time, prothrombin time (PT) and activated partial thromboplastin time (APTT) may all be prolonged. See *PROTHROMBIN TIME* and *ACTIVATED PARTIAL THROMBOPLASTIN TIME (APTT)*. In many cases PT and APTT can be in or below the normal range due to activated factors affecting these tests.[48]

Treatment

1 Resuscitate the patient, ensuring an adequate airway and ventilation. Maintain the patient's circulation with appropriate fluids, i.e. crystalloid/colloid/blood ± inotropic support. See *BLOOD TRANSFUSION*.

2 Identify the pathological process triggering DIC and treat definitively if possible.

3 Attempt to reverse the coagulopathy and reduce blood loss. Organise urgent consultation with a haematologist. A combination of blood, platelets, fresh frozen plasma, cryoprecipitate and clotting factor concentrates will be required. Aim to maintain APTT in the normal range and platelet count $> 50 \times 10^9$/L. In general PT should be ignored.[49]

4 Cryoprecipitate infusion should be targeted towards a fibrinogen level of 100–150 mg/dL.

5 Prostacyclin may be helpful by decreasing platelet activation.

6 Heparin therapy may be helpful. The rationale is that DIC is driven by the pathological production of thrombin, and heparin inhibits thrombin. At the 'right dose' it is hypothesised that heparin will inhibit the low concentration of thrombin in the circulation without preventing appropriate haemostatic plugs forming at extravascular sites. Several heparin regimens are suggested.

Horne[49] recommends heparin 20 U/kg bolus, then 5 U/kg/h. Measure platelet count and fibrinogen levels which should both increase with treatment. (APTT cannot be used to monitor therapy and PT should be helpful). Increase dose by 25% every 4–6 h until the platelet and fibrinogen levels stabilise at a satisfactory level. If bleeding worsens stop heparin or decrease infusion rate.

Feinstein[50] suggests giving IV heparin at a rate of 7.5 U/kg/h. After 1–2 h give platelets to increase levels to 50×10^9/L, and cryoprecipitate to increase fibrinogen levels to 150 mg/100 mL. Measure platelet and fibrinogen levels 30–60 min after transfusion. If adequate counts and levels are not achieved or maintained, increase the rate of heparin infusion by 2.5 U/kg/h. Repeat this sequence of evaluation.

D

The Role of Recombinant Activated Factor VII (rFVIIa)

This drug appears to be a major breakthrough in the management of intractable haemorrhage. There are many case reports in the literature of rFVIIa being used successfully to treat severe haemorrhage in pathological conditions likely to lead to DIC. For example Bouwmeester et al. reported a 30-year-old female with severe intractable postpartum haemorrhage due to uterine atony and vaginal lacerations in whom haemorrhage could not be controlled with conventional therapy.[51] rFVIIa was used successfully to control haemorrhage within 10 minutes of administration.

rFVIIa has also been used successfully to treat bleeding in documented cases of DIC.[52,53] See *RECOMBINANT ACTIVATED FACTOR VII*.

Dobutamine

Synthetic isoprenaline derivative. Dobutamine is used for its positive inotropic effects in situations where there is low cardiac output due to such causes as myocardial infarction, cardiac surgery or cardiomyopathy.

Acts mainly on β1 adrenergic receptors, with a slight action on β2 and α adrenergic receptors. Dobutamine's main effects are to increase cardiac contractility and heart rate, with a modest decrease in systemic vascular resistance.

Dobutamine has similar properties to a combination of dopamine and sodium nitroprusside, i.e. a fixed combination of inotropic drug and vasodilator.

Preparation and Administration

Mix 250 mg dobutamine with 100 mL of 5% glucose. Administer preferably via a central line, but as there is little vasoconstrictor activity, it can be given via a peripheral cannula temporarily.

Dose

Titrate to desired effect.

Dose range: 0.5–15 μg/kg/min[54]

Table D5 Rate of infusion of dobutamine for a 70 kg patient	
Rate of infusion	Dose
1.7 mL/h	1 μg/kg/min
4.2 mL/h	2.5 μg/kg/min
25.5 mL/h	15 μg/kg/min
Alternatively:	Mix (3 × body weight) mg in 50 mL N/S.
1 mL/h = 1 μg/kg/min	

Dolasetron Mesylate

Long-acting single daily dose anti-emetic, which acts through selective 5-HT$_3$ receptor antagonism. No dosage adjustment is required in the presence of renal or hepatic impairment.

Adult Dose

For the *prevention* of nausea/vomiting (N/V) give 12.5 mg IV over 30 s or 50 mg PO daily. For the *treatment* of N/V give 12.5 mg IV over 30 s daily. Not currently approved for use in children.

Dopamine

Naturally occurring catecholamine used for its positive inotropic and chronotropic actions, and its effects on systemic vascular resistance, via its actions on α and β adrenergic receptors. Dopamine also has the ability to increase renal blood flow via its action on specific dopamine receptors and to increase urine output. This traditional view is oversimplified and has been greatly challenged by recent research. It is believed by many investigators that dopamine increases renal blood flow through its cardiac inotropic effects.[55] The diuretic and natriuretic effects of dopamine are now thought to be due to a direct tubular action.[55]

Dopamine also causes inhibition of noradrenaline release by stimulation of dopamine 2 receptors on the presynaptic sympathetic nerve terminals.[56]

Uses

1 Positive inotropic agent in low cardiac output states.
2 Impending renal failure to improve renal perfusion and urine output. This is a controversial and unresolved issue.[55] To date there is an absence of properly controlled studies supporting the hypothesis that low dose dopamine alters renally related mortality or morbidity.[56,57]

Dose

Depends on desired effect, dose range 1–20 µg/kg/min:

▶ Low Dose (1–5 µg/kg/min)

Stimulates mainly dopamine receptors, causing renal vasodilatation and increased renal blood flow and urine output.

▶ Medium Dose (5–10 µg/kg/min)

β adrenergic effects predominate with increased cardiac output mainly due to increased stroke volume. Blood pressure may fall due to β2 adreno-receptor mediated vasodilatation causing decreased systemic vascular resistance.

▶ High Dose (> 15 µg/kg/min)

α adrenergic effects predominate with increased systemic vascular resistance and subsequent increased blood pressure. May get baroreceptor-mediated reflex bradycardia. Renal blood flow is decreased.

Preparation and Administration

Mix 200 mg dopamine with 100 mL 5% glucose. Administer only by a central venous line.

µg/kg/min (mL/h)	Used for
Table D6 Rate of administration of dopamine (2 mg/mL) for 70 kg patient	
3 (6.3 mL/h)	Improving renal function
8 (17 mL/h)	Mainly β effects
16 (34 mL/h)	Mainly α effects
Alternatively:	Mix (3 × body weight) mg with 50 mL N/S.
1 mL/h = 1 µg/kg/min	

Other Effects of Dopamine

1 Increased Na^+ excretion by the kidney.
2 Emetic effect.
3 Increased prolactin release.
4 Tachycardia and tachydysrhythmias.
5 Depressed respiratory drive (hypoxic and central).
6 Increased intrapulmonary shunt.
7 Gut ischaemia may occur.[57]

Dopexamine

Dobutamine analogue, agonist at dopamine (DA) 1 and β2 adreno-receptors with lesser effect on DA2 and β1 adreno-receptors. Dopexamine has minimal α adreno-receptor effects.

Uses
Improving cardiac output (CO) in low CO states, e.g. post cardiac surgery and acute heart failure.

Main Effects
Dopexamine increases CO and heart rate. It decreases systemic vascular resistance with little change in blood pressure. Gives increased renal blood flow due to its DA1 receptor stimulation effects with increased urinary output.

Dose
Given by IV infusion 0.5–6 µg/kg/min, titrate to desired clinical effect.

Double Lumen Endotracheal Tubes

See *ONE-LUNG VENTILATION*.

Doxacurium

Benzylisoquinolinium type non-depolarising neuromuscular blocking drug. It is long acting and 2.5–3 × more potent than pancuronium.

Dose
For intubation, give 50–80 µg/kg. 'Top up' dose: 5–10 µg/kg. Duration of action ≈ 100 min. Doxacurium is not metabolised; it is excreted in bile and urine unchanged. The drug does not release histamine and is very cardiovascularly stable.

Doxapram

Respiratory stimulant drug, which acts by stimulating peripheral carotid chemoreceptors and the medullary respiratory centres. Used for:

- counteracting postanaesthetic respiratory depression
- treating laryngospasm.

Dose

1 mg/kg IV, acts in 20–40 s and lasts 5–12 min.

Can also be given by infusion; 1–3 mg/min (in the adult).

Note: Doxapram should not be used in patients with epilepsy, thyrotoxicosis, ischaemic heart disease or hypertension.

Drixine

See *OXYMETAZOLINE*.

Droperidol

Butyrophenone derivative useful for its anti-emetic effects and in the antiquated technique termed 'neuroleptanalgesia'. Droperidol exerts its effects by dopamine 2 receptor blockade, post synaptic GABA antagonism and some α adrenergic receptor blocking effects. It may be more effective for preventing nausea than vomiting.

Dose for Anti-emesis in Adult

1.25 mg IV.[58] Its duration of action is limited by its elimination half-life of ≈ 2 h.

Points to Note

1 Droperidol causes dose-dependent sedation and drowsiness. Droperidol can cause neuroleptic malignant syndrome (see entry).[59]

2 Droperidol may be particularly useful for morphine PCA induced PONV in adults, e.g. consider adding droperidol 2.5 mg to 100 mg of morphine for PCA use.[60]

Dynastat

See *PARECOXIB*.

D

Dystonic Reaction, Acute

This syndrome is characterised by tonic muscular contractions such as torticollis, oculogyric crisis and opisthotonis. Exaggerated posturing of the head, neck and/or jaw and laryngo-pharyngeal spasm may also be seen. It occurs as an idiosyncratic reaction to drugs such as metoclopramide and prochlorperazine. This side-effect is due to the central dopaminergic 2 receptor blockade effect of these drugs.

Treatment

Give benztropine mesylate 0.5–2 mg IV or IM or procyclidine 5–10 mg IV.

Ee

Ebstein's Anomaly

See *TRICUSPID REGURGITATION AND EBSTEIN'S ANOMALY*.

ECG Monitoring

See *ELECTROCARDIOGRAPHY* and *MYOCARDIAL ISCHAEMIA, INTRA-OPERATIVE*.

Eclampsia

See *PRE-ECLAMPSIA/ECLAMPSIA*.

EDLA

Stands for an extended duration LA preparation consisting of poly-lactico-glycolic acid polymer microspheres 25–125 μm in diameter, which contain bupivacaine ± dexamethasone. These microspheres biodegrade over 7 days, thus prolonging the LA effects.

Eisenmenger's Syndrome

More than a brief outline of this complicated condition is beyond the scope of this manual. Evidence from the literature is mainly anecdotal and theoretical due to the rareness of this condition.

Definition

In this syndrome, an atrial or ventricular septal defect or other congenital cardiac abnormality causes a left to right shunt. This results in an increased load on the pulmonary circulation, causing pulmonary hypertension and right ventricular hypertrophy. In time the pulmonary vascular resistance increases to the point where

E

pulmonary pressure is equal to or greater than systemic pressure and the shunt becomes bidirectional or reversed (right to left shunt). This causes cyanosis.

Although regional and general anaesthesia are associated with considerable risk in patients with Eisenmenger's syndrome, many types of anaesthetic have been used successfully in this condition.

Management Aims

The main aim is to minimise the degree of right to left shunt. Right to left shunt will be increased by factors that:

- increase pulmonary vascular resistance (PVR)
- decrease systemic vascular resistance (SVR).

Towards this main aim:

1 Prevent further elevation of PVR. See *PULMONARY HYPERTEN-SION*. Factors which increase PVR include hypoxia, hypercarbia, acidosis, hypothermia, lung hyperinflation and positive end expiratory pressure.

2 Maintain pre-operative levels of SVR.[1]

3 Keep systemic blood pressure and cardiac output well maintained throughout the peri-operative period.

4 Maintain optimal intravascular fluid volume and replace fluid losses promptly. Unreplaced extracellular fluid loss is poorly tolerated.[2]

5 In some Eisenmenger's patients, the PVR decreases with O_2 therapy and the degree of right to left shunt is reduced.[3] (Note that hypoxaemia due to right to left shunt is not usually reversible by O_2 therapy.)

6 Administration of an α adrenergic receptor agonist may increase SVR more than PVR and produce a reduction in right to left shunting, and thus be beneficial.[3]

7 Consider the use of selective pulmonary vasodilator drugs such as nitric oxide and inhaled prostacyclin.

8 Provide antibiotic prophylaxis against bacterial endocartis. See *BACTERIAL ENDOCARDITIS PROPHYLAXIS*.

9 These patients are at increased risk of thrombo-embolic disease due to an elevated haematocrit and require appropriate anti-coagulant therapy. Venesection for polycythaemia may be required for haematocrits over 65%.

10 Bradycardia must be prevented.

Anaesthetic Management

▶ *Preinduction Phase*

1 Ensure the patient's intravascular volume is optimal.

2 In addition to routine monitoring, insert an arterial cannula for invasive blood pressure readings.

3 Use of a pulmonary artery catheter is not advised because:[2,3]
   (a) There is an increased risk of pulmonary artery rupture due to pulmonary hypertension.
   (b) Dysrhythmias, thrombosis and embolism (including para-doxical embolus) risks are increased.
   (c) Interpretation of PA catheter readings in the presence of a bidirectional shunt is extremely difficult.

4 Central venous pressure (CVP) monitoring is useful to measure right ventricular (RV) filling pressure. Optimal RV filling may help minimise right to left shunt and an excessive elevation in CVP may indicate that the RV is failing.[3]

▶ *Induction Phase*

Agents used successfully for induction of anaesthesia include the following:

1 Ketamine is useful as it does not cause a reduction in SVR.[2] However, it may increase PVR thus precipitating cyanotic spells.[4]

2 Etomidate appears appropriate for use in this condition as it has the least cardiovascular effects.[5]

E

3   Sammut and Paes suggest the use of a noradrenaline infusion to maintain satisfactory SVR.[6]

▶ Maintenance Phase

1   Several different inhalation agents have been used successfully in this syndrome (halothane, enflurane).[5,6] It is not clear whether one agent in particular should be recommended. Maintaining SVR is of utmost importance

2   N_2O can cause reduced ventricular function and pulmonary vasoconstriction, which may be detrimental.

3   Use IPPV with low inflation pressures. Plan for early extubation.

4   There is an increased risk of paradoxical embolism of gas, fat, clot or amniotic fluid.[6]

▶ Postoperative Phase

These patients should be monitored closely for postoperative deterioration in ICU or the high dependency ward. Many patients with this disease may survive surgery, only to die soon after the operation from thromboembolic disease,[7] heart failure and other complications.

▶ Obstetric Implications

Pregnancy is contraindicated in this condition, and termination is frequently recommended. The mortality of termination is about 7%.[8]

1   The combination of Eisenmenger's syndrome and pregnancy is associated with a mortality of about 40–50%.[9] The foetal loss rate is about 8%.[7]

2   Caesarean section maternal mortality rate in Eisenmenger's syndrome is between 46% and 70%.[8]

3   It is unclear whether patients with Eisenmenger's syndrome should be allowed to labour and deliver vaginally or whether elective CS should be performed. A decision about the preferred mode of delivery must be made for each individual case well before term.

4 Well-managed epidural anaesthesia has been successfully used for labour and delivery in these patients.[10] The main concern is reduction in SVR, which must be avoided. Do not use adrenaline-containing solutions due to the potential for peripheral vasodilating β adrenergic receptor effects.[11]

5 Syntocinon may cause a dramatic reduction in arterial O_2 tension due to vasodilatation.[12]

▶ *Laparoscopic Surgery*

Can be hazardous in these patients due to the effects of pneumoperitoneum, including decreased venous return. Other problems include the following:

1 PVR may be increased by elevation of airway pressure as intra-abdominal pressure rises.

2 Hypercarbia/acidosis, due to CO_2 gas insufflation, can also increase PVR.

Recommendations:

1 Intra-abdominal pressure should be < 15 mmHg.

2 Avoid the Trendelenburg position.[6]

3 Gasless laparoscopy with mechanical abdominal wall elevation may be preferable.[2]

Ejection Fraction

See *CARDIAC INVESTIGATIONS*.

Elbow Blocks

Anatomy

▶ *Ulnar Nerve (C7, 8, T1)*

A branch of the medial cord of the brachial plexus, it passes along the posterior surface of the medial epicondyle at the elbow. It enters the forearm between the two heads of flexor carpi ulnaris.

E

Supplies

Sensory to the dorsal and palmar aspects of the little and half the ring finger and ulnar side of hand. Motor to the medial two lumbricals and the interossei, adductor pollicis, flexor carpi ulnaris and the medial half of flexor digitorum profundus.

▶ Median Nerve (C5, 6, 7, 8, T1)

Arises from the medial and lateral cords of the brachial plexus. The nerve crosses the elbow in the antecubital fossa, lying on the brachialis medial to the brachial artery.

Supplies

Sensory to the thenar eminence and palmar aspect of the lateral three and a half digits and the skin on the dorsal tips of the same fingers. Motor to all the intrinsic muscles of the thumb except adductor pollicis, the lateral two lumbricals and some of the forearm muscles.

▶ Radial Nerve (C5, 6, 7, 8, T1)

Arises from the posterior cord of the brachial plexus. The radial nerve winds around the lower end of the humerus to end in front of the lateral epicondyle. Here it divides into the superficial radial nerve and the posterior interosseous nerve.

Supplies

Skin over posterior arm, postero-lateral lower arm and forearm, dorsal aspect of thumb base and the back of the lateral three and a half digits except for the tips. Motor to triceps, brachialis, brachioradialis and extensor carpi radialis longus.

▶ Lateral Cutaneous Nerve of Forearm

The continuation of the musculocutaneous nerve. In the antecubital fossa it lies just lateral to the biceps tendon at the elbow crease.

Supplies

Skin on the lateral half of the forearm as far as the wrist and a variable area on the dorsum of the hand.

E

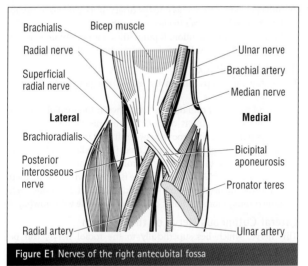

Figure E1 Nerves of the right antecubital fossa

Ulnar Nerve Block

1 Flex the elbow to 30° and identify the ulnar nerve in the sulcus of the medial epicondyle.
2 Insert a 25 G 38 mm needle 1–2 cm proximal to this position and elicit paraesthesia. Inject 2 mL lignocaine 1% with adrenaline over 10–20 s.

Median Nerve Block

1 Extend the elbow and identify the medial and lateral epicondyles. Draw a line between them, which should be ≈ 3–4 cm proximal to the flexion crease.
2 Palpate the brachial artery and insert a 25 G 38 mm needle on the epicondylar line about 0.5 cm medial to the brachial artery

and elicit paraesthesia deep to the artery. It may be necessary to fan the needle in order to elicit paraesthesia.

3   Inject 5 mL of LA solution. If paraesthesia is not obtained inject a wall of LA alongside and deep to the brachial artery.

Radial Nerve Block

1   Identify the biceps tendon by asking the patient to flex the elbow.

2   Extend the elbow and draw a line between the medial and lateral epicondyles. Insert a 25 G 38 mm needle just lateral to biceps tendon in the groove between it and the brachioradialis muscle on the epicondylar line. Direct the needle slightly cephalad and medial to contact the lateral condyle of the humerus.

3   Inject 2–4 mL of LA while the needle is withdrawn ≈ 0.5 cm, then withdraw the needle almost to the skin. Reinsert 2 × more, each time aiming more medially, and injecting while withdrawing.[13]

Lateral Cutaneous Nerve of the Forearm

This nerve, which lies superficially to the radial nerve, can be blocked by injecting 5 mL of LA subcutaneously in the groove between the biceps tendon and brachioradialis.

Electrocardiography

Topics Covered in this Section

▶ Lead Placement for Standard 12 Lead ECG Recording
▶ Lead Positions for Monitoring
▶ Normal ECG Values
▶ Some Important Diagnostic ECG Patterns

Lead Placement For Standard 12 Lead ECG Recording

There are four limb leads and six chest leads. The chest leads are positioned as follows:

- *V1*: 4th intercostal space (ICS) at the right sternal border (SB)
- *V2*: 4th ICS, left SB
- *V3*: between V2 and V4
- *V4*: 5th ICS in the midclavicular line (MCL)
- *V5*: 5th ICS in the anterior axillary line
- *V6*: 5th ICS in the midaxillary line.

Lead Positions for Monitoring

▶ *Standard 3 Lead Monitoring*

Right arm lead (white) on the right shoulder, left arm lead (black) on the left shoulder, left leg lead (red) on left lower chest. Usually monitor lead II.

▶ *CM5 Configuration*

This is a means of optimising the 3 lead system in order to detect ischaemia. This is achieved by placing the left arm electrode (black) on the V5 position and right arm lead (white) over the manubrium. The 3rd (indifferent) lead is placed on the left shoulder. Monitor lead I (not II).

▶ *5 Lead ECG Monitoring*

Place the right arm lead (white) on the right shoulder and the left arm lead (black) on the left shoulder. Place the right leg lead (green) in the mid-axillary line low on the chest. Place the left leg lead (red) in the same position on the left side. Place the chest lead (brown) in the V5 position (see above). Monitor leads II and V. See also *ST SEGMENT ANALYSIS*.

Normal ECG Values

Standard running speed 25 mm/s. Therefore 0.5 cm (one large square) = 0.2 s, and 1 mm = 0.04 s. 1 cm (two large squares) amplitude = 1 mV

PR interval   NR 0.12–0.2 s
QRS   NR $\leq$ 0.12 s

QT *interval*   Corrected QT interval (QTc) = $\dfrac{Q - T}{\sqrt{(R - R \text{ interval})}}$

NR QTc = 0.39 s ± 0.04 s. See *QT Interval Abnormalities* below.

Normal axis –30° to +120°

J point is the end of the QRS complex.

Some Important Diagnostic ECG Patterns

▶ Axis Abnormalities

A significant left axis deviation is indicated by a negative QRS complex in lead II. A significant right axis deviation is indicated by a negative QRS complex in lead I.

▶ Abnormal ECG Waves

- *U wave*—occurs after the T wave. An inverted U wave in leads I, II and V5 may be seen in ischaemic heart disease (IHD) and hypertension.
- *Delta wave*—slurred upstroke on the R wave. Classically seen in Wolff-Parkinson-White syndrome. See *WOLFF-PARKINSON-WHITE SYNDROME*.
- *J wave*—a rounded hump-like wave on the down stroke of the R wave. Also called an Osborne wave. Seen in hypothermia.

▶ P Wave Abnormalities

- *P mitrale*—a bifid P wave is associated with left atrial hypertrophy, as can occur with mitral stenosis.
- *P pulmonale*—a tall peaked P wave. This pattern is associated with right atrial enlargement as can occur with pulmonary hypertension and tricuspid valve stenosis.

▶ Strain Pattern

Depression of the ST segment and T wave inversion. This pattern may be seen with myocardia ischaemia.

▶ QT Interval Abnormalities

- *Prolonged QTc interval* is associated with hypocalcaemia, myocarditis, myocardial infarction, certain drugs (e.g. quinidine) and sympathetic stimulation as can occur with head injury. Anaesthetic drugs that prolong the QTc interval include isoflurane and sevoflurane. Halothane and propofol do *not* prolong the QTc interval.

* *Shortened QTc interval* can occur with digoxin therapy, hyperthermia, hypercalcaemia and vagal stimulation.

▶ Electrolyte Disturbances

* *Hyperkalaemia*—prolonged PR interval, widened QRS, flattening of the P wave, tall and peaked T waves, deep S wave. Ultimately get a sine wave ECG pattern, which precedes asystole.
* *Hypokalaemia*—prolonged PR interval, T wave amplitude diminishes and then becomes inverted, development of U waves.
* *Hypermagnasaemia*—prolonged PR interval and widened QRS due to a non-specific intraventricular conduction system delay. Sino-atrial and atrioventricular node block may occur. See *Magnesium Therapy* in *PRE-ECLAMPSIA ECLAMPSIA* for more information.
* *Hypomagnasaemia*—increased PR and QT interval and myocardial irritability.
* *Hypercalcaemia*—increased PR and QRS intervals and a shortened QT interval. T wave flattening and widening and AV nodal block (which may progress to complete heart block).
* *Hypocalcaemia*—prolonged QT interval.
* *Hyponatraemia*—Na < 115 mmol/L, widened QRS and ST segment elevation. Na < 100 mmol/L may cause ventricular dysrhythmias such as ventricular tachycardia or fibrillation.

▶ Bundle Branch Conduction Defects

* *Right bundle branch block (RBBB)*—rSR pattern in V1 and a broad and slurred S wave in V5 and V6. With *incomplete* RBBB the QRS

complex duration is between 0.10 s and 0.12 s. With *complete* RBBB the QRS duration is > 0.12 s.

- *Left BBB*—QRS > 0.12 s. A wide, notched M-shaped QRS complex is seen in leads V5 and V6.
- *Fascicular blocks*—these include left anterior and left posterior hemiblocks.
- *Left anterior hemiblock*—left axis deviation, tall R wave in AVL, deep S wave in II, III and AVF. QRS widened but < 0.12 s.
- *Left posterior hemiblock*—right axis deviation and prominent S wave in I and AVL. Tall R waves in II, III and AVF (but especially III).
- *Bifascicular blocks*—include combinations of RBBB and fascicular blocks.
- *RBBB and left anterior hemiblock*—right bundle branch block pattern with a left axis deviation.
- RBBB and left posterior hemiblock—right bundle branch block pattern, right axis deviation, prominent S wave in I and AVL. Tall R waves in II, III and AVF.
- *Trifascicular block*—consists of a right bundle branch block plus a fascicular block and a type of atrioventricular conduction block (see below).

▶ Heart Block or Atrioventricular Block
See *HEART BLOCK (HB)*.

▶ Ventricular Hypertrophy
- *Right ventricular hypertrophy*—right axis deviation, large R wave in V1, V2 with initial slur. May also see inverted T wave in V2, V3 and a strain pattern V1–V4 with prominent S wave in I, II, III.
- Left ventricular hypertrophy—left axis deviation. Tall R wave in V5, V6. Deep S wave in V1, V2. S wave in V1 + R wave in V5 or V6 > 35 mm.

▶ *Myocardial Ischaemia*

Is suggested by horizontal or down-sloping depression of the ST segment (1 mm or more) with an upright T wave or T wave inversion. Left bundle branch block may occur with significant left axis deviation. Sharply pointed symmetrical T waves that may become taller than on non-ischaemic ECG may occur.

▶ *Myocardial Infarction (MI)*

ECG changes include:

1 ST segment elevation—occurs in minutes
2 tall and widened T waves—occurs in minutes
3 inversion of T waves
4 appearance of pathological Q waves, i.e. > 0.04 s wide and > 0.2 mV deep. These appear over hours to days.

Localising the Site of Infarction

1 *Inferior*—changes in leads II, III, AVF.
2 *Posterior*—tall R waves and tall, wide asymmetrical T waves in V1–V3.
3 *Anteroseptal*—V1–V4 changes.
4 *High anterolateral*—I, AVL, V5, V6 changes.
5 *Extensive anterior*—I, AVL, V1–V5 changes.

▶ *Pulmonary Embolus*

May cause an acute strain on the right ventricle with right bundle branch block, right axis deviation, prominent S wave in I, Q wave in III and inverted T wave in III. May also see non-specific ST changes and T inversion in anterior leads, P pulmonale and atrial dysrhythmias.

▶ *Pulmonary Hypertension*

See right axis deviation, ECG changes of right ventricular hypertrophy and P pulmonale. A right bundle branch block pattern is common.

Electroconvulsive Therapy

1   Full pre-anaesthetic assessment, monitor ECG, blood pressure, pulse oximetry.
2   Pre-oxygenate, then induce with methohexitone 1 mg/kg IV. Propofol or thiopentone can also be used.[14]
3   Suxamethonium 0.3–0.5 mg/kg IV.
4   When the patient is paralysed insert a mouth guard (if the patient has teeth) and instruct the psychiatrist to give the 'shock'.
5   After the seizure has terminated, give 100% O_2 and assist ventilation until the patient is breathing spontaneously, then place the patient in the left lateral position.
6   Continue to supply O_2 via a Hudson mask until the patient is fully awake.

Electromechanical Dissociation

See *CARDIAC ARREST*.

EMLA

Topical anaesthetic agent useful for anaesthetising intact skin. EMLA stands for Eutectic Mixture of Local Anaesthetic Agents. A eutectic mixture is one in which the melting point is lower than the constituents of the mixture. EMLA is a mixture of equal parts lignocaine and prilocaine.

The resulting mixture has a melting point of 16ºC. The LA agents are emulsified with water to give a final concentration of 25 mg lignocaine and 25 mg prilocaine per gram of EMLA.

Dose

For venipuncture, apply over a suitable vein and cover with an occlusive dressing for at least 1 h.

For superficial skin surgery such as harvesting of skin grafts, apply over the donor site and cover with an occlusive dressing for at least 2 h prior to the procedure.

Note: There is a risk of toxic blood levels if the cream is swallowed, especially by small children.

Endocarditis

See *BACTERIAL ENDOCARDITIS PROPHYLAXIS*.

Endotracheal Tube Sizes

All sizes quoted are for the internal diameter of the endotracheal (ET) tube in mm.

Table E1 ET tube sizes for different ages of patient	
Age	Tube size (mm)
Premature neonate	2.5
Term neonate	2.5–3.0
1–3 months	3–3.5
3–6 months	3–3.5
6–9 months	3–3.5
9–14 months	3.5–4
15 months–2 years	4–4.5
3–4 years	4.5–5
5–6 years	5–5.5
7–9 years	6–6.5
10–12 years	7–7.5
13–15 years	7–7.5 cuffed

E

Adult

▶ *Male*

8.0–8.5

▶ *Female*

7.0–7.5

Formula for Calculating Tube Size in the Child

$$\frac{\text{Age (years)}}{4} + 4$$

Formula for Tube Length at Lips When Tube is in Good Position in the Child

$$\frac{\text{Weight (kg)}}{2} + 7 \text{ cm or } 2 \times \text{tube size} + 3 \text{ cm}$$

Formula for Calculating Length of Tube at the Nares For a Nasal Tube in Good Position in the Child

$$\frac{\text{Age (years)}}{2} + 15 \text{ cm}$$

Some Important Lengths

Neonates: Gums to vocal cords 5 cm, vocal cords to carina 5 cm

Adults: Tracheal length 10–12 cm, cords to carina 14–15 cm.

Enoxaparin (Clexane)

A low molecular weight heparin drug used for its anticoagulant effect.

Dose

▶ *DVT Prophylaxis*

- *Moderate risk patient*: 20 mg subcutaneously daily. Give the first dose 2 h before surgery.
- *High risk patient*: 40 mg subcutaneously on the evening before surgery, then 40 mg daily (beginning with the evening

after surgery). Continue for 7–10 days or until DVT risk has diminished.

▶ *DVT Treatment*

1 mg/kg 12 h subcutaneously or 1.5 mg once daily subcutaneously until warfarinised.

See *HEPARIN, UNFRACTIONATED AND LOW MOLECULAR WEIGHT HEPARINS and DEEP VENOUS THROMBOSIS (DVT) PROPHYLAXIS.*

Enoximone

Phosphodiesterase (PDE III) inhibitor useful for the treatment of:

1 acute (and chronic?)[15] heart failure
2 weaning from and post cardiac bypass
3 patients awaiting heart transplant.[16]

The main actions of enoximone are positive inotropism and peripheral vasodilatation. Cardiac output and left ventricular stroke work index are increased without an increase in myocardial O_2 consumption.[15]

Dose

Infusion of 90 µg/kg/min over 10–30 min then reduce infusion rate to 5–20 µg/kg/min.[17] Onset of effect 10–30 min, duration of effect 4–6 h.[17]

Advantages of Enoximone Compared to Other PDEIII Drugs[18]

1 Available as an oral agent.
2 Low incidence of associated dysrhythmias.

Ephedrine

Sympathomimetic drug derived from the Ma Huang plant. Ephedrine stimulates α and β adrenergic receptors directly, and also causes endogenous release of noradrenaline. It is useful for the treatment of:

1 hypotension associated with regional and GA
2 nasal decongestion.

Dose

▶ *Adult*

3–6 mg IV boluses titrated to the desired clinical effect. Onset of effect is rapid and effects last for about 1 h. Can also give 15 mg IM when a sustained effect on blood pressure is required.

Note: Ephedrine has a long duration of action due to its resistance to metabolism by COMT and MAO. Tachyphylaxis occurs with prolonged use.

Epidural Abscess

The incidence of epidural abscess associated with epidural anaesthesia is difficult to estimate. A figure of 2 per million epidurals is suggested.[19] The rate of spontaneous epidural abscess in the general hospital population is calculated to be in the range of 1–2 per 10 000 hospital admissions.[20] The mean time of onset of symptoms and signs is 2 weeks after epidural or spinal anaesthesia.

Clinical Presentation

Symptoms and signs of epidural abscess include:

- back pain
- spinal tenderness, swelling and erythema
- fever (absent in 30–40%)
- sphincter incontinence and paresis (late signs).

Investigations

1 The definitive investigation for epidural abscess is a gadolinium MRI scan.[21]
2 ESR and WBC are usually raised.

3   Positive blood cultures are usually obtained. In the majority of cases the causative organism is *Staphylococcus aureus or Staphylococcus epidermidis.* Gram negative bacilli and anaerobic bacteria may also be causative.

4   Send pus obtained from the abscess site for Gram stain and culture.

5   Remove the epidural catheter if it is still in situ and send the tip for culture.

6   Lumbar puncture should not be done as it may cause meningitis or neurological deterioration.[22]

Treatment

1   Urgent neurosurgical consultation. Emergency surgical decompression and drainage of pus is usually required if neurological signs are present.

2   IV antibiotics depending on Gram stain and sensitivities. For urgent antibiotic treatment while awaiting sensitivities a reasonable choice of agents would be timentin and gentamicin.

Prognosis

Mortality is about 7%.[23] Development of paralysis is irreversible in up to 50% of cases, and this is especially likely to occur if paralysis is present for more than 48 h.[24,25]

Epidural Anaesthesia

Topics Covered in this Section

▶ Anatomy of the Epidural Space

▶ Contraindications to Epidural Anaesthesia

▶ Technique for Lumbar Epidural Insertion

▶ Epidural Anaesthesia for Labour Pain

▶ Epidural Anaesthesia for Caesarean Section

Anatomy of the Epidural Space

The epidural space extends from the foramen magnum to the sacral hiatus and surrounds the dura. It is bounded anteriorly by the posterior longitudinal ligaments of the spinal column. Laterally the epidural space is bounded by the intervertebral foramina and pedicles, and posteriorly by the ligamentum flavum. The epidural space contains nerve roots, fat, lymphatic and blood vessels, and areolar tissue.

The structures encountered when inserting a Tuohy needle into the epidural space, using a midline approach, are: skin, supraspinous ligament, interspinous ligament and ligamentum flavum.

Contraindications to Epidural Anaesthesia

The absolute contraindications to epidural anaesthesia are:

* patient refusal
* coagulopathy
* infection at the site of insertion

Technique for Lumbar Epidural Insertion

1 Assess the patient adequately and identify possible contra-indications to the procedure.

2   Ensure that the patient gives informed consent and is cooperative.

3   Insert 16–18 G IV cannula and commence IV N/S or Hartmann's solution. Adjust rate of IV fluid infusion to maintain normovolaemia.

4   Ask the patient to fully flex the lumbar spine in the sitting or lateral position. Identify a suitable intervertebral space, usually L3–4 (see *SPINAL ANATOMY*). Sterilise and drape the site using a strict aseptic technique.

5   Inject 1% lignocaine into the skin and deeper structures of the chosen intervertebral space, use 38 mm 23 G needle.

6   Insert the Tuohy needle into interspinous ligament, remove the trocar, and attach a low resistance syringe filled with either saline or air.

7   Identify the epidural space by the sudden loss of resistance as the syringe and Tuohy needle are slowly and carefully advanced with pressure on the syringe plunger. Resistance to needle advancement will increase just prior to entering the epidural space because of the ligamentum flavum. Do not advance the needle during a uterine contraction in a labouring patient. In 80% of cases the space will be at a depth of between 4 and 6.5 cm.[26]

8   Insert the epidural catheter through the Tuohy needle and remove the needle over the catheter. Pull the catheter back so that only about 3–4 cm remains in the epidural space. Do not insert the catheter during a uterine contraction. *Never pull the catheter out through the needle as this may shear the catheter.*

9   Attach the filter connector to the catheter and use a syringe to attempt to aspirate cerebrospinal fluid or blood. If nil aspirated, flush the filter with LA agent and attach it to the filter connector. Secure the epidural catheter to the patient with sterile adhesive dressings.

Epidural Anaesthesia for Labour Pain

▶ Test Dose

Inject a test dose through either the Tuohy needle or the catheter. Use 3 mL of 2% lignocaine. Addition of adrenaline to the test dose may or may not result in a tachycardia and is not reliable for detecting intravascular injection in the obstetric patient.[27]

▶ Establishing the Block For Patient in Labour

1   Give 500 mL to 1 L of Hartmann's solution or N/S prior to initiating epidural blockade.

2   Inject 15–20 mL of bupivacaine 0.125% with 1:400 000 adrena-laline and fentanyl 5 µg/mL. Inject slowly and incrementally. Ask the patient to report any ill effects such as tinnitus, tingling in lips and tongue or dysphoria (suggesting IV injection). Alternatively, ropivacaine 2 mg/mL with fentanyl 2 µg/mL can be used in similiar volumes to bupivacaine 0.125%.

3   Ensure ephedrine and/or aramine is available at all times to treat hypotension.

▶ 'Top Up' Doses

Give 15–20 mL of the same mixture used to establish the block up to every 1–2 h as required to treat the patient's distress. Alternatively the patient can be given an infusion of bupivacaine 0.125% with fentanyl 2.5 µg/mL run at an initial rate of 10 mL/h with 10 mL boluses as required up to each h.

▶ Epidural Anaesthesia and Chorioamnionitis

With covering antibiotic therapy the risk of epidural abscess associ-ated with chorioamnionitis appears to be very low.[28]

Epidural Anaesthesia for Caesarean Section

Lignocaine 2% + 1:200 000 adrenaline with fentanyl 5 µg/mL. Give 20–25 mL, slowly titrating dose to effect. It is necessary to block to a dermatomal level T4–6. Can alternatively use a mixture of ligno-caine 2% and bupivacaine 0.5% + fentanyl 100 µg. About 1.5–2 mL of LA is required per dermatomal segment.

Technique for Thoracic Epidural Insertion and Dosage Recommendations

Thoracic epidural anaesthesia can provide excellent postopera-tive analgesia following abdominal or chest surgery, rib fractures, pancreatitis and unstable angina. It is a considerably more diffi-cult technique to perform than lumbar epidural placement.

▶ Site of Thoracic Epidural Insertion

The epidural space for insertion of the catheter should correspond to the mid-dermatomal innervation of the surgical incision. Some examples are:

1 abdominal aortic aneurysm surgery: T7–T8 or T8–T9
2 upper abdominal surgery: T6–T7 or T7–T8
3 lower abdominal surgery: T9–T10.

▶ Anatomical Considerations

The vertebral prominence at the base of the neck corresponds to the C7 level and the inferior angle of the scapula corresponds with T7 level. The thoracic dorsal spines are angulated and this angulation is maximal in the mid thoracic region (T5–T8). A paramedian approach may thus be more successful than a midline approach in this region. The ligamentum flavum in the thoracic region is thinner than in the lumbar region and may also be softer.

The epidural space is much thinner in the thoracic region compared with the lumbar region. See Table E2.

There is a significant risk of spinal cord damage if the needle passes through the epidural space. The spinal cord becomes the cauda equina at the L1–2 disc space in the adult and at the L3 ver-tebra in the newborn.

E

Table E2 Width of the epidural space at various spinal levels	
C5	1.0–1.5 mm
T6	1.5–3 mm
L3	5–6 mm

▶ *Midline Approach to Thoracic Epidural Placement*

1 Position the patient either sitting or laterally with maximal spinal flexion. Little flexion of the thoracic spine is possible because the intervertebral joints allow mainly for rotational movements.

2 Sterilise and drape the site of entry as for lumbar epidural insertion. Anaesthetise the skin and deeper structures with a 32 mm 23 G needle. While infiltrating, use this needle to evaluate the correct angle of epidural needle insertion to pass it between the spinous processes.

3 Insert the epidural needle and use a 'loss of resistance' technique to identify the epidural space.

4 When the epidural space is identified insert the epidural catheter. Aim to leave about 3–4 cm of epidural catheter in the epidural space. Remove the needle and secure the catheter.

▶ *Paramedian Approach to Thoracic Epidural Placement*

1 Prepare the patient as described above.

2 At the selected vertebral level palpate the spinous process. The insertion point is ≈ 1.5 cm lateral to the spinous process.

3 Use a 32 mm 23 G needle to anaesthetise the skin and deeper structures. Insert the needle perpendicularly to the skin and attempt to contact the vertebral lamina.

4 Insert the Tuohy needle through the initial puncture wound, then walk the needle, aiming for ≈ 10–45° medial angulation

E

and ≈ 45–55° of cephalad angulation (in the mid-thoracic region). These angles will vary greatly from patient to patient and between thoracic levels. The aim is to identify the cephalad medial edge of the lamina. At this site bone will not be encountered at the expected depth.

5   The Tuohy needle is then advanced with extreme care through the thin ligamentum flavum and into the epidural space.

6   Once the epidural space is identified proceed as described above.

▶ *Thoracic Epidural Dose*

Give a test dose of 3 mL of lignocaine 2%. Subsequent doses depend on the type and duration of surgery and the patient's size and cardiovascular stability. As a rough guide thoracic epidural dosages are generally 30–50% lower than lumbar dosages to block the same number of dermatomes. For example, for a large bowel resection give ≈ 0.1 mL/kg bolus of bupivacaine 0.25% with fentanyl 5–10 µg/mL prior to surgical incision.

Alternatively, ropivacaine 5 mg/mL with fentanyl 5–10 µg/mL can be used. Give further 2.5–5 mL boluses intra-operatively depending on the patient's physiological responses to surgery and the epidural itself, to a total of ≈ 15 mL.

Epidural Anaesthesia for Postoperative Pain Management

▶ *Epidural Infusions of LA + Opioid*

Bupivacaine and Fentanyl

Use a solution of bupivacaine 0.125% + fentanyl 2.5 µg/mL.

Adults: Run the infusion at 6–20 mL/h for a lumbar catheter and 4–12 mL/h for a thoracic catheter.

Children: The maximum theoretical infusion rate for children is 0.3–0.4 mL/kg/h of this solution.

Bupivacaine and Morphine

Mix 4 mg of morphine with 200 mL of bupivacaine 0.125%.
Adult: Run the infusion at 4–12 mL/h. This type of epidural infusion is particularly useful for abdominal wounds extending over many dermatomes, e.g. from xiphisternum to pubis.

Ropivacaine and Fentanyl

Use a solution of ropivacaine 2 mg/mL with fentanyl 2–4 µg/mL. Run the infusion at 4–12 mL/h for a thoracic epidural.

▶ *Pethidine Epidural Patient Controlled Anaesthesia (PCA)*

Adults

Give 50 mg pethidine loading dose epidurally. Use a solution containing 300 mg pethidine in 60 mL N/S. Set the PCA pump to give 20 mg boluses (4 mL) with a 10 min lockout and a background infusion of 5 mg/h (1 mL).

▶ *Epidural Morphine Boluses*

Morphine provides excellent analgesia lasting about 16 h.

Dose

Adult: 1–5 mg, depending on the size and fitness of patient (average dose 3 mg).

▶ *Morphine Epidural Infusion*

Give morphine at a rate of 0.2–0.6 mg/h. A morphine infusion may be safer than intermittent bolusing.[29]
Note: Epidural morphine use is associated with an increased risk of late respiratory depression.

Troubleshooting Problems with Epidural Infusions

▶ *Inadequate Epidural Anaesthesia*

1 Check the dermatomal level of the block with ice. Identify which dermatomes are analgesed and whether the epidural blockade is partially or fully unilateral. Give the patient a bolus of the

usual hourly rate of the infusion and assess the response. If there does not appear to be any significant epidural blockade, check that the catheter has not fallen out and that the infusion pump is working.

2   If the catheter is in place and a dermatomal level cannot be identified, give a bolus of 5–10 mL of lignocaine 2% (the dose depending on the site of the epidural catheter) to re-establish the block. If an epidural block cannot be re-established, abandon the epidural and substitute with an alternative analgesia regimen opioid technique or resite the epidural catheter.

3   If the lignocaine bolus is effective, increase the epidural infusion rate by 2–3 mL/h and reassess the patient in 2–3 h or sooner if the patient becomes uncomfortable.

4   If analgesia is still inadequate despite demonstrating that some epidural blockade is occurring, treatment options include the following:

(a) Increase the fentanyl in the epidural solution to 5 µg/mL.

(b) Continue the epidural infusion with opioid free bupivacaine or ropivacaine solution and provide the patient with IV opioid PCA.

(c) Change the patient over to epidural PCA pethidine and cease the epidural LA agent (see above).

(d) Give an epidural bolus dose of morphine (or infusion). This will take ≈ 1 h to provide effective analgesia. During this time analgese the patient with an appropriate dose of IV opioid.

(e) If the pain problem is due to a 'missed segment' or asymmetrical dermatomal blockade, pulling back the catheter slightly using an aseptic technique may help improve the quality of the block.

▶ *Blocked Epidural Catheter*

Flush the epidural catheter with 1 mL N/S or LA solution. Check that connection between the filter and filter connector is not too tight.

▶ Hypotension

1 Establish the clinical urgency of situation, i.e. is patient symptomatic, is there evidence of a 'high block'? (See *Total Spinal* below.)

2 Elevate the patient's legs.

3 Give a vasopressor drug such as ephedrine, or metaraminol. See *EPHEDRINE* and *METARAMINOL.*

4 IV fluid loading with colloid such as Haemaccel or gelofusine 250–1000 mL rapidly, depending on the urgency of the situation.

5 Cease the epidural infusion if the level of epidural blockade is excessive.

6 Exclude/diagnose/treat other causes of hypotension, e.g. haemorrhage, sepsis.

Dural Puncture (Spinal) Headache and Blood Patching

CSF can be distinguished from saline used to find the epidural space. CSF feels warm on the gloved hand, and is positive for glucose and protein on using urine test sticks.[30] The pH of CSF is 7.5 or greater whereas the pH of saline is usually less than 7.5.[30] The incidence of postdural puncture headache with an 18 G Tuohy needle is approximately 75–85%.[31]

▶ Initial Management of Dural Puncture

If dural puncture occurs inform the patient, and discuss the implications fully and frankly. There are various options of management. For patients in labour one approach is to reattempt epidural insertion one intervertebral space higher. Once the epidural catheter is sited:

1 Give a test dose as described above, then give the full epidural dose slowly and incrementally looking for any evidence of subarachnoid block.

2 Subsequent 'top up' bolus doses for labour pain should be given by the anaesthetist and any evidence of subarachnoid block sought.

3 Another approach is suggested by Kuczkowski and Benumof.[32] These authors aimed at maintaing CSF volume by the following steps:

   (a) Reinjection of CSF seen in a loss of resistance syringe attached to the Tuohy needle.
   (b) Injection of 3–5 mL of preservative-free normal saline intrathecally.
   (c) Insert the epidural catheter through the Tuohy needle into the subarachnoid space.
   (d) Establish SAB anaesthesia for labour with 1 mL of bupivacaine 0.25% plus 10 µg fentanyl.
   (e) To maintain analgesia, an intrathecal infusion of bupivacaine 0.625% with fentanyl 2 µg/mL is run at 2 mL/h.
   (f) The intrathecal catheter is left in situ for 8–12 h post delivery.

   This approach resulted in an incidence of PDPH of only 14%.

▶ *Treatment of PDPH*

There is no evidence that bed rest or keeping the patient excessively hydrated will prevent the development or reduce the severity of headache.[33] If headache occurs:

1 Treat the headache initially with simple oral analgesics such as paracetamol and codeine. Use IM pethidine or morphine if oral analgesics are inadequate. Consider giving stool softener therapy (e.g. lactulose) if opioids are used, to reduce the risk of constipation and straining.

E

2   Caffeine 300 mg PO or theophylline 300 mg PO are reported to be effective in some patients.[33] Sumatriptan has also been used successfully to treat postdural puncture headache.[34] The dose is 6 mg subcutaneously, with repeat dose given in 24 h if the headache recurs. Relief occurred in 30 min in one series.

3   If severe headache persists after 24–48 h, perform an epidural blood patch (EDBP) unless there is a contraindication, e.g. the patient is anticoagulated or septic. The success rate for epidural blood patching is estimated to be ≈ 90% and a further 8% are successfully treated by a second EDBP.[35] This high rate of success is reduced if the procedure is undertaken in the first 24 h after dural puncture or if ≤ 10 mL of blood is used.[36] The following technique is suggested:

(a) After preparing and anaesthetising the same intervertebral level as the site of dural puncture, insert a Tuohy needle into the epidural space. If unable to identify the epidural space at this level, reattempt 1 space caudad rather than more cephalad. This is because blood in the epidural space tends to spread in a cephalad direction.[37]

(b) An assistant aseptically withdraws 20 mL of blood and this is injected slowly into the epidural space. 15–20 mL of blood is injected. Discontinue the injection if the patient complains of discomfort such as back or leg pressure. Send the remaining blood for blood culture.

(c) The patient should lie flat for 2 h after the procedure.[33]

(d) The patient should avoid straining or lifting for 4–5 days and seek medical attention if headache recurs.[38]

(e) Patients should be followed up in the out-patient clinic until full recovery has occurred.

Intravenous Injection of Bupivacaine

See *BUPIVACAINE*.

'Total Spinal'—Unintentional Extensive Subarachnoid Blockade

May result in ascending sensation loss and weakness, leading to respiratory compromise. The patient may lose consciousness. Cardiovascular effects include hypotension, bradycardia and cardiac arrest.

▶ Treatment

1 *Airway*: Optimise the airway. If the patient loses consciousness and there is a risk of aspiration (e.g. pregnant), apply cricoid pressure, give IV suxamethonium and intubate the trachea. If the patient is conscious, but unable to self-ventilate, perform a rapid sequence induction with thiopentone, cricoid pressure and suxamethonium.

2 *Breathing*: Ventilate with 100% O_2.

3 *Circulation*: Support blood pressure aggressively with IV fluid loading and vasopressor agents such as ephedrine, metaraminol and, if necessary, adrenaline. Treat brady-cardia with atropine. *Maintain left lateral tilt if the patient is pregnant.*

4 If a patient with an epidural in situ is progressing to total spinal anaesthesia, aspiration of CSF from the epidural catheter (20–30 mL) may prevent 'total spinal' from occurring, or reduce its effects.[39] In addition, after aspirating CSF, consider injecting 20 mL of N/S or a combination of N/S and Hartmann's solution through the epidural catheter. This may be of further benefit by diluting the remaining intrathecal LA.[40]

Anticoagulant Therapy and Epidurals

▶ Heparin

Do not attempt epidural anaesthesia if the patient is fully heparinised. If the patient is receiving subcutaneous heparin in prophylactic doses, do not attempt epidural anaesthesia within 6 h of the last dose.[41] In addition, do not remove the epidural catheter within 6 h of the last dose, or within 2 h of next dose of subcutaneous heparin. If the patient is to be fully heparinised intra-operatively or postoperatively, defer heparinisation for at least 1 h after the epidural is inserted.[42] If a 'bloody tap' occurs and the patient is to be fully heparinised some practitioners advise rescheduling surgery for 24 h later, without reattempting epidural blockade.[42]

▶ Low Molecular Weight (LMW) Heparin

For patients on prophylactic LMW heparin therapy, e.g. clexane 40 mg, do not use epidural anaesthesia within 12–24 h of the last dose. If patients are on therapeutic LMW heparin, e.g. clexane 1 mg/kg, do not use epidural anaesthesia within 24 h of the last dose. If epidural anaesthesia is used, give the first postoperative dose of LMW heparin 12 hours after needle placement. If blood is seen in the epidural catheter, resite and delay the first dose of LMW heparin for 24 h.[43]

An epidural catheter should not be removed within 12 h of the last dose of prophylactic LMW heparin and 24 h if therapeutic doses are used. If the epidural catheter is removed the next dose of LMW heparin should not be given for at least 2 h.

Additional antiplatelet drugs such as aspirin or non-selective NSAIDs should be avoided in patients receiving LMW heparin and regional anaesthesia.

▶ Aspirin

Probably safe to proceed if there is no clinical evidence of increased bleeding tendency.[44]

▶ NSAIDs

Probably safe to proceed unless other complicating factors are present.[45]

▶ *Platelet Adenosine Diphosphate (ADP) Receptor Antagonists, e.g. ticlopidine and clopidogrel*

These drugs inhibit the binding of platelets to fibrinogen and platelet–platelet interaction. The risk of epidural haematoma in the presence of these drugs is unknown. It is advisable to delay regional anaesthesia until drug effects have dissipated, i.e. clopidogrel 7 days, ticlopidine 14 days. See *PLATELET ADENOSINE DIPHOSPHATE (ADP) RECEPTOR ANTAGONISTS.*

▶ *Platelet Glycoprotein IIb/IIIa Receptor Antagonists, e.g. abciximab (RePro), eptifibatide and tirofiban.*

The risk of epidural haematoma in the presence of these drugs is unclear from the literature. Do not use epidural anaesthesia until the effects of these drugs have fully dissipated. See *PLATELET GLYCOPROTEIN IIb/IIIa RECEPTOR ANTAGONISTS.*

Combined Spinal Epidural Anaesthesia
See *SUBARACHNOID BLOCK.*

Complications of Epidural Anaesthesia
1 Headache (see above). The overall risk of dural puncture followed by headache is about 1:200 epidurals.
2 Epidural haematoma (see below).
3 Epidural abscess (see entry).
4 Cranial nerve palsies. These occur in 1–3.7 per 100 000 obstetric epidurals and the abducens nerve is the most commonly affected causing diploplia.[46]
5 Chronic back pain? There is probably no increased risk of chronic back pain after epidural anaesthesia for labour.[47]

Epidural Haematoma

Description
Epidural haematoma is a rare complication of epidural or spinal

anaesthesia. The incidence of epidural haematoma associated with epidural anaesthesia is estimated to be about 1 in 150 000–190 000.[48,49] Predisposing factors include:

- anticoagulant therapy (see *EPIDURAL ANAESTHESIA, Anticoagulant Therapy and Epidurals*)
- haemostatic abnormalities such as thrombocytopaenia
- elderly patients.

Presentation and Diagnosis

Typically patients present with:

- neurological deficit such as paralysis of the lower limbs, decreased leg sensation
- back pain.
  MRI is the diagnostic test of choice.

Treatment

Epidural haematoma with neurological deficit is a neurosurgical emergency requiring urgent decompression. A relatively good outcome is expected if decompression laminectomy is performed within 8 h of the onset of neurological symptoms.[50]

Epiglottitis

This disease is typically seen in children 2–6 years but can occur at any age. The usual causative organism is *Haemophilus influenzae* (type B).

Presentation

The usual presentation is a child with:

- drooling, sitting up
- tachypnoea, stridor and suprasternal recession
- absent cough
- possible complete airway obstruction
- fever, tachycardia.

Treatment

1 Stay with the child until the airway is secure. Do not examine the pharynx or insert an IV cannula or upset the child in any way.
2 Notify the on-call ENT surgeon and paediatrician.
3 Before induction of anaesthesia, ensure a surgeon is available who is competent to perform an urgent tracheostomy.
4 Perform a gaseous induction with O_2 and sevoflurane. Use halothane if sevoflurane is not available. When the patient is deeply anaesthetised obtain IV access and give atropine 10 µg/kg. If the airway is difficult to maintain, try pulling the tongue forward to disimpact the epiglottis.
5 Intubate the patient orally with an endotracheal tube that is 0.5 mm smaller than normal. Inspect epiglottitis to make the diagnosis, and obtain throat swab and take blood for blood culture and full blood count. Post obstructive pulmonary oedema may occur, requiring intermittent positive pressure ventilation.
6 Give cefotaxime 50 mg/kg/12 h IV.
7 When the situation is completely controlled change the oral endotracheal tube to a nasal tube under direct vision.
8 Secure the patient's arms with splints to prevent self-extubation and transfer the patient to ICU.
9 Give rifampicin antibiotic prophylaxis to all family members and other close contacts.

Epilepsy, Status

Definition

Status epilepticus is defined traditionally as an epileptic 'condition' (seizure or seizures) lasting more than 30 min.[51] Experimental research suggests that seizure or seizures lasting more than 60 min can result in:[51]

- permanent brain cell damage
- lactic acidosis

E

- hypoglycaemia
- myoglobinuria, renal failure
- cardiac arrest.

The longer status epilepticus goes on untreated, the harder it is to treat with drugs.[52]

Aetiology

Possible causes include the following.

▶ Intracerebral Disorders

- Epilepsy, especially if anticonvulsant withdrawal is occurring.
- Cerebral tumour, haemorrhage, infection, trauma.
- Hypoxic brain damage.

▶ Metabolic Causes

- Electrolyte disturbances such as hyponatraemia
- Alcohol withdrawal
- Hypoglycaemia

▶ Systemic Illness

- Eclampsia. See *PRE-ECLAMPSIA/ECLAMPSIA*.
- Severe sepsis.

Treatment

1 *Airway*: Ensure adequate airway; intubate the patient if required.
2 *Breathing*: Ensure adequate ventilation and consider hypoxia/hypercarbia in the differential diagnosis of seizure aetiology.
3 *Circulation*: Provide adequate circulatory support. Consider a cardiovascular cause for the seizure, e.g. dysrhythmia.
4 Check BSL, FBC, UEC, calcium, magnesium, phosphate, ABG, and if relevant anticonvulsant levels, blood alcohol, drug screen.
5 If hypoglycaemia is the possible cause of seizures, give 50 mL of 50% glucose. If there is *any* possibility of thiamine deficiency, give thiamine 100 mg IV prior to the glucose. This is to avoid the precipitation of Wernicke's encephalopathy.

6 *Benzodiazepines—diazepam. Adult*: 5–10 mg IV increments to a maximum dose of 20–30 mg. *Child*: 0.2 mg/kg IV—repeat as necessary. If unable to site IV give 0.5 mg/kg PR. Alternatively, lorazepam 0.1 mg/kg IV can be used.[53]

7 *Paraldehyde.* Should be considered in children with status epilepticus (100 µg/mL) 0.2 mL/kg IM (maximum 10 mL). Use a glass syringe.

8 *Phenytoin. Adult/Child*: 15–20 mg/kg IV in N/S no faster than 50 mg/min. May get hypotension or heart block—slow infusion if these occur. Use ECG monitoring during infusion. If seizures persist give an additional phenytoin dose of 5 mg/kg.

9 For ongoing seizures give phenobarbitone 20 mg/kg IV at 100 mg/min.

10 If status epilepticus continues despite the above treatment, perform a rapid sequence induction with thiopentone 3–5 mg/kg, cricoid pressure, suxamethonium 1.5 mg/kg and intubation. See *RAPID SEQUENCE INDUCTION.*

11 Consider an infusion of thiopentone 1–5 mg/kg/h.[54]

12 Seek urgent ICU/neurologist consultation. Search for a precipitating cause through history, physical examination and relevant investigation.

Eptacog Alfa (Activated)

See *RECOMBINANT ACTIVATED FACTOR VII.*

Ergometrine Maleate

Contains ergonovine, an ergot alkaloid, which causes uterine contractions superimposed on tonic contraction and peripheral vasoconstriction. Used to prevent/treat postpartum haemorrhage and haemorrhage associated with incomplete abortion. Ergometrine can cause hypertension.

E

Dose

200–500 µg IM. Onset of action takes 5–7 min and effects last ≈ 45 min.

Dose for Emergency Control of Haemorrhage

100–500 µg IV

Note: IV ergometrine can cause vasoconstriction and severe hypertension especially in the pre-eclamptic patient.

Syntometrine is a combination of ergometrine 500 µg and oxytocin 5 units in a volume of 1 mL.

Esmolol

Relatively selective β1 adreno-receptor blocker, particularly useful for its rapid onset and offset of effects (elimination half-life 10 min).

Metabolised by hydrolysis via plasma esterases.

Uses

1   Acute supraventricular dysrhythmias, including atrial fibrillation and flutter.
2   Control of peri-operative hypertension.
3   Treatment of myocardial infarction.
4   Reduces the hypertensive response to intubation.

Dose

Give 500 µg/kg over 1 min, then an infusion of 50–150 µg/kg/min, titrated to response. Given in a concentration of 10 mg/mL, preferably via a peripheral line. In 70 kg man give 20–60 mL/h. Onset of effect occurs in 5–10 min; effects cease after ≈ 20 min.

Bolus Dose (to Blunt the Response to Intubation)

2–3 mg/kg 2 min prior to intubation or 1–2 mg/kg + opioid 4 min before intubation.[55]

Esmolol may not be effective for treating pregnancy-induced hypertension.[56] See *HYPERTENSIVE RESPONSE TO INTUBATION (ATTENUATION OF)*.

Etomidate

Carboxylated imidazole IV anaesthetic drug.

Dose for Induction of Anaesthesia

0.3 mg/kg

Advantages

1 Excellent cardiovascular stability. Etomidate is indicated for IV induction in patients wih unstable CVS status, e.g. shocked patients, and patients with known cardiovascular disease.
2 Etomidate causes a reduction in ICP and intra-ocular pressure (IOP).

Disadvantages

1 May get pain on injection (25–50%). This is reduced by the addition of lignocaine.
2 Involuntary movement.
3 Causes adreno-cortical suppression and is not suitable for prolonged use by IV infusion because of this effect.
4 Etomidate is contraindicated in patients with porphyria. See *PORPHYRIA*.
5 Causes nausea and vomiting (more than thiopentone).[57]
6 Dissolved in propylene glycol, which causes a high incidence of thrombophlebitis.
7 Etomidate should be avoided in patients with known seizure disorders.

Eye Blocks

These are used for procedures such as cataract surgery.

Innervation of the Eye

Afferent fibres from the cornea and conjunctiva pass through the ciliary ganglion in the retrobulbar space and thence to the *ophthalmic division* of the *trigeminal nerve*. The lateral rectus muscle is supplied by the *abducent nerve (VI)*, the superior oblique by the *trochlear nerve (IV)* and the remainder by the *oculomotor nerve (III) ($LR_6SO_4R_3$)*.

Two types of block are described. With each type first establish IV access.

Peribulbar Eye Blocks

▶ *Two-injection Technique*

1   Use a mixture of bupivacaine 0.5%, 4 mL + lignocaine 2% and hyaluronidase 150–300 units. Alternatively, use ropivacaine 10 mg/mL with hyaluronidase. Use a 25 G 33 mm orbital block needle. Although adrenaline-containing solutions are frequently used,[58] they are not without risk. Adrenaline does not prolong the effects of bupivacaine and results in a reduction of ophthalmic artery pressure.[59] Adrenaline should not be used if orbital vascular pathology is suspected.[58,59]

2   Surgically prep the skin with a suitable antiseptic. Ask the patient to fix the eye on an object on the ceiling so that the eye does not move and is in the neutral position. Anaesthetise the conjunctiva with amethocaine 1%. Consider sedating the patient prior to LA injection with a small dose of propofol, e.g. 10–40 mg IV.

3   *First injection*: Insert percutaneously into the lower outer quadrant of the orbit at the junction of the lateral third and medial two-thirds of the inferior orbital rim. Direct the needle posteriorly. Once past the equator of the eye, angle the needle superomedially so that the tip lies near the apex of the orbital cone, at a depth of about 2.5 cm. Ensure that the eye moves freely, and that it has not been penetrated. If aspiration is negative, inject 4–6 mL of LA. The upper eye lid should drop almost immediately. Inject another 1 mL while withdrawing the needle.

4   *Alternatively for first injection—inject transconjunctivally*. Retract the

lower eyelid, and insert the needle into the inferior fornix at the 7:30 clock position in the right eye and 4:30 clock position for the left eye, 2 mm lateral to the limbus.[58] Advance the needle tangentially between the rim of the orbit and the globe. When the needle tip is past the equator, angle the tip medially and cephalad, and insert to a depth of 2.5 cm. Inject as above.

5   *Second injection*: Insert needle percutaneously 2 mm inferior and 2 mm medial to the supraorbital notch. Direct the needle posteriorly and slightly superiorly to a depth of 2 cm, then 0.5 cm medially.[60] Inject 2–3 mL of LA.

6   After the above injections, tape the eye closed, and apply pressure via a Honan balloon or similar mercury-filled device. Aim to apply 20–30 mmHg pressure for 5–10 min.[58] Do not apply for more than 20 min.[58]

7   If the block is inadequate after 10 min, 'top up' the block with 2–5 mL of 2% Lignocaine via the first injection site.

▶ *Single Injection Technique*

In this variation a relatively large volume of ropivacaine plus hyaluronidase is used.

• The site of injection is identical to the first injection site described above.

• For the averaged-sized orbit inject 8 mL of ropivacaine 10 mg/mL plus hyaluronidase 750 units over 30–45 s.[61] Inject an additional 2–4 mL if a 'top-up' injection is required 10 min after the initial injection.[61]

Sub–Tenon's Block (Single Quadrant Approach as Described by Guise)[62]

Tenon's capsule is a dense layer of connective tissue surrounding the eye and the extraocular muscles at the front of the orbit.

1   Anaesthetise the conjunctiva as above.

2   Position the lid speculum to keep the eye open.

3 Instil 1–2 drops of 5% povidone to sterilise the conjunctiva.

4 Direct the patient to look upwards and outwards, and instil amethocaine 1% onto the medial portion of the bulbar conjunctiva.

5 Using small, sterile forceps, pick up the conjunctiva and anterior Tenon's capsule at the infer-nasal point 7–10 mm from the limbus (7:30 clock position for the left eye).

6 With a curved pair of spring scissors make a small cut 1–2 mm long through the conjunctiva and Tenon's capsule so that bare sclera is visible.

7 Using blunt dissection with the curved spring scissors develop a plane posteriorly between sclera and Tenon's capsule. After 5–10 mm the posterior sub-Tenon's space is reached.

8 Insert a sterile lacrimal cannula along sub-Tenon's space to the posterior part at the back of the eye.

9 Inject 2–3 mL of LA solution over 15–30 s. Consider changing the cannula tip position slightly after each mL to make injection easier.

10 Apply Honan balloon or similar device for 5 min.

11 Consider a facial nerve block, achieved by infiltration with 1.5 mL of LA into the lateral aspect of each eyelid deep to orbicularis oculi.

Eye Injury, Penetrating

If the patient is not fasted, surgery is urgent and the eye is salvageable, the first priority is to prevent aspiration of gastric contents. The second priority is to prevent loss of intra-ocular contents. The most appropriate technique in the 'open eye, full stomach' scenario is controversial, as discussed below.

1 Consider the following drugs to reduce the risk and effects of aspiration:

    (a) ranitidine 50 mg IV

    (b) metoclopramide 10 mg IV

    (c) sodium citrate 0.3 M 30 mL PO

2 Preoxygenate for 5 minutes, and consider the following drugs to attenuate the effects of laryngoscopy and intubation on intra-ocular pressure (IOP):

    (a) lignocaine 1.5 mg/kg IV.

    (b) fentanyl 2 µg/kg.

    Give both drugs 3–4 min prior to intubation.

3 Consider giving a small dose of a non-depolarising neuromuscular blocking drug such as vecuronium 1 mg to attenuate the effects of suxamethonium on IOP. See the discussion in step 5 below.

4 Thiopentone 3–5 mg/kg. Apply cricoid pressure with the onset of anaesthesia.

5 Suxamethonium 1.5 mg/kg (immediately after thiopentone). Suxamethonium is known to increase IOP in the normal eye and theoretically could cause further damage to the open eye. However, despite its widespread use in this situation there have been no reports of additional eye damage.[63] In contrast, if the patient coughs, loss of intra-ocular contents is likely. Clinical studies involving the use of suxamethonium in the open eye injury involved pretreatment with a non-depolarising muscle relaxant so this must be at least considered.[64]

6 Intubate, ventilate and maintain anaesthesia with O_2, N_2O and volatile agent + non-depolarising muscle relaxant.

7 Extubate in the lateral position only when the patient is able to protect his or her own airway.

Alternatively: If suxamethonium is contraindicated or considered unsuitable, a modified rapid sequence technique can be used, utilising rocuronium 0.6–0.9 mg/kg. However, suxamethonium remains the muscle relaxant of choice in this situation. See *RAPID SEQUENCE INDUCTION.*

Ff

Failed Intubation

See *DIFFICULT AIRWAY MANAGEMENT*.

Failure to Regain Consciousness after General Anaesthesia

See *CONFUSION, DECREASED LEVEL OF CONSCIOUSNESS, POST ANAESTHETIC*.

Fasting Pre-operatively

These guidelines relate to elective surgery. See also *ASPIRATION, PREVENTION AND TREATMENT*.

Adult

Fast for solid food for 6 h, and for clear fluids for 4 h pre-operatively. Clear fluids more than 2 h before anaesthesia are probably acceptable.[1] Alcoholic beverages delay gastric emptying and are not acceptable as clear fluids.[2] One study of gum chewing before surgery did not suggest an increased risk of aspiration.[2]

Children

Fast for solid food and formula milk for 6 h pre-operatively. Clear fluids and breast milk can be given up to 4 h pre-operatively. Clear fluids more than 2 h before anaesthesia are probably acceptable.[3]

Fastrach Device

A laryngeal mask type device used as an aid to intubation. See *LARYNGEAL MASK AIRWAY (INCLUDING PROSEAL AND FASTRACH)*.

Fat Embolism Syndrome and Bone Cement Implantation Syndrome

Fat Embolism

▶ Description

In this condition fat globules and bone marrow elements cause potentially life-threatening clinical effects on the lungs and brain. The source of the fat emboli may be long bone fractures, and orthopaedic techniques associated with knee and hip replacements. However, the syndrome may also occur with bone marrow transplant and liposuction.[4] The presence of intra-vascular fat globules is probably very common with long bone fractures or instrumentation but only a small percentage of such patients develop the syndrome.[5] These fat globules cause acute lung and brain injury through as yet unexplained mechanisms. Fat may enter the systemic circulation and travel to the brain via a patent foramen ovale. There is evidence that fat embolisation to the brain can occur even in the absence of a patent foramen ovale.[6] Fat may be able to traverse the pulmonary circulation and enter the systemic circulation.

▶ Clinical Manifestations

1 Hypoxia, bilateral pulmonary infiltrates, ventilation–perfusion mismatch and shunting. Florid pulmonary oedema may occur.
2 Pyrexia.
3 Confusion and restlessness, coma.
4 Petechial rash particularly affecting the upper half of the body, conjunctiva and mucous membranes of the mouth.
5 Retinal examination may reveal exudates and haemorrhages. Fat droplets may be seen traversing the retinal vessels.
6 Coagulopathy, thrombocytopaenia and coagulopathy may occur.

F

▶ *Diagnosis*

1 The diagnosis can be made on the clinical picture with manifestations occurring within 48 h of a relevant procedure or injury.[7]

2 CXR may show poorly defined diffuse pulmonary infiltrates.

3 ECG may show a right ventricular strain pattern with right bundle branch block, right axis deviation, prominent S wave in I, Q wave in III and inverted T wave in III.

4 ABG may show a severe alveolar–arterial oxygen tension gradient of greater than 100 mmHg.

5 Examination of urine and sputum may reveal the presence of fat globules.

6 A fall in $ETCO_2$ during surgery may indicate that fat embolism is occurring.

▶ *Treatment*

1 Treatment is largely supportive and predominantly aimed at improving oxygenation. Death is usually due to respiratory complications. Consider high concentration O_2 therapy, CPAP, or intubation and IPPV ± PEEP.

2 Neurological damage may be considerable and cause long-term disability.

3 The mortality is between 10 and 45% in florid cases.[7]

Bone Cement Implantation Syndrome

▶ *Description and Pathophysiology* [8]

This syndrome occurs in association with cemented total hip replacement surgery. A combination of methylmethacrylate, bone cement, air, fat and bone marrow produces the syndrome at the time of hip prosthesis implantation. This syndrome thus overlaps with fat embolism syndrome. Embolised material is thought to cause a sudden increase in pulmonary vascular resistance, increased pulmonary artery pressure, right ventricular dilatation with reduction in the compliance and cavity size of the left ventricle. This leads to decreased left ventricular filling, reduced cardiac output and myocardial ischaemia.

▶ *Clinical Manifestations[7]*

Clinical features include:

- hypotension
- hypoxaemia
- pulmonary hypertension
- cardiac dysrhythmias, pulseless electrical activity
- cardiac arrest and death.

▶ *Treatment*

The syndrome may last seconds to minutes, particularly in patients with healthy hearts. Treatment is supportive. Cardiac output and blood pressure must be maintained with:

1 IV fluid loading
2 vasoactive drugs such as metaraminol
3 inotropes such as adrenaline, if required
4 oxygenation.

Fatty Liver of Pregnancy, Acute

This very rare condition of unknown aetiology occurs in ≈ 1:13 000–16 000 pregnancies.[9] The liver abnormalities may be confused with, or overlap with, pre-eclampsia. Mortality is between 10% and 20% and liver transplant may be required.[10]

Clinical Picture

The main symptoms, signs and biochemical abnormalities are:

- nausea, vomiting, heartburn, oesophagitis, gastric erosions and haematemesis
- upper right abdominal pain
- jaundice, which is often mild

F

- coagulopathy, DIC
- elevated liver transaminase values
- leukocytosis, hyperuricaemia, hypoglycaemia
- renal failure
- fulminant hepatic failure with hepatic coma.

Diagnosis

Definitive diagnosis is by liver biopsy or typical findings on CT scan.

Treatment

Delivery provides the only definitive treatment, resulting in reversal of the condition unless liver damage is very severe.[10]

1 Monitor BSL frequently. A continuous infusion of 10% glucose to prevent/treat hypoglycaemia may be required.

2 Correct clotting abnormalities, if present, with FFP, vitamin K, platelets.

3 Optimise intravascular volume.

4 Epidural anaesthesia is probably preferable to GA for Caesarean section but is contraindicated if a significant coagulopathy is present.

Femoral Nerve Block and Three-In-One (Triple Nerve) Block

The three-in-one block aims to block the femoral and obturator nerves and the lateral cutaneous nerve of the thigh.

Anatomy

▶ *Femoral Nerve (L2, 3, 4)*

Arises from the lumbar plexus and is sensory to the anterior thigh. Through the saphenous nerve branch it also supplies sensation to the medial leg, ankle and foot. The motor supply of the femoral nerve is to the muscles of the anterior thigh, including the quadriceps. The nerve enters the thigh beneath the inguinal ligament just lateral to the femoral artery.

◗ Obturator Nerve (L2, 3, 4)

Also arising from the lumbar plexus, the obturator nerve innervates the skin on the medial side of the thigh and the knee and hip joint.

◗ Lateral Cutaneous Nerve of Thigh (L2, 3)

Supplies the skin over the antero-lateral thigh to the knee.

◗ Technique for Femoral Nerve Block

1 Secure IV access, and sterilise the skin at the injection site.
2 Insert a short bevelled 22 G block needle in a 30° cephalad direction just lateral to the femoral artery and just below the inguinal ligament.
3 Feel for two 'pops' as the needle passes first through the fascia lata and then the fascia iliaca. The tip of the needle should lie just lateral to, and slightly deeper than, the femoral artery and preferably the needle should be seen to pulsate slightly. A nerve stimulator can also be used, looking for contractions of the quadriceps, with a stimulating current of ≈ 0.3 mA.
4 Inject 15 mL of bupivacaine 0.5% incrementally, ensuring negative aspiration prior to, and during, injection.

◗ Technique for Three-In-One Block

The site of injection is identical to above but a greater volume of LA is used. Inject 30 mL (2–2.5 mg/kg) of bupivacaine 0.5% while applying pressure distal to the injection site to encourage LA spread towards the lumbar plexus.

◗ Comments

The femoral nerve block provides analgesia for femoral shaft and neck fractures and surgery on the anterior thigh. Three-in-one (triple nerve) block additionally aims to block the obturator nerve. This second technique, combined with sedation and a separate block of the lateral cutaneous nerve of thigh, has been used for hip replacement surgery.[11]

Fenoldopam Mesylate

Fenoldopam is a selective dopamine 1 receptor agonist. Its effects include:[12]

- renovascular vasodilatation (3.5 × more potent than dopamine)
- natriuresis.

Dose

0.1 μg/kg/min by IV infusion.

Fentanyl

Synthetic phenylpiperidine derivative (like pethidine) with opioid type analgesic properties. 60–80 × more potent than morphine, with a more rapid onset of action.[13] Fentanyl has a high margin of safety, producing little cardiovascular depression but may cause bradycardia. It also has a short duration of action at low dose (< 10 μg/kg) but becomes a long-acting drug at high dose (50–100 μg/kg). Elimination half-life 1.5–6 h.

Dose

▶ *Non-cardiac Surgery*

Dose depends on the duration and nature of surgery.

▶ *Adult Dose*

For minor surgery 50–100 μg is a reasonable dose in the adult with effects lasting 30–60 min. Higher doses will cause more prolonged effects.

▶ *Child Dose*

1–2 μg/kg

▶ *Cardiac Surgery*

50–100 µg/kg IV. Effects last ≈ 6 h.

▶ *IV Infusion (for Postoperative Analgesia)*

50 µg/kg in 50 mL N/S run at 1–4 mL/h (equivalent to 1–4 µg/kg/h).

▶ *Epidural*

50–100 µg. See *EPIDURAL ANAESTHESIA* and *PATIENT-CONTROLLED ANALGESIA*.

▶ *Intrathecal*

25 µg is effective and safe to supplement LA used for SAB.[14]

▶ *Topical Fentanyl*

Applied in the form of fentanyl patches, which are currently available in four different strengths (25, 50, 75 and 100 µg/h) delivered to the systemic circulation. The patches are applied for 72 h and are used in the treatment of chronic cancer pain. Fentanyl 50 µg/h is ≈ 135–244 mg/day of oral morphine (transdermal fentanyl product information).

▶ *Intranasal Fentanyl*

See *PATIENT-CONTROLLED ANALGESIA*. Intranasal fentanyl is about 70% as effective as IV fentanyl.[15]

Fibre-optic Intubation

See *AWAKE FIBRE-OPTIC INTUBATION*.

Fibrin Degradation Products (FDPs)

NR < 10 µg/mL. Plasmin causes the breakdown of fibrin into FDPs. FDP levels therefore reflect fibrinolysis. The effects of FDPs include:[16]

- possibly inhibit clot formation by competing with fibrin polymerisation sites

- interfere with platelet function and inhibit thrombin
- may damage vascular endothelium.

FDPs thus inhibit coagulation and FDP levels are increased by syndromes involving increased fibrinolysis and defibrination such as disseminated intravascular coagulation (DIC), in which FDP levels increase to > 40 µg/mL.

Fibrinogen

NR 200–400 mg/100 mL. Low levels occur in conditions such as disseminated intravascular coagulation.

Fitting

See *EPILEPSY, STATUS*

Flecainide

This fluorinated analogue of procainamide is a Class 1c antiarrhythmic drug useful for the treatment of:

1 life-threatening ventricular dysrhythmias (2nd line therapy)
2 conversion of atrial fibrillation, atrial flutter and ectopic atrial tachycardia to sinus rhythm
3 termination of AV nodal re-entrant tachycardia, and SVTs associated with Wolff-Parkinson-White syndrome.

Dose In Adults

Oral dose: 50–100 mg 8–12 h
IV dose: 2 mg/kg over 30 min

Precautions

1 Due to its ability to cause dysrhythmias, flecainide is recommended for oral treatment only if life-threatening ventricular arrhythmia occurs that is not responsive to other therapy.

2 Markedly decreases ventricular function. Effects are additive to β blockers and calcium channel blockers. Flecainide should be avoided in patients with impaired ventricular function and/or ischaemic heart disease.

Fluid Replacement Therapy

F

Paediatric Patient: Maintenance Fluid Requirement per Hour

4 mL/kg first 10 kg + 2 mL/kg for next 10 kg + 1 mL/kg for rest of weight. For example, a 32 kg child requires 40 + 20 + 12 mL/h = 72 mL/h maintenance. Standard fluid in child up to 1 year; N/4 saline + 5–10% glucose. Older child N/4 saline + 3.75% glucose.

Potassium requirements are 3 mmol/kg/day. Add 10 mmol KCl per 500 mL bag of fluid. Ensure urine output is established before giving potassium. See Table F1.

Adult Maintenance Fluid Requirements

Healthy 70 kg patient requires ≈ 125 mL/h maintenance fluid.

Table F1 Insensible losses occurring intra-operatively in adults	
Surgery type	Insensible loss/3rd space loss
GA alone	1–2 mL/kg/h
Small incision	3–4 mL/kg/h
Large incision	5–6 mL/kg/h
Bowel drawn out of wound	7–8 mL/kg/h
Major viscus or vascular surgery	9–10 mL/kg/h[17]

Points to Note

Blood loss (up to the point of requiring transfusion) should be replaced in the following ratios:

- with colloid: 1 mL blood:1 mL colloid
- with crystalloid: 1 mL blood:3–5 mL crystalloid.

Flumazenil

An imidazobenzodiazepine used as a competitive antagonist of benzodiazepine drugs.

Dose

▶ Adult

200 μg IV over 15 s, then 100 μg at 60 s intervals, titrate to response. Max. total dose in adult 1 mg (2 mg in ICU). Effects last 15–140 min and resedation may therefore occur.

IV infusion: 100–400 μg/h

▶ Child

5 μg/kg bolus, repeat dose at 60 s intervals to max. 40 μg/kg total dose.

IV infusion: 2–10 μg/kg/h

Foetal Death in Utero

See *INTRA-UTERINE FOETAL DEATH*.

Forehead Block

Requires the blocking of the *supraorbital nerve,* which supplies the upper eyelid medially and the forehead and scalp to the vertex, and the *supratrochlear nerve*, which supplies the conjunctiva and the skin of the medial upper eyelid and skin of the medial orbit and the root of nose.

Technique

Raise a wheal of LA just above the orbital ridge (5 mL). Also inject 2 mL of LA just above the supraorbital notch. Extend the wheal to the midline to block the supratrochlear nerve.

Fresh Frozen Plasma (FFP)

Most of the information following was obtained from the Australian Red Cross Blood Service (with permission).[18]

Description and Storage

A unit of FFP is collected from a single unit of whole blood. It contains all the coagulation factors found in plasma, including 200 units of Factor VIII, 200 units Factor IX and 400 mg of fibrinogen. The FFP bag also contains citrate. The total volume is 150–300 mL, which is stored at –25°C. FFP is considered expired 1 year after the collection date. If thawed, FFP can be stored at 2–6°C for up to 24 h (or up to 5 days if treating a condition other than Factor VIII deficiency).[19]

Compatibility

Compatibility tests prior to transfusion are not required. Give ABO group compatible FFP but in an emergency non-group compatible FFP can be used. Only group O FFP should be given to group O blood type recipients.

Indications

1   Coagulopathic patients with blood loss. In adults 4–8 units of FFP is required for a significant clinical effect. See *BLOOD TRANSFUSION*. In children give 10–20 mL/kg over 1 h.
2   Reversal of warfarin. Sufficient FFP (depending on the degree of warfarinisation) will reverse the effects of warfarin for ≈ 6–8 h.[20]

Gg

Gas Embolism, Venous

Due to venous entrainment of air or other gas such as CO_2 or N_2O used for laparoscopy. In the adult, 100–300 mL of air embolised rapidly can be fatal.[1] The effect of intravenous air embolism is greater in the child than in the adult on a mL/kg basis.[1] Larger volumes of air can be tolerated if it is infused slowly.

Clinical Effects and Diagnosis

1 Decrease in end-tidal CO_2 concentration (by > 2 mmHg) unless CO_2 is the causative gas.
2 Increased end-tidal N_2 concentration by 2–3% with air embolus.[2]
3 Loud, coarse continuous 'millwheel' heart murmur.
4 Hypotension, bradycardia.
5 Gasping respiration (if patient is breathing spontaneously).
6 Changes in sound detected by a precordial Doppler (described as an irregular roaring noise).
7 Bubbles of gas are easily detected by transoesophageal echocardiography.

Treatment

1 Notify the surgeon immediately.
2 Cease administration of N_2O, give 100% O_2.
3 Stop all pressurised gas administration, such as CO_2 for laparoscopy. The physiological disturbance from CO_2 insufflation is 6.5 times less than air due to the higher blood solubility of CO_2.[3]
4 Check that central venous access lines are not entraining air.
5 If cardiac arrest, resuscitate as per section on *CARDIAC ARREST*.

6 Direct the surgeon to flood the surgical field, and provide a Valsalva manoeuvre by squeezing the reservoir bag, to reveal the vascular entry site of air. In neurosurgical cases, compress jugular veins bilaterally to reveal the site of bleeding.

7 Position the patient so that the surgical site is *below* the heart level, and preferably place the patient in the left lateral decubitus position, tilted head down 15°. This manoeuvre may reduce the amount of air entering the heart.

8 Attempt to aspirate air from a central venous line. The optimal site for the tip of the catheter for this purpose is in the right atrium 2 cm below the junction of the right atrium and the SVC.[1]

9 The patient may require inotropic support of the cardiovascular system.

10 Add positive end-expiratory pressure of 5 cm H_2O, to reduce the pressure gradient favouring air entrainment. This may cause a further decline in cardiac output.

11 Cardiopulmonary bypass may be lifesaving in extreme cases, if available.

12 Thoracotomy and direct aspiration of air from the heart and great vessels may be needed.

13 Consider using hyperbaric oxygen, if available.

Gelofusin

Description and Composition

Gelofusin is a synthetic colloid solution with an average molecular weight of 35 000 daltons and contains 4% succinylated bovine gelatin in saline. Gelatin is obtained through the hydolysis of collagen creating a purified protein.

Gelofusin contains:

- sodium 154 mmol/L
- chloride 120 mmol/L

- pH 7.4 ± 0.3
- osmolarity 274 mOsm/L.

There are minimal amounts of potassium and calcium. It has a shelf life of 3 years at room temperature.

Uses

Gelofusin is used to treat hypovolaemia and for isovolaemic haemodilution. The plasma half-life is less than 4 h. The product information recommends giving the first 20–30 mL slowly, as anaphylaxis can occur with this solution.

Problems

In patients on angiotensin converting enzyme inhibitors under anaesthesia who are hypotensive, the hypotension may be worsened by gelofusin.[4]

The emergence of bovine spongioform encephalomyopathy (mad cow disease) has raised concerns regarding the use of bovine gelatin and the risk of prion contamination.

Glasgow Coma Scale (GCS)

Originally developed for grading severity and outcome for head injury.[5]

Eyes open	Score
Spontaneously	4
To speech	3
To pain	2
Nil	1

Best motor response	
Obey commands	6
Localise pain	5
Withdraw to pain	4
Abnormal flexion	3

| Extensor response | 2 |
| Nil | 1 |

Verbal response

Orientated	5
Confused	4
Inappropriate words	3
Sounds other than words	2
Nil	1

G

Glucose-6-Phosphate Dehydrogenase (G6PD) Deficiency

G6PD deficiency results in episodic haemolytic anaemia due to accumulation of methaemoglobin and deficiency of reduced glutathione in red blood cells.[6] These episodes can be precipitated by certain drugs, including primaquine and chloroquine, sulphonamides, nalidixic acid, nitrofurantoin, nitrates, aspirin in high doses, phenacetin, vitamins K and C and methylene blue.

Other drugs to avoid include penicillin and probenecid.[7] Occurs most commonly in male blacks and people of Mediterranean origin (X-linked disorder).

Anaesthetic Implications[6]

Do not exceed the maximum safe doses of drugs such as prilocaine and sodium nitroprusside, which can result in haemolysis. If methaemoglobinaemia occurs methylene blue is ineffective in treatment and may cause haemolysis.

Glyceryl Trinitrate

Organic nitrate which produces venodilation at low doses and arterial vasodilatation at higher doses. Acts by increasing production of nitric oxide in vascular smooth muscle cells, causing relaxation.

Results in redistribution of coronary blood flow to ischaemic myocardium and is less likely to produce coronary steal than sodium nitroprusside.[8]

Uses

For treatment of:

- myocardial ischaemia.
- left ventricular failure associated with myocardial infarction.
- treatment of hypertension.
- induction of hypotension.
- for producing uterine relaxation in situations such as retained placenta and uterine inversion. See *UTERINE RELAXATION FOR RETAINED PLACENTA.*

Dose for IV Infusion

1 Add 250 mg glyceryl trinitrate to 500 mL 5% glucose in a glass container.
2 Administer via a GTN-approved administration set (to reduce absorption into plastics).
3 *Usual dose range*: 0.5–6 µg/kg/min, equals 4–50 mL/h of the above solution.

Dose for Uterine Relaxation

▶ *IV Dose*

Remove 1 mL from an ampoule containing 50 mg of glyceryl trinitrate in 10 mL (5 mg) and dilute to 10 mL with N/S. Take 1 mL (500 µg) from this solution and dilute to 10 mL, resulting in a final concentration of 50 µg/mL. Give 1 mL boluses as required. The dose required is variable but 100–200 µg is usually effective.[9]

▶ *Sublingual Dose*

Two sprays of sublingual glyceryl trinitrate (800 µg) has been reported as effective and well tolerated.[10]

Glycopyrronium (Glycopyrrolate)

Quaternary ammonium anticholinergic compound with similar actions to atropine, but does not cross the blood–brain barrier and thus has no central actions. Glycopyrronium causes less tachycardia than atropine.[11]

Uses

Antisialogogue, treatment of bradycardia, and for protection against the muscarinic effects of anticholinesterase drugs such as neostigmine.

Dose

10 µg/kg IV

Hh

Haemaccel

Contains polygeline, a polypeptide manufactured from urea-linked bovine gelatin, with an average molecular weight of 30 000. Gelatin is obtained through the hydrolysis of collagen from animals creating a purified protein. Haemaccel also contains:

- sodium 145 mmol/L
- potassium 5.1 mmol/L
- calcium 6.25 mmol/L
- chloride 145 mmol/L
- pH 7.4 ± 0.3
- osmolarity 301 mOsm/L.

Uses

Colloid plasma volume expander. Stays in the intravascular space longer than crystalloid solutions but for a shorter time than dextrans.[1] Plasma half-life of haemaccel ≈ 4 h.[1]

Problems

1. May cause clotting of citrated blood used for transfusion due to haemaccel's calcium content.
2. Reactions to haemaccel occur in 0.04% of administrations, ranging from minor to severe allergic responses.[2]
3. Haemaccel administration can result in increased bradykinin production, resulting in hypotension. Bradykinin production is inhibited by angiotensin converting enzyme (ACE). Patients on ACE inhibitors appear to be more susceptible to haemaccel-induced hypotension for this reason.
4. The emergence of bovine spongioform encephalomyopathy

(mad cow disease) has raised concerns regarding the use of bovine gelatin.

Haemoglobin

See Table H1.

Table H1 Normal Hb levels for age in g/100 mL	
Age in months/years	Hb (g/100 mL)
Birth	13.6–19.6
3 months	10–11
1 year	11.2
10 years	12.9
Adult male	13.5–18
Adult female	11.5–16.4

Haemoptysis, Massive

Massive haemorrhage into the airway is an anaesthetic and surgical emergency. It can be defined as > 600 mL in 24 h.[3] Death can result from asphyxia due to flooding of the airways and alveoli. Emergency surgical consultation should be sought.

Management

1 *Airway*: Clear the airway and optimise the patient's position. Suction the airway to remove blood and place the patient head down. If the side of bleeding is known, e.g. known left lung carcinoma, place the patient lateral with the bleeding side down. If bleeding does not diminish rapidly, or the patient is in extremus, intubate the trachea. Consider an awake intubation if possible;

otherwise perform a rapid sequence induction. Have two or more working suction units available.

2   Ideally a double lumen tube should be inserted to isolate the non-bleeding lung. Otherwise a single lumen tube can be used and the lumen advanced into the bronchus of the non-bleeding lung. If the ET tube enters the bleeding bronchus, consider placing a Fogarty catheter through the ET tube. The balloon on the catheter is inflated in the bronchus; then the ET tube is removed.

3   *Breathing*: Give supplementary oxygen, 100% O_2 concentration. IPPV may be required. Avoid high airway pressures if possible due to the risk of air embolism. Do not use jet ventilation, which may cause blood in the airway to dry and solidify, exacerbating airway obstruction.[3]

4   *Circulation*: Optimise intravascular volume and provide blood transfusion if required (uncommon).

5   *Diagnose source of blood loss:* Investigations include CXR, ABG, pulse oximetry, bronchoscopy (flexible/rigid), arteriography.

6   *Manage blood loss*: Treatment strategies include the following:
    (a)   correcting any underlying coagulopathy
    (b)   bronchoscopic manoeuvres, including iced saline lavage, injection of adrenaline at the bleeding site, placement of bronchial blockers
    (c)   selective embolisation of the bleeding segment
    (d)   definitive surgical resection if the bleeding site can be identified.

Haemorrhage

See *BLOOD LOSS ASSESSMENT AND INITIAL MANAGEMENT* and *BLOOD TRANSFUSION*.

Halothane

Halogenated hydrocarbon volatile inhalational anaesthetic agent.

Physical properties and MAC

Blood:gas solubility coefficient	2.3
Oil:gas solubility coefficient	224
Saturated vapour pressure at 20°C (32 kpa)	244 mmHg
Boiling point	50.2°C
MAC	0.75

Advantages
Sweet, non-irritating odour suitable for inhalational induction. Potent agent.

Disadvantages
1 Requires preservative, 0.01% thymol, accumulation of which can interfere with vaporiser function.
2 Risk of halothane hepatitis.
3 Sensitises myocardium to catecholamines more than other modern inhalational agents.
4 Causes prolongation of the QT interval, predisposing the patient to ventricular tachycardias such as torsade de pointes.
5 Produces vagal stimulation, which can result in marked brady-cardia.
6 Halothane is a potent trigger for malignant hyperpyrexia.

Recommendations
1 Avoid repeated exposure. Do not use halothane within 6 months of previous halothane anaesthetic unless there is an overriding clinical indication.
2 A history of unexplained jaundice or pyrexia after previous halothane anaesthetic is an *absolute contraindication* to repeat halothane exposure.
3 Caution with adrenaline because of the risk of cardiac dysrhythmia such as ventricular ectopic beats and ventricular tachycardia. Avoid using concentrations of adrenaline > 1:100 000 and volumes of this concentration > 10 mL in 10 min or > 30 mL/h.

4 Do not use halothane in patients with a prolonged QT interval or patients taking drugs known to prolong the QT interval.

Hartmann's Solution (Ringer's Lactate)

Crystalloid solution containing sodium 131 mmol/L, potassium 5 mmol/L, calcium 2 mmol/L, chloride 111 mmol/L, lactate 29 mmol/L, osmolarity 274 mOsm/L (hypotonic), pH 5–7. Lactate is metabolised by both gluconeogenesis and oxidation (mainly in the liver) to bicarbonate and glucose. Hartmann's solution should not be given to diabetic patients as it may increase glucose levels and cause elevated ketone levels.[4]

Heart Block (HB)

HB (atrioventricular block) can be divided into three main types.

1 *first degree HB*: P–R interval > 0.20 s (5 mm)
2 *second degree HB*: subdivided into:
   (a) *Wenckebach or Morbitz 1*: Gradual lengthening of P–R interval until a dropped beat occurs, then the cycle repeats.
   (b) *Morbitz 2:* Fixed ratio of P waves to QRS complexes, e.g. 2:1, 3:1.
3 *third degree HB:* No relationship between P waves and QRS complexes.

Treatment

First degree and Morbitz type 1 second degree HB usually require no treatment. Morbitz type 2 and third degree HB require treatment if cardiovascular compromise is present. For emergency management:

1 *Isoprenaline:* 2 mg in 50 mL 5% glucose. In the adult start at 1.5 mL/h. Infusion range 1–10 µg/min (1.5–15 mL/h). Can also give boluses of 20 µg (0.5 mL).[5] Child dose: 0.02–0.15µg/kg/min.
2 Use an adrenaline infusion if isoprenaline is not available. See *ADRENALINE*.

3   External transcutaneous pacing.
4   Temporary pacing wire.
5   Permanent pacemaker. See *PACEMAKERS AND ANAESTHESIA*.

Heart Transplant Patients, Anaesthesic Considerations for Non-cardiac Surgery

Physiological Considerations

1   The transplanted heart is denervated and is paced by the donor atrium at a resting rate of 90–100 beats per minute. Systemic vascular resistance is increased in these patients and ventricular hypertrophy is usual.[6]
2   The donor heart is responsive to volume loading by increasing stroke volume via the Frank-Starling mechanism.[7] In addition, heart rate increases over 5–6 minutes in response to the release of endogenous catecholamines.[7] The transplanted heart is pre-load dependent and responds poorly to hypovolaemia and decreased systemic vascular resistance.

Pathophysiological Considerations

1   There is accelerated coronary artery atheromatous disease.[8] However, the patient will not experience chest pain due to myocardial ischaemia.
2   There is an increased incidence of dysrhythmias such as ventricular ectopic beats. First degree atrioventricular block, right bundle branch block and bradyarrhythmias are common.[6] Episodes of dysrhythmia may indicate rejection. Note that the ECG often contains 2 P waves due to the presence of residual recipient atrial tissue. About 10% of recipients require a permanent pacemaker. See *PACEMAKERS AND ANAESTHESIA*.
3   Immunosupressive drugs result in an increased susceptibility to infection. About 75% of patients develop hypertension secondary to cyclosporin A therapy.

4 Renal impairment may occur due to the nephrotoxic effects of cyclosporin A.

Pharmacology and the Transplanted Heart

1 The donor heart rate will have no response to drugs with autonomic activity such as *anticholinergics (atropine, glycopyrrolate)* and *anticholinesterases (neostigmine)*, but will increase with sympathomimetic amines such as *adrenaline, isoprenaline, ephedrine, dobutamine and dopamine.*

2 Reflex tachycardia with vasodilators such as *sodium nitroprusside* is absent and the hypotensive effects of these drugs may be exaggerated.

3 The transplanted heart is usually exquisitely sensitive to adenosine and this drug should be used with extreme caution. Use a starting dose of 1 mg rather than 3 mg.[9] See *ADENOSINE.*

4 Digoxin is ineffective on the transplanted heart.[9]

Pre-operative Assessment and Preparation

1 Liaise with the patient's cardiologist and the transplant team if possible.

2 Look for any evidence of rejection, such as increasing symptoms of heart failure, dysrhythmias, low voltage ECG and deteriorating ventricular function on echocardiograghy.[6]

3 Avoid procedures that may result in infection, such as nasal intubation and invasive monitoring. Use strict asepsis when performing invasive procedures.

4 Use appropriate antibiotic prophylaxis, including antistaphylococcal cover (e.g. flucloxacillin).

5 Continue immunosuppressive therapy throughout the perioperative period. Azathioprine can be given IV at the same dose as PO. Patients will require peri-operative steroid coverage. See *STEROID 'COVER'.*

6 Establish monitoring as appropriate for the procedure and the patient's physiological condition. If central venous pressure monitoring is required do not use the right internal jugular vein. This is because this vein is used for cardiac biopsies.[8]

7 Ensure adequate preload prior to the induction of anaesthesia and at all other times.

8 Ensure isoprenaline and/or transcutaneous pacing is readily available to treat bradycardia. See *ISOPRENALINE*.

Intra-operative Care

1 General and/or regional anaesthesia has been used successfully in heart transplanted patients.

2 Significant hypotension may occur with epidural or spinal anaesthesia if preload is not maintained.[6]

3 Maintain preload at all times.

4 Avoid myocardial depressant drugs.

5 Hypotension can be treated with ensuring adequate preload and vasoconstrictors such as mataraminol or phenylephrine.

Postoperative Care

1 Liaise with the patient's cardiologist and transplant team regarding postoperative management, including immunosuppressive therapy while the patient is nil by mouth.

2 Remove all unnecessary intravascular lines, drains and other invasive equipment to reduce the risk of infection.

HELLP Syndrome

This term describes a form of severe pre-eclampsia/eclampsia with Haemolysis, Elevated Liver enzymes and Low Platelets. See *PRE-ECLAMPSIA/ECLAMPSIA*.

Heparin, Unfractionated and Low Molecular Weight Heparins

Heparin (Unfractionated)

Anticoagulant drug. Acts by binding reversibly to antithrombin III and enhancing its ability to inhibit certain coagulation proteases such as XIII, plasmin and thrombin. Also inhibits platelet aggregation by fibrin.

▶ Uses

1 Prevention and treatment of venous and arterial thromboembolic disease.
2 Anticoagulation for cardiac bypass surgery.
3 Priming dialysis and cardiopulmonary bypass machines to prevent extra-corporeal clot formation.

▶ Dose in Adults

1 *Prevention of deep venous thrombosis (DVT) and pulmonary embolus (PE)*: 5000 U subcutaneously 8–12 h.
2 *Treatment of DVT*: 5000 U IV loading dose, then IV infusion 1250 U/h. Check APTT after 4 h. Aim for therapeutic APTT range of 60–85 s. Increase or decrease the infusion rate accordingly.
3 *Treatment of PE*: See PULMONARY EMBOLISM.
4 *Reversal of heparin*: See PROTAMINE.

Low Molecular Weight (LMW) Heparins

Anticoagulant drugs that act by catalysing the inhibition of activated factors IX, X, XI and XII by antithrombin III.

▶ Advantages of LMW Heparins

1 These drugs inhibit platelets less than heparin and may produce less intra-operative bleeding.[10]

2 They have a longer duration of action than heparin, making administration easier.

3 LMW heparins have less risk of producing heparin-induced thrombocytopaenia.

4 LMW heparins are more effective in reducing mortality from pulmonary embolus than heparin.[10]

5 Less monitoring of the anticoagulant effect of LMW heparin is required compared with heparin.

▶ *Disadvantages of LMW Heparins*

1 Measuring the anticoagulant effects of LMW heparin is more difficult. This is done by measuring anti-Xa activity, the therapeutic range for treatment of established DVT/PE being 0.3–0.8 anti-Xa units/mL at 3–5 h after the dose.

2 In cases of bleeding LMW heparin is more difficult to reverse than heparin. See below.

▶ *Dose in Adults*

1 *Prevention of DVT and PE:* See *DEEP VENOUS THROMBOSIS (DVT) PROPHYLAXIS.*

2 *Treatment of DVT and PE:*

   (a) *Dalteparin* 100 U/kg/12 h subcutaneously or 200 U/kg/day.

   (b) *Enoxaparin* 1 mg/kg/12 h subcutaneously or 1.5 mg/kg/day. Therapy with LMW heparin should be continued for at least 5 days, overlapping with oral warfarin therapy from day 1. INR must be in the therapeutic range (2.0–3.0) for at least 2 days before ceasing LMW heparin.

3 *Reversal of LMW heparin activity*: LMW heparin can be ≈ 60% neutralised by protamine and fresh frozen plasma is also effective. See *PROTAMINE.*

Hepatitis B and C

See *NEEDLE-STICK INJURY.*

Hepato-renal Syndrome

Describes the syndrome of renal impairment secondary to severe liver disease, usually cirrhosis. It is thought to be due to intrarenal vasoconstriction despite systemic vasodilatation.[11] Once established, renal failure is resistant to treatment unless liver function improves, e.g. by liver transplant.

Preventative strategies include:

1   adequate hydration, with IV fluids for at least 12 h pre-operatively.
2   mannitol 20% 100 mL immediately pre-operatively. Give a second dose postoperatively if urine output < 50 mL/h.[12]
3   Consider sodium taurocholate 1 g PO 8 h for 48 h.[13]

Herbal Medicines and Anaesthesia

It is advisable to ask all patients if they are taking herbal or other non-prescribed medication. Although most herbal medicines are probably harmless, it may be prudent to ask the patient to cease all herbal remedies for at least 2 weeks prior to surgery.[14] Adverse effects of specific herbal medicines include:

- *Echinacea* is contraindicated in patients taking immunosuppressive drugs, with autoimmune disease and with human immunodeficiency virus infection.[15]
- *Ephedra* has been associated with hypertension, tachycardia, seizures, intracranial haemorrhage, myocardial infarction and psychosis.[15]
- *Feverfew (Tanacetum parthenium)* can cause platelet dysfunction.
- *Garlic (Allium sativum):* Anecdotal reports suggest heavy garlic intake can cause an increased bleeding tendency with unexpected surgical bleeding and a report of a spontaneous epidural haematoma.[16,17] Garlic should not be taken with warfarin, aspirin or other NSAIDs.[18] The effects of garlic last about 7 days.
- *Ginger (Zingiber officinale)* may potentiate the effects of warfarin.

- *Ginkgo biloba* has been associated anecdotally with bleeding tendencies. As for garlic, gingko should not be taken with warfarin, aspirin or other NSAIDs. Gingko effects last about 36 h.
- *Ginseng* can induce tachycardia and hypertension. Ginseng can also interfere with warfarin, decreasing its effect. Patients on antidepressants may develop mania if given ginseng.
- *Goldenseal (Hydrastis canadensis)* can cause hypertension, oedema, or hypokalaemia due to its mineralocorticoid effects.
- *Kava* interacts with levodopa and can potentiate Parkinson's disease. It also causes sedation and an increased risk of suicide in patients with depression.
- *St John's wort* increases uterine tone and should be avoided in pregnancy. St John's wort decreases the efficacy of warfarin, digoxin and anticonvulsants. This herb can potentially interact with tramadol to cause serotonin syndrome. See *SEROTONIN SYNDROME*.[19] St John's wort can also decrease the efficacy of HIV protease inhibitor drugs.
- *Licorice (Glycyrrhiza glabra)* can cause hypertension, low potassium levels or oedema.
- *Valerian (Valeriana officinalis)* causes sedation and thus may enhance the effects of sedative drugs such as benzodiazepines. It can prolong barbiturate induced sleep.

Human Immunodeficiency Virus (HIV)

See *NEEDLESTICK INJURY*.

Hydralazine

A phthalazine derivative that acts directly on vascular smooth muscle, causing arteriolar vasodilation. Used for the treatment of moderate to severe hypertension, and severe heart failure.

Treatment of Hypertension

▶ *Dose*

IV Adult: 5–10 mg IV boluses every 20 min to a max. dose of 20–40 mg. Duration of action 2–6 h.

Hydromorphone (Dilaudid)

This analgesic drug is a semi-synthetic modification of morphine. 2 mg of hydromorphone is equivalent to morphine 10 mg.

Adult Doses

PO: 1–8 mg 4 h
IM/subcut: 1–2 mg 4–6 h
IV: 0.5 mg 4–6 h

Child Doses

PO: 0.05–1 mg/kg/dose
IM/subcut: 0.02–0.05 mg/kg/dose
Slow IV: 0.01–0.02 mg/kg/dose 4–6 h

Advantages

1 Hydromorphone may have a lower incidence of side effects such as nausea and vomiting, sedation and pruritus compared to morphine.[21]

2 Hydromorphone is as effective for analgesia as morphine at equivalent doses.

3 Epidural hydromorphone may produce less respiratory depression, itch and urinary retention than epidural morphine.[23]

Disadvantages

1 Hydromorphone may have a higher incidence of mood and sleep disturbances than morphine when both are used by the PCA route.[24]

2 Hydromorphone and its metabolites are excreted renally. Caution must therefore be used in patients with renal impairment.

Hydroxyethylated Starch (Hydroxyethyl Starch, HES)

Description

These solutions are manufactured by treating starch from maize or sorghum with ethylene chlorohydrin and pyrimidine. Hydroxyethylated starch contains 90% amylopectin. Hetastarch, with an average molecular weight of 450 000 daltons, is the most common form used. It is primarily excreted by the kidneys.

Uses

Hydroxyethylated starch is used for plasma expansion and hetastarch has a half-life in the plasma of less than 24 h.[25] It is the most commonly used colloid in the United States.

Problems

High molecular weight HES solutions can cause a coagulopathy by reducing levels of Factor VIII and von Willebrand Factor. The maximum recommended dose is 33 mL/kg/day.[26]

Hypercapnia

The normal range of arterial $PaCO_2$ is 35–45 mmHg.

Hypercapnia can result from respiratory and non-respiratory causes.

Respiratory Causes of Hypercapnia

1 Hypoventilation.
2 Increased anatomical or non-atomical dead space.
3 Increased ventilation/perfusion (V/Q) mismatch.

Non-respiratory Causes of Hypercapnia

1 Rebreathing of CO_2, e.g. failure of the CO_2 absorber.
2 Exogenous CO_2, e.g. during laparoscopy.

3 Sodium bicarbonate administration.
4 Hypermetabolic state, e.g. fever, sepsis and malignant hyper-pyrexia.

Hyper/Hypocalcaemia

See *CALCIUM.*

Hyper/Hypokalaemia

See *POTASSIUM.*

Hypertension

Causes during anaesthesia include:

1 *physiological*, e.g. nociceptive stimulation, awareness, laryngo-scopy/intubation, volume overload, hypoxia, hypercapnia
2 *pathological*, e.g. raised intracranial pressure, phaeochromocy-toma, pre-eclampsia, renovascular and essential hypertension
3 *pharmacological,* e.g. acute withdrawal of antihypertensive medication, vasopressor drugs.

Treatment

Depends on cause. See *COVER ABCD CRISIS MANAGEMENT ALGORITHM.*

Must exclude hypoxia, ensure that the depth of anaesthesia is adequate and that the blood pressure reading is not artifactual. Consider:

1 *deepening anaesthesia.* Increase inspiratory concentration of inhalational agent, and/or bolus of IV anaesthetic agent, e.g. thiopentone
2 *supplementing analgesia.* Give opioid drug IV or additional LA + opioid via the epidural catheter.
3 *antihypertensive drugs.* Suitable agents include:

(a) β blocker. Especially useful if there is an associated tachycardia or a tachycardia is undesirable. For example, give metoprolol 1–2 mg IV boluses minutely to a maximum total dose of 15–20 mg. Do not use a β blocker if phaeochromocytoma is suspected.

(b) *hydralazine* 5–10 mg IV boluses

(c) *phentolamine* 0.5 mg boluses IV

(d) *glyceryl trinitrate infusion* 250 mg in 500 mL 5% glucose 0.5–6 μg/kg/min

(e) *sodium nitroprusside infusion* 50 mg in 100 mL 5% glucose, run at 0.5–6 μg/kg/min.

See entry for each drug.

Hypertensive Response to Intubation (Attenuation of)

Attenuation of the hypertensive response to intubation is desirable in conditions such as:

- phaeochromocytoma
- cerebral aneurysm
- pre-eclampsia/eclampsia.

Techniques

The following dosages are, in general, quoted for situations in which a single agent is used. If using multiple agents together, lower doses should be used to avoid severe hypotension.

1 Ensure that the patient is well anaesthetised prior to intubation with a judicious dose of IV induction agent or inhalational drug.

2 *Opioids*: Consider fentanyl 5–10 μg/kg IV or sufentanil 0.5–1.0 μg/kg IV, 3–5 min before intubation.[27] Alfentanil 25–50 μg/kg IV is also effective. Remifentanil 2 μg/kg with a propofol induction will ablate the haemodynamic response to

intubation.[28] However, a bolus of this magnitude may result in severe bradycardia and hypotension before intubation.[29]

3 Lignocaine 1.5–2 mg/kg IV 90 s before induction.

4 β blocker: Esmolol 2–3 mg/kg[30] or labetalol 0.15–0.45 mg/kg IV.[31]

5 Hydralazine 5–10 mg IV 15 min before induction of anaesthesia.[32]

6 Glyceryl trinitrate infusion 5–50 µg/kg/min just prior to laryngoscopy.[32]

7 Sodium nitroprusside 1–2 µg/kg.[31]

8 Using a nerve stimulator, ensure that the patient is completely paralysed prior to intubation.

Hypertrophic Obstructive Cardiomyopathy (HOCM)

This condition is defined as hypertrophy of the left or right ventricle without dilation in the absence of an identifiable cause.[33] Over 70% of cases are familial with autosomal dominant inheritance and variable penetrance. There may be dynamic left ventricular outflow obstruction due to abnormal forward motion of the mitral valve with impaction of the anterior leaflet against the hypertrophied septum.[34] However, only about 25% of patients with hypertrophic cardiomyopathy demonstrate LV outflow tract obstruction and the term 'hypertrophic cardiomyopathy' (HCM) is replacing HOCM.[35,36] When there is LV outflow obstruction this may be referred to as idiopathic hypertrophic subaortic stenosis. There is a 2–3% annual death risk.[37]

Pathophysiology and Investigations

1 Typically get hypertrophy, mainly of the interventricular septum, but the hypertrophy can be highly variable.

2 There is excessive contractility in systole.

3 Diastolic relaxation is abnormal with decreased left ventricular compliance, high diastolic filling pressures and decreased end-diastolic ventricular volume (i.e. a low capacity stiff ventricle).

4 Mitral regurgitation can occur due to interference to mitral valve leaflet function by the hypertrophied septum.

The above pathology results in a dynamic left ventricular outflow obstruction due to the hypertrophied septum, which is worsened by factors that increase contractility or increase ventricular emptying (decreased preload and/or afterload).

Relevant investigations include the following:

1 *ECG* may indicate left ventricular hypertrophy, ST segment depression and T wave changes.

2 *Echocardiography* typically shows left ventricular wall thickening. If the ratio of intraventricular septal thickness to left ventricular free wall thickness is > 1.3:1, the diagnosis of HOCM must be considered.[38]

Clinical Features

1 Ventricular dysrhythmias, supraventricular tachycardia and atrial fibrillation may occur and can be fatal.

2 The patient may experience dyspnoea, angina, syncope, heart failure and sudden death.

3 A systolic ejection murmur may be present.

Treatment

HOCM patients are frequently treated with β blockers, which relieve angina and dyspnoea. Calcium channel blockers may improve diastolic relaxation and increase exercise tolerance. These patients may also be on anti-arrhythmic therapy, e.g. amiodarone, sotalol, anticoagulants (for atrial fibrillation), and have implantable defibrillators. Other treatments include dual chamber pacemakers, septal myotomy/myomectomy and cardiac transplant.

Anaesthetic Management

It is imperative to avoid factors that increase myocardial contractility, decrease ventricular filling or increase ventricular emptying. Aim for strict haemodynamic stability and modest bradycardia. Consult directly with the patient's cardiologist or obtain cardiology review if the patient is newly diagnosed.

Pre-induction Phase and Throughout all Phases of Anaesthesia

1 *Maintain preload.* Ensure the patient is well hydrated pre-operatively and maintain intravascular volume throughout the peri-operative period. Do not use vasodilators such as sodium nitroprusside.

2 *Maintain afterload,* as a fall in systemic vascular resistance can result in increased ventricular emptying with increased outflow tract obstruction. *Epidural/spinal anaesthesia may be extremely hazardous* in the presence of HOCM and these procedures have been associated with severe bradycardia, hypotension, myocardial infarction and death.[39] However, epidural anaesthesia has been used successfully in labouring patients.[40]

3 *Consider invasive monitoring* (for major operations) such as an arterial line, CVP line, pulmonary artery catheterisation and transoesophageal echocardiography. Pulmonary capillary wedge pressure (PCWP) measurements can help predict optimal fluid loading of the left ventricle without producing pulmonary oedema. Cardiac output monitoring can also help assess the response to therapeutic measures. Also, the PCWP waveform can be observed for evidence of mitral valve regurgitant flow (giant V waves), indicating increased outflow obstruction.[41]

4   *Avoid tachycardia*, which can increase outflow obstruction and decrease cardiac output. Bradycardia can be beneficial by increasing preload. Do not use ephedrine, atropine, ketamine or pancuronium, which may increase heart rate.

5   *Avoid increases in myocardial contractility.* Do not give inotropic drugs such as digoxin, dobutamine.

6   *Bacterial endocarditis* prophylaxis is required.[33] See *BACTERIAL ENDOCARDITIS PROPHYLAXIS*.

7   *Maintain sinus rhythm.* Consider immediate cardioversion if a dysrhythmia occurs.

Induction Phase

1   Propofol or thiopentone are suitable induction agents. Do not use ketamine, which may cause a tachycardia and increase contractility.[38]

2   Use rocuronium or cisatracurium for muscle relaxation. Do not use pancuronium, which may produce a tachycardia.

Maintenance Phase

1   *Avoid intermittent positive pressure ventilation*, as this may decrease preload. If the patient must be ventilated, avoid high airway pressures and the Valsalva manoeuvre.

2   *Halothane* is a good choice for an inhalational agent as it decreases myocardial contractility and produces less of a fall in peripheral vascular resistance than isoflurane.[38] Halothane is also less likely than isoflurane to produce an increase in heart rate.

3   *Hypotension* should be treated with intravascular volume loading. If this is ineffective administer an α1 adreno-receptor agonist such as phenylephrine (50–100 μg increments) or methoxamine (1 mg IV boluses).[34] Do not use ephedrine.

4   *Hypertension* should be treated with increased concentration of inhalational anaesthetic agent. If this is inadequate use esmolol (see *ESMOLOL*). Do not use vasodilators such as sodium nitroprusside.

Treatment of Heart Failure

If heart failure occurs in a patient with HOCM, treatment principles include:

1 Increase preload with IV fluids.
2 Increase afterload with an α adreno-receptor agonist such as metaraminol.
3 Decrease heart rate and contractility with a β adreno-receptor blocker drug.
4 Give frusemide if pulmonary oedema occurs.[42]

HOCM and Obstetric Anaesthesia

▶ Preterm Labour

If there is LV outflow obstruction betamimetic tocolytic agents for premature labour are absolutely contraindicated.[37]

Magnesium sulphate would probably be safer.[37]

▶ Epidural Analgesia for Labour

Epidural anaesthesia has been used successfully in HOCM patients in labour.[40,43] Recommendations include:

1 Consider starting epidural infusion early in labour.
2 Use low concentrations of LA agent, e.g. bupivacaine 0.125%. Titrate dose gradually.
3 Do not use adrenaline-containing solutions in order to avoid any adrenaline-induced increase in myocardial contractility or heart rate.
4 Arterial line to monitor blood pressure closely.
5 ECG monitoring.
6 Oxytocin may cause adverse effects due to relaxation of vascular smooth muscle. It must be administered slowly and carefully. Boccio et al. recommend ergonovine as an alternative.[44]

Anaesthesia for CS

Opinion regarding optimal anaesthesia for CS in HOCM patients favours GA.[44,45] Minnich et al. argue that, for patients with HOCM with an epidural for labour pain already present, it would be reasonable to gradually and carefully 'top up' the epidural for CS.[43] Their recommendation is to revert to GA if there is significant CVS deterioration that is not responsive to fluids and vasopressors. Autore reported three cases of successful epidural anaesthesia for CS.[46]

Hypocapnia

Is defined as $PaCO_2$ < 35 mmHg. Hypocapnia can result from:
- hyperventilation
- reduced CO_2 production.

Hypotension

Specific treatment depends on cause. Causes can be divided into:

1   *inadequate preload*, e.g. hypovolaemia, supine hypotensive syndrome
2   *cardiac impairment,* e.g. tamponade, dysrhythmia, ischaemia, drug-induced myocardial depression
3   *reduced afterload*, e.g. sepsis, anaphylactic/anaphylactoid reactions.

Treatment

Urgency and aggressiveness of treatment depends on the severity of hypotension and the cause. Principles of management are:

1   *optimise preload.* Give IV fluids of appropriate type and volume (crystalloid, colloid, blood).
2   *correct cardiac impairment*, e.g. reduce/cease administration of volatile anaesthetic agent. If no palpable pulse, commence immediate external or internal cardiac massage.
3   *optimise afterload.* Give vasoconstrictor drug, e.g. ephedrine 3–6 mg boluses IV, metaraminol 0.5–1 mg IV boluses, adrenaline 10 µg–1 mg IV, depending on severity of situation ± IV infusion (see *ADRENALINE*).

Diagnosis of Hypotension Using COVER Algorithm (Search for Cause Simultaneously with Treatment)

- *C (Circulation and Colour)*: Feel pulse for rate, rhythm and character. Pulse quality may indicate that the blood pressure measurement is artifactual, or a dysrhythmia is present. Assess the patient's colour, looking especially for cyanosis, or erythema suggesting an allergic reaction. Look at the ECG tracing and treat significant dysrhythmias if present.

- *O (Oxygen supply, Oxygen analyser)*: Ensure that the patient is adequately oxygenated. Ventilate with 100% O_2 if severe hypotension is present. Look at the pulse oximetry trace. The presence of a pulse waveform suggests that some output is present.

- *V (Ventilation and Vaporiser)*: Assess ventilation. Examine the chest for tension pneumothorax/bronchospasm. Listen to the heart sounds. May hear muffled valve sounds in tamponade or 'mill wheel murmur' with gas embolus. Check the capnograph trace. The presence of expired CO_2 indicates some cardiac output is present. Check the vaporiser setting. An overdose of volatile anaesthetic agent may be the cause of the hypotension. Reduce delivered concentration or cease volatile administration.

- *E (Endotracheal tube and Elimination)*.

- *R (Review monitors and equipment)*: Recheck pulse oximetry, capnography, ECG and any other monitors in use, such as CVP. Check equipment such as drug infusion pumps, e.g. is inotropic drug failing to reach patient due to infusion pump or IV line problems? Check the surgeon's positioning of instruments as this may be causing decreased venous return. Assess the degree of blood loss (check suction bottles). Excessive insufflation of gas during laparoscopy may also be a cause.

- *A (Reassess Airway)*.

- *B (Reassess ventilation)*.

- *C (Reassess Circulation)*, i.e. preload (blood loss?), cardiac function (myocardial ischaemia?) and afterload (total spinal?). Optimise the above.
- *D (Drug effects)*: Review intended, possible/actual unintended drug administration or substance administration, e.g. bone cement, accidental rapid infusion of vancomycin. Reconsider failure of a drug to reach the patient, e.g. kinked cannula.

If the cause of hypotension still not apparent move onto *A SWIFT CHECK* algorithm.

See *COVER ABCD CRISIS MANAGEMENT ALGORITHM*.

H

Hypoxia/Hypoxaemia

Hypoxaemia can be defined as a PaO_2 < 60 mmHg or O_2 saturation < 90%. Causes include the following.

Above the Airway
1 Inadequate inspired FiO_2.
2 Inadequate ventilation, e.g. ventilator failure or switched off.
3 Disconnection.

Airway Problems
1 Oesophageal intubation.
2 Blocked ET tube.

Patient Problems
1 Ventilation–perfusion mismatch, e.g. bronchial intubation.
2 Shunt.
3 Diffusion block, i.e. impaired transfer of O_2 across alveolar wall to pulmonary capillary as can occur with pulmonary oedema.
4 Inadequate cardiac output.
5 Decreased O_2 carrying capacity of blood, e.g. anaemia, carbon monoxide poisoning.

Hypoxia Management 'Drill'

1 Check that the pulse oximeter is properly attached to the patient. *Always assume the pulse oximeter reading is correct until proven otherwise.*

2 Check the oxygen analyser; ensure that O_2 is being delivered to the patient. Look at the other monitors, especially capnography, ECG and blood pressure.

3 Perform a rapid screen of the anaesthetic circuit from the wall oxygen outlet to the patient, looking for causes of inadequate ventilation such as disconnections.

4 Eliminate the ventilator by hand-ventilating the patient with the reservoir bag. Increase the inspired O_2 concentration of the delivered gas (to 100% if necessary) and make sure the oxygen analyser shows a rising O_2 concentration in the inspired gas. Feel lung compliance and look at the capnography trace and other monitors. *Get help early if the situation is not resolving rapidly.*

5 Ensure the patient has an adequate pulse and check blood pressure. Attempt to exclude a circulatory cause for hypoxaemia. Examine the patient for any other obvious abnormality such as rash, swelling of the lips and eyelids, or subcutaneous emphysema.

6 Auscultate the chest and look at chest expansion, ensuring that chest expansion is equal on both sides. If ventilation is difficult the cause may be:

(a) circuit causes, e.g. blocked filter due to secretions. Disconnect the circuit from the patient and check patency. Substitute a self-inflating bag for the anaesthetic circuit if a circuit problem is suspected.

(b) tube problems. Consider tube blockage, kinking. Pass a suction catheter down the endotracheal tube to check for patency. Have a low threshold for changing the tube. Exclude endobronchial intubation.

(c) patient pathology, e.g. bronchospasm, pulmonary oedema.

7 If no apparent lung pathology or anaesthesia circuit problems are identified, consider other causes such as gas embolism, aspiration. Consider anaemia, methaemoglobinaemia and other blood causes of hypoxia. Obtain an urgent chest X-ray. If the cause is still not apparent consider other investigations such as fibre optic bronchoscopy.

Diagnosis of Hypoxia Using the COVER ABCD Crisis Management Algorithm

The COVER ABCD A SWIFT CHECK crisis management algorithm should be immediately applied with simultaneous diagnosis and treatment. If patient is undergoing mask anaesthesia, begin with A B.

- *A*: Ensure patent airway.
- *B*: Ensure patient is breathing; if not, ventilate with 100% O_2.
- *C (Circulation and Colour):* Feel pulse, ensure circulation is adequate; if not, treat as per *HYPOTENSION* above. Check patient's colour for cyanosis or erythema (suggesting allergic reaction).
- *O (Oxygen supply and Oxygen analyser):* Increase FiO_2 (to 100% if hypoxia severe) and ensure the O_2 analyser shows a rising concentration of O_2 distal to the common gas outlet. Always consider a contaminated O_2 supply. If contamination is suspected, use cylinder O_2. If no cylinder O_2, use your own expired O_2.
- *V (Ventilation and Vaporiser):* Ventilate lungs by hand to assess lung compliance, circuit integrity, and airway patency. Look at chest expansion and perform auscultation to detect wheezing/asymmetrical breath sounds. If unilateral chest expansion, consider endobronchial intubation, pneumothorax or sputum plugging of bronchus. Consider urgent chest X-ray/fibre-optic bronchoscopy. See *PNEUMOTHORAX*. Check capnography trace. If expired CO_2 low consider pulmonary embolus or decreased cardiac output. Check vaporiser setting.

H

- *E (Endotracheal tube and Eliminate)*: Check ET tube for patency/kinks. Pass suction tubing down the ET tube and suck out secretions. Consider ET tube cuff herniation (deflate cuff), bronchial/oesophageal intubation, tracheal tear (tube passes through cords but tip of tube lies outside trachea). 'When in doubt, take it out', i.e. replace tube. 'Eliminate' the anaesthetic machine if a contaminated O_2 supply is suspected, or undiagnosed equipment problem is occurring. Use self-inflating bag and cylinder O_2 to ventilate the patient. For example, a near-fatal tension pneumothorax occurred at Westmead Hospital due to kinked expiratory limb tubing.
- *R (Review Monitors and Equipment)*: Review all monitors, especially pulse oximetry, capnography ECG, BP. Check for hyperthermia and exclude malignant hyperpyrexia. Review all equipment, including surgical equipment, e.g. gas insufflation for laparoscopy may be causing embolus.
- *A (Reassess Airway)*
- *B (Reassess ventilation)*
- *C (Reassess Circulation)*: Must ensure adequate pulse and blood pressure.
- *D (Drug effect)*, e.g. formation of methaemoglobin by drugs such as prilocaine. If the cause of hypoxia is still not apparent move onto *A SWIFT CHECK* algorithm. See *COVER ABCD CRISIS MANAGEMENT ALGORITHM.*

Ii

Infraorbital Nerve Block

Anatomy

Supplies sensory innervation to the lower eyelid, cheek, upper lip and side of nose. Emerges from the infra-orbital foramen 1.5 cm below the inferior orbital rim. This foramen lies ≈ 2 cm from the lateral border of the nose and is in line with the pupil when the eye is in the neutral position.

Technique

The nerve can be blocked by passing a 23 G needle through the skin 0.5 cm below the foramen and injecting at the orifice. Alternatively, the needle can be inserted through the mucosa adjacent to the upper gum and aimed towards the palpating finger of the opposite hand held over the foramen. Inject 2 mL of LA solution (e.g. lignocaine 2% solution).

Inguinal Field Block

Used for inguinal hernia repair. Inguinal region supplied by:

1 *iliohypogastric nerve (L1)*. Innervates the suprapubic skin and the skin immediately above the inguinal ligament.

2 *ilioinguinal nerve (L1)*. Supplies the skin of the scrotum (or labium) and adjacent upper thigh.

3 *genitofemoral nerve*. The genital branch supplies the skin over scrotum (or labium) and adjacent thigh while the femoral branch supplies the skin over the upper part of the femoral triangle.

Technique (as described by Dr C. Sparkes et al.)[1]

1 Draw a line between the anterior superior iliac spine (ASIS) and the umbilicus.

2 2 cm from the ASIS along this line, sterilise and anaesthetise the skin and puncture the skin with a 19 G needle.

3 Insert a 22 G short bevelled (SB) needle at this point 90° to skin. After ≈ 1 cm a 'pop' is felt.

4 Inject 7 mL of lignocaine 1% + 1:200 000 adrenaline (to anaesthetise *iliohypogastric nerve*). Insert the needle another 0.5 cm. A second 'pop' is felt and there is 'loss of resistance' (LOR) to injection. Inject 8 mL of LA (to anaesthetise the *ilioinguinal nerve*).

5 Next, identify the mid-inguinal point, anaesthetise the skin 1 cm cephalad to this point, and make a hole in the skin as above. Insert the SB needle until two 'pops' are felt and there is again LOR to injection (at a depth of ≈ 4 cm). Inject 25 mL of LA solution (to block *genitofemoral nerve*).

6 Ask surgeon to mark the line of incision on the patient's skin and infiltrate along this line with 20 mL of 0.5% lignocaine + adrenaline using a 9 cm 22 G spinal needle. At the lateral end of the incision line inject a further 3 mL of LA subcutaneously in the direction of umbilicus.

7 The surgeon may need to supplement the block with additional LA intra-operatively.

8 Consider an additional 5–10 mL of LA injection around pubic tubercle percutaneously.

Insulin/Glucose Infusion

See *DIABETES MELLITUS, PREPARATION FOR SURGERY*.

Intercostal Drain

See *CHEST DRAIN*.

Intercostal Nerve Block

Anatomy

The *intercostal nerve* lies in the intercostal groove at the lower edge of each rib. T2–T6 supply the chest and T7–T11 the abdomen (sensory and motor innervation).

Technique

The best access to the intercostal nerve is behind the mid-axillary line.

1   Using a sterile technique, pull the skin cephalad over the rib and insert a 23 G sharp-bevelled needle at 90° to the skin. Anaesthetise the skin, then walk the needle off the lower border of the rib.
2   At edge of the rib, angle the needle cephalad and insert the needle no more than 2 mm so that the point is in the intercostal groove.
3   If aspiration is negative inject 3–5 mL of bupivacaine 0.5% + adrenaline 1:200 000. The block will last 6–10 h.

Note: The blocks are done more easily with the patient prone or sitting.

Complications

1   Pneumothorax.
2   Inadequate ventilation due to intercostal muscle paralysis.
3   Systemic LA toxicity due to intravascular injection.
4   Inadvertant subdural or epidural injection producing hypotension and/or extensive blockade.

Multilevel Intercostal Blockade with a Single Injection

Extensive intercostal blockade can be achieved with a single injection with a similar effect to intrapleural blockade. In a technique described by Murphy, local anaesthetic is deposited in a tissue plain

between the internal intercostalis aponeurosis and the deeper intercostalis intimus muscles.[2]

▶ Technique

1 Identify the intercostal site appropriate for the surgical incision.

2 Insert a 23 G sharp-bevelled needle at the angle of the rib
   ($\approx$ 6 cm from the midline posteriorally).

3 Contact the rib, then walk the needle off the lower border.
   Insert the needle a further 3–5 mm under the rib. The needle
   should have pieced the aponeurosis of the internal intercostalis muscle.

4 Inject 10–15 mL of LA e.g. ropivacaine 10 mg/mL.

Internal Jugular Vein Catheterisation

Anatomy

The internal jugular vein (IJV) originates from the jugular foramen
at the base of the skull and terminates between and behind the clavicular and sternal heads of the sternomastoid muscle where it joins
the subclavian vein. At its origin the IJV lies posterior to the internal
carotid artery but as it descends it becomes lateral to the common
carotid artery (CCA). The vagus nerve lies between and posterior to
the two vessels.

Technique

Position the patient supine without a pillow and with the head
turned slightly to the contralateral side with the bed tilted 10–20°
Trendelenburg. There are two main approaches. Use strict aseptic
technique + LA infiltration in the awake patient.

▶ High Approach

1 Identify the midpoint between the mastoid process and the ipsilateral sternoclavicular joint. Palpate the carotid artery at this
   level. The IJV should lie just lateral to this pulsation.

2　Use a 23 G 'seeker' needle to identify the IJV. Be careful not to compress the vein while palpating the carotid pulse. Aim in the direction of the ipsilateral nipple.

3　After identifying the IJV with the seeker needle leave this needle in place and insert an 18 G cannula or a needle suitable for insertion of the guide wire. Insert this cannula/needle parallel and alongside the seeker needle. Insert the guide wire through cannula/needle and remove the latter.

4　After using a scalpel to nick the skin insert the dilator over the wire and dilate the tract to the IJV. Remove the dilator and then insert the central venous catheter over the wire. Never lose sight of the distal end of the wire. *Never insert the catheter without holding the distal end of wire.*

5　Ensure blood can be aspirated from each lumen and flush each lumen with heparinised saline, then *close off each lumen.*

6　Suture the catheter into position. For an adult this will be at ≈ 15 cm for a right IJ line and ≈ 17 cm for a left IJ line. Apply a sterile dressing.

7　Perform a postprocedure chest X-ray to check the position of the catheter tip. The tip should lie in the SVC, above the level of the carina.[3]

▶ Low Approach

1　Position the patient as above and identify the sternal and clavicular heads of the sternomastoid muscle.

2　Insert the 23 G 'seeker' needle at 45° to the skin, parallel with the long axis of the body, at the apex of the triangle formed by these two muscle heads. Use a stabbing motion to penetrate the IJV, which normally lies in this gap closer to the clavicular than the sternal head. The IJV usually lies at a depth of 0.5–2 cm.

3　Once the vein is identified leave the seeker needle in place. Insert an 18 G cannula or a needle suitable for insertion of the guide wire parallel and alongside the seeker needle. Then proceed as above.

▶ *Aids to Success*

1 The diameter of the internal jugular vein can be increased by a Valsalva manoeuvre, IPPV, PEEP and increasing head down tilt.[4]

2 Hand-held Doppler probes or larger ultrasound machines can be used to identify vein position. In 5.5% of patients the internal jugular vein is positioned remotely from the usual landmarks described above.[4]

▶ *Complications of Internal Jugular Vein Catheterisation*

1 If the tip of the central venous catheter lies within the pericardium, cardiac tamponade may occur.[5]

2 Carotid artery puncture.

3 Haemorrhage with possible airway compromise.

4 Infection.

5 Pleural puncture.

International Normalised Ratio (INR)

The INR was developed to improve comparability of measures of prothrombin time (PT) between laboratories. INR thus correlates with PT, which measures the effectiveness of the *extrinsic* clotting pathway. Normal range (NR) for PT is 10–12 s, NR for INR is 0.8–1.2. Both INR and PT are elevated by deficiencies or abnormalities of clotting factors II, V, VII, X such as in the presence of warfarin therapy. The recommended INRs for standard and high dose anticoagulant therapies are 2.0–3.0 and 2.5–3.5 respectively.

Interosseous Puncture

Useful for obtaining immediate access to intravascular space when venous cannulation has failed, in children less than 5–6 years old. A 16 G bone marrow biopsy needle or a Cook interosseous needle is used.

Technique

1 Surgically prep the insertion area, which lies on the anteromedial surface of the tibia ≈ 2–3 cm below the tibial tuberosity.

2 Use LA to anaesthetise skin and deeper structures.

3 Insert the needle with a screwing motion through the bony cortex, angling away from the joint and epyphyseal plate. There is a sensation of 'loss of resistance' as the marrow cavity is entered.

4 Aspiration of bone marrow confirms proper placement. Inject a test dose of saline 10 mL. This should inject freely.

5 Injection of certain drugs such as sodium bicarbonate via the interosseous route is controversial because of the increased risk of tissue necrosis and osteomyelitis associated with hypertonic solutions.[6]

Note: Other sites of insertion that have been utilised include the distal tibia, distal femur, iliac crest and sternum.

Intra-arterial Injection

Effects of Intra-arterial Drug Injection

The effects of intra-arterial drug injection depend on the type of drug injected. Examples from the literature include:

1 *Buprenorphine*: Intra-arterial injection produced peripheral cyanosis.[7]

2 *Diazepam*: Intra-arterial diazepam has resulted in effects similar to thiopentone with ischaemia and tissue necrosis.

3 *Etomidate*: No significant effects from intra-arterial injection.[8]

4 *Flucloxacillin*: Intra-arterial flucloxacillin can produce severe reactions with arterial vasospasm and peripheral gangrene.[9]

5 *Midazolam*: Does not appear to be hazardous.[10,11]

6 *Morphine*: Does not appear to be hazardous.

7 *Propofol*: Intra-arterial propofol has resulted in pain, local blanching and a transient decrease (5 min) in blood flow to the

distal limb. Significant limb morbidity appears less likely than with thiopentone.[12]

8   *Thiopentone*: Can also cause severe vasospasm and gangrene.

Treatment of Intra-arterial Drug Injection Producing Sequelae

1   Remove any residual drug from the line, leave the arterial cannula in situ and flush with saline.

2   Look for any evidence of vascular spasm. If this does occur, consider the following vasodilators:[10]

   (a) Papaverine 40–80 mg in 20 mL N/S intra-arterially

   (b) Tolazoline 25–50 mg intra-arterially

   (c) Reserpine 1.25 mg IV

   (d) Phenoxybenzamine 0.5 mg IV.

3   Intra-arterial guanethidine has been used effectively. The dose is 5 mg in 5 mL N/S.[9]

4   Iloprost, a thromboxane inhibitor. This was used to treat a buprenorphine arterial injection (combined with a dextran 40 infusion).[7]

5   Dextran 40 infusion to improve microcirculation in the ischaemic area.[7] See *DEXTRAN*.

6   Consider urokinase intra-arterially.

7   Stellate ganglion block, brachial plexus block.

Flushing the cannula with procaine, phentolamine or heparinised saline is *not* of proven benefit.[13]

Intracranial Pressure (ICP) and Treatment of Raised ICP

ICP is defined as the pressure in the lateral ventricle or in the subarachnoid space over the convexity of the cerebral cortex. Normal ICP is $\approx$ 13 cmH_2O or 10 mmHg. 20–25 cmH_2O ICP is equivocal while > 25 cmH_2O (18 mmHg) is 'high'.

Methods of Reducing Raised ICP

1 Exclude hypoxia and hypercapnia and ensure optimal patient oxygenation.

2 Elevate the head 15–30°. Keep the head in the neutral position. Ensure that there is no venous obstruction at the neck due to e.g. endotracheal tube tied around the neck too tightly.

3 Ensure adequate muscle relaxation, as increased thoracic and abdominal muscle tone may increase ICP.

4 Hyperventilate the patient to an end tidal expired CO_2 concentration of 30 mmHg. Check $PaCO_2$ on arterial blood gas analysis. Excessive hyperventilation may lead to cerebral ischaemia.[14]

5 Mannitol 20% 0.25–1.5 g/kg IV. The dose given depends on the severity of the situation. Give mannitol over 20 min, as it may cause hypotension if given faster.[14] Its effects start within 10 min and peak at about 1 h. If ICP remains persistently raised, give 0.25–0.5 g/kg mannitol every 6 h. Effects of mannitol are enhanced by the addition of frusemide 0.3 mg/kg IV.[14] Frusemide can also be used instead of mannitol in a dose of 1 mg/kg.

6 Give steroids if raised ICP is due to a brain tumour. Give dexamethasone 16 mg IV LD, then 4 mg 6 h.

7 Cease N_2O and volatile anaesthetic agent as these drugs may contribute to raised ICP.[15] Substitute N_2O and volatile anaesthetic agent with a propofol infusion for maintenance of anaesthesia.

8 Consider boluses of thiopentone.

9 Removal of CSF may produce a marked improvement.

Intra-operative Myocardial Ischaemia

See *MYOCARDIAL ISCHAEMIA, INTRA-OPERATIVE.*

Intrapleural Anaesthesia

This technique involves repeated injection of LA into the pleural space via a catheter, and can be used for postoperative analgesia and for the treatment of pain associated with chest drains.

Technique

1   Place the patient lateral with the side to be anaesthetised uppermost.
2   Aseptically prep the skin around the point of insertion, which is 10 cm lateral to the spinous processes at the sixth, seventh or eighth ribs.
3   Anaesthetise the skin and deeper tissues if the patient is awake, then insert an 18 G Tuohy needle to contact the superior surface of the rib. Remove the stylet and attach a 10 mL syringe (without the piston) filled with sterile saline.
4   Advance the needle slowly over the superior surface of the rib. When the pleural space is penetrated the saline will be sucked into the pleural space. Usually a 'pop' sensation is felt.[16]
5   Insert an epidural catheter 5–6 cm into the pleural space and secure.
6   Check postprocedure chest X-ray for pneumothorax.
7   Kits are available for pleural anaesthesia, such as the Arrow Intrapleural Set.

Dose

For adults, inject 20 mL of 0.5% bupivacaine with adrenaline 1:200 000 every 4–6 h. Inject with the patient in the supine position for 30 min.

For Patients Requiring a Chest Drain For Pneumothorax[17]

1   Insert an epidural catheter 5–10 cm into the pleural space dorsal to, and in the same intercostal space as, the chest drain.

2   Use the Tuohy needle for insertion as described above.
3   Inject bupivacaine through the pleural catheter as above, with the patient in a supine position for 30 min and the chest drain clamped for 10 min if on suction.

Intrapleural Catheter

See *CHEST DRAIN*.

Intrathecal Anaesthesia

See *SUBARACHNOID BLOCK*.

Intra-uterine Foetal Death

Intra-uterine foetal death can be associated with disseminated intravascular coagulopathy (DIC), probably due to the release of foetal thromboplastin. DIC rarely occurs unless the dead foetus has been retained for days or weeks, and delivery soon after foetal death will usually prevent DIC occurring.[18]

Intravenous Regional Anaesthesia

See *BIER BLOCK*.

Intubating Laryngeal Mask

See *LARYNGEAL MASK AIRWAY (INCLUDING PROSEAL AND FAST-RACH)*.

Isoflurane

Halogenated methyl ether inhalational anaesthetic agent.

Physical Properties and MAC

Blood:gas solubility coefficient	1.4
Oil:gas solubility coefficient	91

Saturated vapour pressure at 20°C	239 mmHg (32 kPa)
Boiling point	48.5°C
MAC	1.15

Advantages

Potent anaesthetic agent suitable for virtually all types of surgery.

Disadvantages

1 May have a 'coronary steal' effect, but the clinical significance of this is unclear.
2 Pungent odour makes isoflurane unsuitable for gaseous induction.
3 Isoflurane, like sevoflurane, significantly prolongs the QT heart rate corrected (QTc) interval.[19] It should not be used in patients presenting with a prolonged QTc interval due to the risk of precipitating torsade de pointes.

Isoprenaline

Synthetic catecholamine used for the treatment of complete heart block until transvenous pacing can be arranged. Acts on β adreno-receptors, thus causing positive cardiac inotropy and chronotropy. There are no significant α adreno-receptor effects.

Preparation

Mix 2 mg of isoprenaline with 50 mL of 5% glucose resulting in a concentration of 40 µg/mL.

Dose

Adult: 20 µg bolus IV. Repeat according to the clinical response. If an infusion is required, give 1–10 µg/min (1.5–15 mL/h of the above solution).
Child: 0.02–0.15 µg/kg/min.

Jj

Jehovah's Witnesses (JW)[1]

> 'Therefore I say, unto the children of Israel, ye
> shall eat the blood of no manner of flesh: for the
> life of all flesh is the blood thereof: whoever eateth
> it shall be cut off' (Levictus;17:10–16.)

Due to their religious beliefs, Jehovah's Witness (JW) patients may
absolutely refuse blood transfusion and transfusion of blood derivatives. At the time of writing there are about 62 000 JWs in Australia,
plus another 50 000 associates. Associates are people who are participating in JW activities, but who have not yet fully decided to
adopt all JW beliefs.

Jehovah's Witness Hospital Liaison Committees
These committees are international and there are, at the time of
writing, 15 in Australia, providing extensive national coverage.
Representatives from these committees can provide useful mediation
between JW patients and medical care providers.

JW Patients Will Accept
Non-blood IV fluids such as N/S, Hartmann's solution and volume
expanders such as haemaccel and dextran.

JW Patients Will *Not* Accept
- Whole blood or packed cells.
- Platelets.
- Plasma.
- Predonation of patient's own blood for later use.
- Intra-operative storage of the patient's own blood for later transfusion.

JW Patients *May or May Not* Accept (Depending on Personal Beliefs)

- Immunoglobulins.
- Haemophiliac preparations such as Factor VIII albumin.
- Systems involving a continuous extracorporeal blood circuit, including cardiac bypass systems, haemodilution, renal dialysis, blood salvage and reinfusion systems. There *must be* a continuous connection between the patient and the extracorporeal blood. There must be no storage. When cardiac bypass is used there should be non-blood prime.
- Organ transplant
- Cell saver devices (noting that these do not maintain circulation continuity).[2]
- Epidural blood patch, provided there is a connection between the venous blood and the epidural space by tubing.[3]

JW Adults and the Law

Competent adult patients have an absolute right to refuse any aspect of medical treatment. The reasons for this refusal are irrelevant. If a competent adult is treated against his or her will then the tort (civil wrong) of battery is committed.[2] For an elective case, the anaesthetist can refuse to be involved. In an emergency case the anaesthetist is bound ethically, medicolegally and contractually to treat the JW (or any other) patient. The anaesthetist should discuss with the JW patient alone exactly what he or she will or will not accept related to blood and blood products and the possible consequences of such refusal, including death. This discussion should be clearly documented in the medical record, signed by the patient, and this should be witnessed by another doctor.

In an emergency, if the specific wishes of the unconscious patient are not known, then the patient must be treated according to the clinical judgment of the doctors involved and the defence of medical necessity applies.[2] Under these circumstances a life-saving blood transfusion could be given. If the patient is semiconscious and refuses blood the attending doctor must decide whether the patient is competent. If the decision is made that the patient is not competent then emergency treatment, including life-saving blood transfusion, is defensible.

JW Children

In broad terms, medicolegally in Australia, a child is defined as being under the age of 18 years. For JW parents, it is extremely distressing and disturbing to their religious values for their child to have a blood transfusion or receive blood products.

If blood transfusion or blood products (or any other treatment) are required for a *life-threatening indication* for a JW child, then such treatment should be instituted and there should not be a negative medicolegal result. Such actions are covered by the *Children and Young Persons (Care and Protection Act) 1998*. The medical superintendent should be involved in this type of situation.

If blood or blood fractions are required but such treatment is not 'necessary as a matter of urgency', such treatment cannot be administered without parental consent or an order of the court. Again, the Jehovah's Witness Hospital Liaison Committee representative can be an invaluable mediator in these situations.

See *BLOOD LOSS PREVENTION*.

Jet Ventilation

See *TRANSTRACHEAL JET VENTILATION*.

Kk

Ketamine

Phencyclidine derivative, used as an intravenous, intramuscular or oral anaesthetic agent and for its analgesic effects. It is particularly useful:

1 for induction of anaesthesia in patients with compromised CVS function, e.g. shocked patients, elderly patients
2 as a sole anaesthetic agent for brief procedures such as change of burns dressings
3 for anaesthesia in developing countries with limited resources
4 for analgesia
5 as an oral premedication drug.

Ketamine is a NMDA receptor antagonist and probably has agonist effects at opioid receptors.[1]

Advantages

1 Causes cardiovascular system stimulation due to sympathetic nervous system enhancement. Baroreceptor function is well maintained.
2 Causes bronchodilation and has been used successfully in the treatment of asthma. Mild respiratory stimulation occurs and airway reflexes are relatively preserved (compared to other IV anaesthetic agents).
3 Ketamine has potent analgesic properties even at sub-anaesthetic doses.
4 Can be given IM, which is particularly useful for situations such as the uncooperative patient.

Disadvantages

1 Ketamine has a slow onset of action, and pain may occur on injection (IV and IM).
2 Sudden jerky movements or hypertonus may occur, interfering with surgery.
3 Disturbing emergence reactions, such as unpleasant dreams and hallucinations, may be experienced.
4 Excessive salivation may occur (alleviated by antsialogogue premedication), and postoperative nausea and vomiting are common.
5 Causes increased intra-ocular pressure and intracranial pressure.
6 Subject to abuse.

Dose for Anaesthesia

1.5–2 mg/kg IV. Onset of action takes about 30 s and lasts 5–10 min. IM dose is 10 mg/kg. Onset of action 2–8 min; effects last 10–20 min. For brief, painful procedures in adults, such as movement of a fractured limb, 10–20 mg IV boluses can be given, titrated to effect.

IV Infusion for Anaesthesia

Ketamine can be used to maintain anaesthesia in a dose of 10–30 µg/kg/min. However, other agents such as propofol will usually be more appropriate.[2]

Use for Analgesia in Patient Controlled Analgesia

Mix ketamine and morphine on a mg for mg basis. See *PATIENT-CONTROLLED ANALGESIA*.

Use by Continuous Infusion for Analgesia

Use with a morphine infusion. Give ketamine 0.5 mg/kg as a bolus, then an infusion of 2–10 µg/kg/min.

Subcutaneous Infusion for Analgesia

Ketamine has been used for pain relief for musculoskeletal trauma at a dose of 0.1 mg/kg/h.[1]

K

Oral Dose as a Premedication Drug

6–7 mg/kg is an effective pre-operative sedative in children, taking effect in 15–30 min.[3] Ketamine should be mixed with a sweet liquid due to its awful taste. It is claimed that emergence problems with ketamine are less frequent in children.[4] Oral secretions may be excessive and an antsialogogue is recommended.[5] In children having upper airway procedures, there may also be an increased incidence of stridor and laryngospasm in the recovery room.[5]

Ketorolac

Non-steroidal anti-inflammatory drug with strong analgesic activity.

Dose

Over 65 years old: 10–15 mg IM, then 10–15 mg IM 4–6 h. Maximum daily dose 60 mg

Under 65 years old: 10–30 mg IM, then 10–30 mg 4–6 h. Maximum daily dose 90 mg

Advantages

Potent analgesic drug in a parenteral form.

Disadvantages

1 Non-selective COX inhibitor.
2 There have been several reports of renal failure associated with its use, even in young patients without other risk factors.[6]
3 There is an increased risk of peptic ulcer disease and GIT haemorrhage, particularly in older patients on prolonged therapy.

Precautions

Do not use for more than 5 days. Do not use in patients with dehydration, hypovolaemia, moderate to severe renal dysfunction, bleeding diatheses, anticoagulant therapy or hypersensitivity to ketorolac. See *NON-STEROIDAL ANTI-INFLAMMATORY DRUGS*.

Westmead Hospital Policy on Ketorolac

Due to the potential for significant side effects with ketorolac, the lowest effective dose is recommended. For adults this is 10 mg IM as required up to 6 h for 48 h.

K

Ll

Labetalol

Selective antagonist at β1 and β2 adreno-receptors and to a lesser extent at α1 receptors. It is used for the treatment of all grades of hypertension and is useful in the treatment of pre-eclampsia. Can be given IV or PO.

Dose

Adult: 5–20 mg boluses IV injected over 2 min, up to a total dose of 200 mg. Acts in 5–30 min and is effective for about 50 min. Can also be given by infusion (in glucose or glucose/saline) at a rate of 20–160 mg/h IV.

Child: 1–2 mg/kg IV dose (max. 100 mg). See *HYPERTENSIVE RESPONSE TO INTUBATION (ATTENUATION OF)*.

Lactate

NR 0.3–1.3 mmol/L. Elevated serum lactate levels can occur with tissue hypoxia. Serum lactate correlates well with the degree of hypovolaemic shock due to haemorrhage. A level of over 9 mmol/L is associated with a 75% mortality in ruptured abdominal aortic aneurysm patients.[1]

Laparoscopic Surgery

Laparoscopic cholecystectomy was first described in 1989.[2] An ever-increasing number of procedures are being carried out this way, including fundoplication, nephrectomy and oesophagectomy.

The main issues in laparoscopic surgery are:
- the physiological effects of pneumoperitoneum
- complications associated with the insertion of Verres needle blindly into the peritoneal cavity
- complications due to gas insufflation into the tissues or a blood vessel.

Induction Phase—To Intubate or Not Intubate

There is an increased risk of regurgitation with pneumoperitoneum.[3] In the past almost all patients having laparoscopic surgery were paralysed, intubated and ventilated. LMAs have been used successfully for laparoscopic procedures but it is recommended that they only be used for short procedures (e.g. laparoscopic sterilisation) in patients without other aspiration risks.

Since its introduction in 2000, the LMA-ProSeal is being used increasingly for laparoscopic surgery as it offers greater protection against aspiration compared to the LMA-Classic. Although most patients are still being paralysed and intubated, this is an evolving area and each individual anaesthetist must decide on a technique they feel is safe in their hands.

For patients having laparoscopic cholecystectomy insert an orogastric tube to deflate the stomach.

Gas Insufflation Phase

For abdominal surgery gas is insufflated into the peritoneal cavity to provide physical and visual access.

Insertion of the Verres needle may cause trauma to blood vessels or other structures.

Gas insufflation is provided by high-flow insufflators with gas flows of 4–6 L/min. Complications that can occur at this stage include:

1 gas embolism due to placement of the Verres needle into a blood vessel. See *GAS EMBOLISM, VENOUS*.

2   Subcutaneous emphysema, pneumothorax and/or pneumome-
    diastinum may occur. The surgeon must cease insufflation
    immediately. Subcutaneous emphysema can result in increased
    end tidal CO_2 measurements but without increased airway pres-
    sure, unless a pneumothorax is also present. Management of
    subcutaneous emphysema includes increasing minute ventila-
    tion to maintain acceptable end tidal/$PaCO_2$ levels, ceasing
    N_2O in the inhaled gas mixture and reassuring the patient after
    surgery.

3   A vagally mediated bradycardia may occur as the peritoneum
    is stretched. This can be severe enough to produce asystole.[4] In
    this situation tell the surgeon to stop insufflation and let out all
    the gas. Give atropine 0.6 mg. If asystole persists see *CARDIAC
    ARREST*.

Intra–operative Phase

1   There is a potential risk of the tip of the endotracheal tube
    migrating into a bronchus with pneumoperitoneum, especially
    with Trendelenburg positioning.[5]

2   Avoid high pressure IPPV and PEEP as this can result in a
    marked reduction in cardiac output in the presence of pneumo-
    peritoneum.[6]

3   Do not allow intra-abdominal pressure (IAP) to rise above 20
    mmHg. This can result in a severe reduction in venous return,
    causing reduced cardiac output. Renal function may also be
    impaired with decreased renal blood flow and glomerular filtra-
    tion rate.[6] An IAP of 15 mmHg is sufficient for most procedures.[6]

4   Functional residual capacity and pulmonary compliance
    are reduced by the pneumoperitoneum.[6] Airway resistance
    is increased.[6] Hypercapnia may occur due to absorption of
    insufflated CO_2. The effects of hypercapnia include tachycar-
    dia, dysrhythmias and reduced systemic vascular resistance.
    Treat with increased ventilation rate.

5 There is an increased risk of embolisation to the cerebral circulation during gynaecological laparoscopic procedures through a patent foramen ovale.[7] A patent foramen ovale is present in about 27% of the population.[8] This predisposition to cerebral embolisation is due to the interaction of pneumoperitoneum, head down tilt and IPPV, resulting in relatively higher pressures in the right atrium than the left atrium.[9] This risk can be reduced by IV fluid loading, e.g. with 500 mL of colloid.[9]

6 Concealed intra-operative haemorrhage can occur at any stage. Have a low index of suspicion for haemorrhage and always have adequate IV access.

7 If N_2O is used for pneumoperitoneum, fire or explosion can occur in the peritoneal cavity with diathermy or laser. CO_2 does not support combustion.

8 If the light cable is disconnected from laparoscope, do not allow the distal end to burn the patient.

9 N_2O in the anaesthetic gas mixture may increase nausea and vomiting postoperatively, especially after gynaecological laparoscopic surgery.[6]

Postoperative Concerns

Up to 62% of patients suffer postoperative nausea and vomiting after laparoscopic cholecystectomy.[10] Consider prophylactic anti-nausea medication such as ondansetron 4 mg + dexamethasone 8 mg given intra-operatively. See *NAUSEA AND VOMITING, PREVENTION AND TREATMENT*. NSAIDs such as parecoxib 40 mg may also be useful by reducing requirements for opioid analgesics.

Laryngeal Anatomy

See *LARYNX, ANATOMY AND INNERVATION*.

Laryngeal Mask Airway (including ProSeal and Fastrach)

Topics Covered in this Section
▶ The LMA-Classic
▶ The LMA-ProSeal
▶ The Fastrach Intubating LMA

The LMA-Classic

The LMA-Classic is a cuffed mask designed to fit over the laryngeal inlet and provide an airway for anaesthesia and resuscitation. It does not protect the trachea from aspiration of gastric contents and is usually used for spontaneously breathing patients. Although it is possible to ventilate patients through the LMA,[11] inflation of the stomach will occur if ventilatory pressures become too high.[12] Therefore, if IPPV is used with the LMA, airway resistance and pulmonary compliance should be normal.[12] See Table L1.

▶ LMA and Difficult Intubation

The LMA can be used to provide a conduit for intubation, by:

1 passing an endotracheal tube through the LMA directly. See *DIFFICULT AIRWAY MANAGEMENT*. The vocal cords will lie about 3 cm from the mask aperture. By using a size 6.0 micro-laryngoscopy tube the extra length of this tube will further ensure correct placement of the endotracheal tube cuff below the vocal cords
   OR

2 passing a Teflon bougie through the LMA blindly into the trachea and then railroading the endotracheal tube over the bougie

Table L1 Appropriate LMA size for different-sized patients

Size	Inflate with	Weight of patient
1	Up to 4 mL	Neonate to 6.5 kg
1.5	Up to 7 mL	5–10 kg
2	Up to 10 mL	6.5–25 kg
2.5	Up to 14 mL	20–30 kg
3	Up to 20 mL	30 kg to small adult
4	Up to 30 mL	Small to medium adult
5	Up to 40 mL	70–100 kg
6	Up to 50 mL	100+ kg

OR

3 passing a fibre-optic bronchoscope through the LMA (with ET tube loaded on the scope) into the trachea, then railroading the tube into the trachea.

LMA-ProSeal

This device is similar to the classic laryngeal mask airway but features a modified cuff, a drainage tube and an integral bite block. The modified double cuff enables an improved seal over the laryngeal inlet to a pressure of ≈ 40–50 cmH$_2$O.[13] This is about twice the seal pressure of the classic LMA. The drainage tube runs from the distal tip of the cuff to the proximal end of the wire-reinforced airway tube. This acts as a channel for gastric fluid and gases, and also facilitates gastric tube placement. This device is designed for positive pressure ventilation. A dedicated introducer tool can be used to aid in correct placement of the LMA-ProSeal. See Table L2 overleaf.

Size	Maximum inflation volume	Weight of patient	Max. diameter of gastric tube
1.5	7 mL	5–10 kg	10 fr
2	10 mL	10–20 kg	10 fr
2.5	14 mL	20–30 kg	14 fr
3	20 mL	30–50 kg	16 fr
4	30 mL	50–70 kg	16 fr
5	40 mL	70–100 kg	18 fr

Table L2 Appropriate LMA-ProSeal size for different-sized patients

Half the inflation volumes quoted may be sufficient.

▶ *Techniques for Insertion of the LMA-ProSeal into the Anaesthetised Patient*

LMA-ProSeal Introducer Tool Insertion Technique[14]

1 Prepare the device by tightly deflating it. A purpose-made LMA ProSeal Cuff Deflator device can be used to achieve the correct wedge shape. Lubricate the posterior tip of the deflated cuff with a water soluble lubricant such as K-Y Jelly.

2 Insert the LMA-ProSeal Introducer. Place the tip of the introducer into the retaining strap at the rear of the cuff. Fold the LMA-ProSeal along the outer curve of the introducer and place the drain tube and airway tube into the appropriate slots.

3 Position the patient's head as for intubation (head extended on the neck, neck slightly flexed).

4 Press the tip of the LMA-ProSeal against the palate and slide the cuff in a rotational movement following the curve of the palate.

Advance the device into the hypopharynx until a definite resistance is felt. The cuff must press against the palate during the insertion manoeuvre.

5 Stabilise the device with one hand while removing the introducer with the other.

6 Inflate the cuff without holding the device, using the volumes described in Table L2. Do not exceed more than 60 cmH$_2$O inflation pressure.

▶ *Index Finger Insertion Technique[14]*

1 The LMA-ProSeal is prepared for insertion exactly as described above but without the introducer tool.

2 The index finger is placed in the strap of the LMA-ProSeal and the device is held like a pen.

3 Under direct vision the tip of the cuff is placed against the hard palate, or a slightly lateral approach can be used.

4 Slide the device inwards, extending the index finger, and pressing it towards the other hand, which holds the back of the head and provides counterpressure.

5 Continue advancing the device until resistance is felt. The index finger should be fully extended and the wrist fully flexed.

6 Grasp the distal end of the airway tube to stabilise the device while removing the hand in the mouth.

▶ *Checking that the LMA-ProSeal is Correctly Positioned*

There is a significant incidence of malposition of the LMA-ProSeal with the first insertion attempt, even in experienced hands. With the introducer tool the failure rate is 16% on the first attempt.[15] With digital insertion the failure rate is 12% on the first attempt.[15] The position of the LMA-ProSeal can be checked by:

1 inserting a small 'blob' of K-Y jelly into the drain tube. If this is expelled by squeezing the ventilation bag, the position is incorrect.

2 performing the suprasternal notch tap test. In this test a finger is tapped over the suprasternal notch. This should compress the distal end of the LMA-ProSeal drain tube and cause a blob of K-Y jelly in the drain tube to move up and down.

3 passing an orogastric tube through the drain tube of the ProSeal. If this passes easily, it suggests good positioning.

4 performing a leak test. In this test the adjustable pressure-limiting valve is closed and fresh gas flow (FGF) adjusted to 3 L/min. The pressure in the anaesthetic circuit connected to the ProSeal is allowed to rise. A rise to 30 mmHg without a leak suggests good positioning.

▶ A New Insertion Technique

This involves inserting the LMA-ProSeal over a gum elastic bougie (GEB).[15] The GEB is passed through the drain tube of the LMA-ProSeal and the distal end of the GEB is inserted into the oesophagus using gentle laryngoscopy with a laryngoscope. This is to prevent the GEB from entering the trachea.

This technique is very effective and prevents the tip of the ProSeal from rolling up. Successful insertion on the first attempt with this technique was 100% in one study.[15] This technique has obvious application to failed intubation management. See *DIFFICULT AIRWAY MANAGEMENT*.

▶ Other Points

1 If a gastric tube is used it must not be stiffened by refrigeration due to the potential for trauma.

2 If regurgitated fluid is expelled through the drain tube and the patient remains well oxygenated, it is advised to leave the LMA-ProSeal in place.[14] This is the intended function of the drain tube. Pass a gastric tube through the drain into the stomach so that it can be emptied.

3 Leave the taping on the device undisturbed until the patient is awake enough to remove the device.

4 The manufacturer recommends deflating the LMA-ProSeal prior to removal although some practitioners remove the device while still inflated.

▶ *The Future*

The role of the LMA-ProSeal continues to evolve. The device appears to be a satisfactory alternative to intubation for laparoscopic chole-cystectomy in selected patients.[16]

Fastrach Intubating LMA

This device is a type of laryngeal mask airway specifically designed as a ventilation device and a guide to tracheal intubation.[17,18] The Fastrach consists of an anatomically curved, short, wide-bore, stain-less steel tube sheathed in silicone. The steel tube is bonded to a laryngeal mask with a single, moveable aperture bar. The laryngeal mask comes in sizes 3, 4 and 5. The stainless steel tube is also bond-ed to a metal guiding bar. Specially designed sizes of silicone ET tube are available in 6, 6.5, 7, 7.5 and 8 mm.

▶ *Technique for Using the Intubating LMA-Fastrach*

1 The head and neck are placed in the neutral position, not the classic sniffing position.

2 The LMA-Fastrach is fully deflated and a bolus of water soluble lubricant (e.g. K-Y jelly) is applied to the posterior saucer shaped tip of the device.

3 The patient should be deeply anaesthetised, or the airway adequately anaesthetised in the awake patient. In most studies of LMA-Fastrach efficacy muscle relaxants were used.[19]

4 While holding the metal guiding bar (handle), the flattened tip of the LMA-Fastrach is placed against the hard palate and then inserted into the oropharynx by using a rotational movement in the sagittal plane.

5   Do not insert LMA-Fastrach to the 'hilt'. Observe for caudal displacement of the prominence of the thyroid cartilage.

6   Inflate the cuff moderately (size 3: 20 mL, size 4: 30 mL, size 5: 40 mL). An intracuff pressure of 60 cmH$_2$O is recommended.

7   The success rate of the LMA-Fastrach as a ventilation device on the first insertion attempt is almost 100%.[18]

8   The well-lubricated silicone ET tube is then passed through the LMA-Fastrach into the trachea. The longitudinal line on the ET tube should be facing the handle.

9   When the ET tube is inserted into the LMA-Fastrach to the transverse line, gently lift the larynx forward a few millimetres using the device's handle (the 'Chandy manoeuvre').

10 Then gently pass the ET tube into the trachea.

11 Intubation through the LMA-Fastrach is successful on the first attempt in about 50% of patients. With one to four adjustment manoeuvres the successful intubation rate is greater than 99%.[18]

12 Adjustment manoeuvres include the following:
    (a) Pull the LMA-Fastrach out 6 cm without deflating the cuff, then re-insert the device (up-down manoeuvre).[18]
    (b) Use a smaller or larger LMA-Fastrach.
    (c) Change the position of the LMA-Fastrach using the handle while the APL valve is closed and while squeezing the bag until optimal effective ventilation is obtained. Then reattempt insertion of the ET tube.
    (d) Rotate the ET tube.
    (e) Adjust the head-neck position.
    (f) Pull the LMA-Fastrach out slightly or inserting it slightly more deeply.

▶ *Points to Note*

1   For patients requiring in-line head and neck stabilisation in the neutral position it is easier to place the LMA-Fastrach than the

LMA-Classic.[20] However, the LMA-Fastrach causes significant segmental cervical spine movement and in patients with cervical spine injury this technique may be inappropriate.[21]

2   Intubation through the LMA-Fastrach is more likely to succeed on the first attempt in patients with predicted or known airway problems.[18]

3   If cricoid pressure is applied the success rate is reduced and cricoid pressure may have to be removed temporarily to allow intubation.

See *DIFFICULT AIRWAY MANAGEMENT*.

▶ *Fibre-optic Intubation and the LMA-Fastrach*

If using a fibre-optic bronchoscope through an intubating LMA, note that the FOB is not stiff enough to push the epiglottic elevation bar out of the way and the tip of the FOB will be deflected to the left or right. Therefore:

1   Pass the specially designed silicone endotracheal tube to just beyond the distal epiglottic elevation bar.

2   Then pass the FOB through the ET tube to visualise the vocal cords and proceed as described above.

Laryngeal Tube (LT)

Ventilatory device for use as an alternative to mask or endotracheal intubation, provided that protection of the airway against regurgitation is not required. This concept is quite similiar to the Combitube airway. The LT consists of a blind-ended, S-shaped tube with a proximal pharyngeal cuff and a distal oesophageal cuff, and a laryngeal ventilation hole. The pharyngeal cuff stabilises the tube and blocks off the naso- and oropharynx. The distal oesophageal tube blocks off the oesophagus. To insert:

1   Fully deflate and lubricate both cuffs.

2   Insert the tube centrally into the mouth until the middle

horizontal 'teeth' line of the tube is aligned with the teeth, or until a distinct resistance is felt.[22]

3 Inflate the cuffs to a pressure of 80 cmH$_2$O, through the single pilot tube, using the cuff pressure gauge provided.

4 When the tube position has settled press the red deflate valve to adjust to the desired pressure (60–70 cmH$_2$O).

5 Ventilate the patient. A ventilation pressure of 30 cmH$_2$O or greater is possible with this device.[23]

6 To remove the LT, deflate both cuffs and remove.

Table L3 Appropriate size of LT	
Patient	LT size
Newborn–6 kg	0
Infant 6–15 kg	1
Child 15–40 kg	2
Child, small adult 30–60 kg	3
Medium adult 50–90 kg	4
Large adult > 90 kg	5

Laryngeal Tube-Suction

This is a new type of laryngeal tube. It incorporates a separate channel from the proximal to the distal end of the device to enable the passage of a gastric tube. This can be used to deflate the stomach and aspirate any gastric fluid.

Laryngoscopy Grading

See Table L4.

Table L4 Cormack and Lehane classification of the view obtained at laryngoscopy[24]

Grade	View obtained
1	Full view of cords
2	Partial view of cords
3	Epiglottis only
4	Epiglottis not visible

Larynx, Anatomy and Innervation

Laryngeal Cartilages
See Figures L1 and L2. The laryngeal cartilages are the:
- thyroid cartilage, which has the thyroid notch anteriorly
- cricoid cartilage, which is shaped like a signet ring with the narrowest part facing anteriorly. Between the thyroid and cricoid cartilages is the cricothyroid membrane.
- the arytenoids cartilages, which are pyramidal in shape and articulate with the supero-lateral aspects of the cricoid cartilage
- the epiglottis, which is a leaf shaped cartilage attached at its lower end to the thyroid cartilage. The vocal cords run from the arytenoid cartilages to the posterior surface of the thyroid cartilage.
- corniculate cartilages, which are small nodules sitting on the arytenoid cartilages
- cuneiform cartilages, which are flakes of cartilage within the aryepiglottic folds.

Innervation of the Larynx
The larynx is innervated by the vagus nerve via the superior laryngeal nerve and the recurrent laryngeal nerve.

L

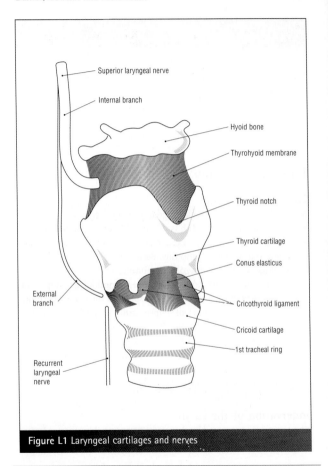

Figure L1 Laryngeal cartilages and nerves

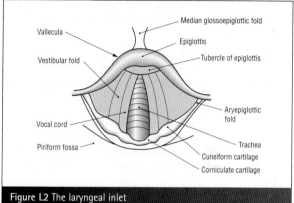

Figure L2 The laryngeal inlet

The superior laryngeal nerve supplies the interior of the larynx as far as the vocal cords.

The recurrent laryngeal nerve supplies the motor supply to the intrinsic muscles of the larynx (apart from the cricothyroid) and the sensory supply to the laryngeal mucosa inferior to the vocal cords.

Laser Surgery

Laser stands for Light Amplification by Stimulated Emission of Radiation.

Examples of Lasers Used Medically

1 CO_2 (wavelength 10 600 nm): used for coagulation and precision cutting.
2 Argon or krypton (wavelength 400–700 nm): used for photocoagulution in eye and skin surgery.

3   Neodymium yttrium-aluminium-garnet (Nd-YAG) (wavelength 1060 nm): used for tumour destruction and photocoagulation.

Precautions for Laser Surgery[25]

1   Protective glasses for staff, with appropriate tint for the type of laser used. CO_2 lasers are more likely to damage the cornea while Nd-YAG lasers are more likely to damage the retina.
2   Moist gauze protection for the patient's eyes.
3   If airway laser is required, use a laser-resistant endotracheal tube (e.g. wrapping the tube with aluminium foil tape), with methylene blue stained saline filling the cuff. Commercially available laser-resistant tubes include the Mallinckrodt Laser-Flex.
4   Use of gas mixtures that support combustion least, e.g. < 30% O_2 in N_2. Alternatively, use jet ventilation.
5   Sterile water/saline should be immediately available in a bucket to extinguish fire. See *TRACHEOSTOMY, ELECTIVE* for management of airway fire.
6   Adequate evacuation of laser plume.
7   All windows should be covered and warning signs displayed.
8   Theatre traffic should be minimised.

Lateral Cutaneous Nerve of Thigh Block

Anatomy

The *lateral cutaneous nerve of thigh* (L2, 3) arises from the lumbar plexus and divides into anterior and posterior branches.

Anterior branch supplies sensation to the skin over the anterolateral aspect of the thigh to the knee.

Posterior branch supplies the skin on the lateral side of the thigh just below the greater trochanter to the mid-thigh level.

Technique

1 Identify the anterior superior iliac spine. Identify the point 2.5 cm medial and 2.5 cm caudal to this landmark. The nerve lies below this point immediately beneath the fascia lata.

2 Sterilise and anaesthetise the skin, then insert a 23 G short bevelled needle in a 45° lateral direction. As the needle pierces the fascia lata a 'popping' sensation is felt.

3 Inject 3–5 mL of LA (e.g. lignocaine 2%) as the needle is slowly withdrawn; then another 3–5 mL is injected as the needle is reinserted more medially. Repeat until 15–20 mL of LA is injected from lateral to medial, above and below the fascia lata in a wall extending for about 5 cm.

Latex Allergy

Latex and Anaphylaxis

Latex accounts for about 12% of anaphylaxis under anaesthesia and is the second most common cause after NMBDs.[26]

Identifying Predisposed Patients

Attempt to identify patients who may be latex allergic and inquire specifically about latex allergy. Predisposed patients include:[27,28]

1 history suggesting latex allergy such as contact dermatitis due to washing up gloves. This is usually a type IV delayed hypersensitivity reaction. Other features on history suggesting latex allergy include tingling and swelling of lips when blowing up balloons, and wheeze and rhinitis in the presence of airborne rubber particles.

2 healthcare workers who routinely wear latex gloves

3 atopic patients and patients with hand eczema

4 spina bifida

5 patients with chronic urological illness requiring repeated catheterisation
6 spinal cord injury
7 patients allergic to exotic fruit such as avocados and papaya
8 patients with myelodysplasia[29]
9 workers in the rubber industry.

Preventing Latex Induced Allergic Reactions

▶ General Measures
1 Remove all latex-containing products from the operating theatre and make this case the first for the day. If emergency surgery, operate in a theatre that has not been in use for some hours.
2 Have latex allergy warning signs on the operating theatre doors and inside the operating theatre. Traffic through the theatre should be minimised.

▶ Gloves
All gloves used by staff must be of non-latex material. The use of non-latex gloves (e.g. neoprene) by the surgeon is the most important preventative measure.[30]

▶ Drug and Fluid Administration
1 Inject drugs via reflux valves and not through latex bungs on IV giving sets. Drugs such as antibiotics should not be drawn up through the rubber bung on the drug ampoule. Use glass syringes rather than rubber tipped plunger syringes.[28] Braun make a two-part, non-latex containing syringe,[30] and Terumo syringes are latex free.
2 Haemaccel containers include a rubber bung and there has been a report of anaphylaxis.[31]

▶ Anaesthetic Circuits and Airways
1 Non-latex containing anaesthetic circuits should be used. Plastic

and silicone products, e.g. a plastic Banes circuit with a silicone bag and mask, should be used.

2 Laryngeal mask airways, PVC endotracheal tubes and plastic Guedel airways are all safe. Do not use black airways.

▶ Ventilators

If a silicone ventilator bellows is not available, use a well-used latex set.[27] Washing the bellows may improve safety.

▶ Monitoring Issues

1 The blood pressure cuff should be placed over a soft cotton wrapping on the patient's skin.

2 Datex pulse oximeter probes contain latex; cover the finger with Tegaderm (3M) prior to application.[30]

3 Use Baxter or 3M ECG electrodes (latex free).[27]

▶ Tapes

Non-latex containing tapes include Micropore, Blenderm, and Steri-strips.[27]

▶ Prevention of Laetx Allergy

There is no evidence that allergy prophylaxis with drugs such as steroids and ranitidine is effective.[30]

Treatment of Latex Allergy

In addition to measures outlined in the section *ANAPHYLAXIS/ ANAPHYLACTOID REACTIONS*, remove all latex contact from the patient.

Investigation of Suspected Latex Allergy

1 Mast cell tryptase levels will often be elevated acutely (normal level 2 μg/L).[28]

2 Skin-prick testing by pricking the patient's skin through a latex glove or a suspension of latex glove particles. If the patient is allergic a wheal develops.[28]

3 Radioallergosorbent testing for latex-specific IgE antibodies is available, but is not as accurate as skin-prick testing.[29]

Left Ventricular Failure, Acute

See *PULMONARY OEDEMA*.

Levobupivacaine

This LA agent is the levo stereoisomer of bupivacaine.

Dose

Equivalent to bupivacaine[32] (see *BUPIVACAINE*). The maximum recommended dose in adults is 150 mg and 400 mg over 24 h.[32]

Advantages

About 30–50% less cardiotoxicity and CNS toxicity than racemic bupivacaine.

Levosimendan

Cardiotonic drug that causes increased cardiac contractility by enhancing the sensitivity of heart muscle to calcium.

Indications

Levosimendan is useful for treating acutely decompensated severe heart failure resistant to conventional therapy (diuretics, ACE inhibitors, digoxin and inotropes).

Contraindications

1 Renal and liver failure.
2 Severe hypotension and tachycardia.
3 History of torsade de pointes.

Dose

1 Mix 10 mL of levosimendan (2.5 mg/mL) with 500 mL of 5% glucose, making a solution of 0.05 mg/mL.

2   Give a loading dose of 12–24 µg/kg infused over 10 min–1 h,
    then an infusion of 0.1 µg/kg/min. If after 30–60 min exces-
    sive hypotension or tachycardia, decrease infusion rate to
    0.05 µg/kg/min. If initial infusion rate is well tolerated consider
    increasing infusion rate to 0.2 µg/kg/min.

Lightwand Intubation

The Trachlight type of lightwand is used as an example of this
technique.

Description of the Trachlight

The device consists of three parts:

1   a reusable handle. A locking clamp is located on the front of the
    handle that secures the ET tube connector.
2   a flexible wand with a bright light bulb at the distal end. This
    wand can be shortened or lengthened by a connecting/locking
    device located on the handle.
3   a stiff retractable stylet encased within the wand. This allows the
    wand to be shaped.

Steps in Lightwand Oral Intubation

1   Prepare the device by inserting the well-lubricated lightwand
    into the chosen ET tube so that the light bulb is positioned at the
    cuff end but not protruding from it. Lock the ET tube connector
    to the handle. Ensure that the stylet which is inserted into the
    lightwand is also well lubricated.
2   The distal end of the lightwand and tube are bent to 90° (the
    stylet keeps this shape).
3   The patient's head and neck are positioned in the neutral posi-
    tion or slightly head-extended position, *not the classic sniffing
    position used for direct laryngoscopy.*[33]
4   The patient must be adequately anaesthetised or have received
    adequate airway topical anaesthesia, prior to insertion of the
    device.

5   Use ambient light conditions unless the patient has a very thick neck.
6   The patient's jaw is lifted forward and the device is inserted exactly in the midline, with a rocking, arcing motion in the sagittal plane, aiming to place the tip at the thyroid prominence.
7   On entering the glottic opening there is a feeling of 'loss of resistance', and a well-defined glow just below the thyroid prominence should be seen. At this point pull the stylet back 10 cm and advance the wand and ET tube into the trachea. The glow should be seen to travel down the trachea and disappear below the sternal notch.
8   Release the ET tube from the connector and remove the wand from the ET tube.

Techniques for Improving Success[34]

1   Using a smaller than usual ET tube (e.g. size 6 mm for an adult female and a size 7 mm for an adult male) may help successful placement.
2   The length of the ET tube beyond the bend should approximate the distance from the pharynx and the cords.
3   The lightwand and ET tube are inserted into the mouth with the right hand, starting on the right side of the mouth (with the angled tip pointing left) and then rotating the wand medially.

Lignocaine

Amino-amide type LA agent and anti-arrhythmic drug. Presented in strengths of 0.5%–2% for local and regional anaesthesia and IV injection. In addition there are topical preparations including a 10% spray and 4% aqueous solution. See also *EMLA*.

Use and Dose as an Anti-arrhythmic

Lignocaine is a Class 1b anti-arrhythmic drug that slows conduction through ischaemic areas of the heart. In therapeutic doses lignocaine usually does not cause a reduction in myocardial contractility and blood pressure. Lignocaine is useful for the treatment of:

1 ventricular tachycardia, fibrillation
2 torsade de pointes.

Dose

Adult: 75–100 mg IV over 2 min, then infusion 4 mg/min for 1 h, then 2 mg/min for 1 h, then 1–2 mg/h subsequently. If initial bolus ineffective give a second bolus after 5 min of 1 mg/kg. The IV infusion rate is 15–50 μg/kg/min. The therapeutic serum level of lignocaine is 1–5 μg/mL.
Child: 1 mg/kg IV, then 15–50 μg/kg/min.

Use of Lignocaine as a Local Anaesthetic

These are approximate guidelines only:

* Maximum dose 4–5 mg/kg
* If adrenaline is added, then a higher maximum dose of 7–8 mg/kg of lignocaine can be given.

Dose for Decreasing the Haemodynamic Response to Intubation

Give 1.5 mg/kg IV 2–3 min before intubating.

Advantages

Lignocaine is suitable for all types of regional anaesthesia including IV limb anaesthesia (see *BIER BLOCK*). It is less cardiotoxic than bupivacaine or ropivacaine.

Disadvantages

1 Lignocaine is shorter acting than bupivacaine or ropivacaine.
2 Lignocaine 5% (+ 7.5% glucose), when used for subarachnoid block, has been associated with transient radicular irritation.[35]

Lorazepam

Benzodiazepine useful for:

1   pre-operative alleviation of anxiety, sedation and profound anterograde amnesia lasting up to 6 h
2   treatment of status epilepticus (IV). See *EPILEPSY, STATUS*.

It has a slow onset of action, taking up to 2–4 h.

Dose

1   For premedication give 50 µg/kg up to a maximum dose of 4 mg PO.
2   For seizures give 0.1 mg/kg IV.

Low Molecular Weight Heparins

See *HEPARIN, UNFRACTIONATED AND LOW MOLECULAR WEIGHT HEPARINS*.

Lower Segment Caesarean Section

See *CAESAREAN SECTION (CS)*.

Ludwig's Angina: Anaesthetic Management

Ludwig's angina is a soft tissue cellulitis of the floor of the mouth and neck, resulting in progressive airway compromise due to massive swelling. The infection source is usually the lower molar teeth. Aspiration of pus into the airways can also occur.

Presentation

The main symptoms and signs are:

- trismus, pain, dysphagia
- fever, septicaemia

- upper airway obstruction with dyspnoea, stridor, cyanosis and asphyxiation.

Anaesthetic Management

The anaesthetic management for securing the airway and surgical drainage involves the following.[36]

▶ Pre-anaesthetic Stage

1. *Antibiotic therapy.* The usual organism(s) are streptococci, staphylococci, *E. coli*, pseudomonas or mixed infections. Recommended antibiotics until the organism is known are clindamycin + penicillin (or ciprofloxacin) and metronidazole.[37]
2. Consider a drying agent such as glycopyrrolate.
3. Consider nebulised adrenaline to reduce airway swelling.
4. An ENT surgeon should be available for immediate tracheostomy.
5. Nasal fibre-optic laryngoscopy can be used to assess airway oedema and predict the difficulty of intubation.

▶ Anaesthetic Phase

Options for securing the airway are:

1. awake tracheostomy using local anaesthesia. A surgical airway risks spreading the infection to deep cervical and mediastinal tissues.
2. Awake fibre-optic intubation (see entry).
3. Gaseous induction using sevoflurane and oxygen. With the patient deep, direct laryngoscopy can be attempted.

Use an armoured (reinforced) tube as the submandibular swelling may compress an ordinary PVC tube.[37]

Blind nasal intubation should not be attempted due to the risk of causing bleeding, and abscess perforation with lung soiling and airway obstruction.

Lumbo-sacral Plexus (Psoas Compartment) Block

This block is useful for postoperative analgesia after surgery on the leg.

Anatomy of the Lumbar Plexus

The lumbar plexus is made up of the anterior primary rami of L1, 2, 3 and part of L4 with a contribution from T12 in 50% of cases. The branches of the lumbar plexus are:

- iliohypogastric and ilioinguinal nerves (L1 ± T12)
- genitofemoral nerve (L1, 2)
- lateral cutaneous nerve of thigh (L2, 3)
- femoral nerve (L2, 3, 4)
- obturator nerve (L2, 3, 4)
- accessory obturator nerve (L3, 4).

Anatomy of the Sacral Plexus

The sacral plexus is made up of the anterior primary rami of L5, S1, 2 and 3 with contributions from L4 and S4. This plexus then gives rise to the following nerves:

- sciatic nerve (L4, 5; S1, 2, 3)
- pudendal nerve (S2, 3, 4)
- pelvic splanchnic nerves.

Technique

1   Position the patient sitting or in the lateral position.
2   Identify the spinous process of L3, then locate the transverse process 3–5 cm laterally using a 22 G spinal needle.
3   Walk the needle off either the upper or lower border of the transverse process.
4   Feel for a 'pop' sensation heralding the passage of the needle through the quadratus fascia into the psoas compartment, or

attempt to elicit paraesthesia. A nerve stimulator can also be used. The correct depth is about 7–10 cm.

5   Inject 20 mL of bupivacaine 0.5% with adrenaline. There should be little resistance to injection. Although anaesthesia of the femoral, obturator and lateral cutaneous nerve of the thigh is expected, the sciatic nerve usually escapes.[38]

Lung Function Tests

See *RESPIRATORY FUNCTION TESTS*.

Lung Volumes

See Table L5.

Table L5 Lung volumes		
Lung volume	mL/kg	For 70 kg patient
Vital capacity	70	5 L
Functional residual capacity	34	2.4 L
Residual volume	14	1 L
Tidal volume	7	500 mL

L

Mm

Magnesium

Most abundant cation in the body after potassium. The normal blood level of Mg^{2+} is 0.75–1.0 mmol/L (1.5–2 mEq/L).

Effects of Hypomagnesaemia
Total body depletion of Mg^{2+} may not be reflected by serum Mg^{2+} levels.[1]

1 Ventricular dysrhythmias.
2 Increased cardiovascular mortality.[1]
3 May lead to intra-cellular potassium depletion.[2]
4 Neuromuscular excitability and, rarely, convulsions.[3]

Effects of Hypermagnesaemia
See *PRE-ECLAMPSIA/ECLAMPSIA*.

Magnesium Sulphate

Mg^{2+} has antidisrhythmic effects, including prolongation of AV nodal conduction and suppression of conduction in accessory pathways.[1] 2.47 g of magnesium sulphate contains 20 mmol or 40 mEq of Mg^{2+}.

Indications and Dosages in Adults

1 *Pre-eclampsia/eclampsia.* Magnesium therapy is used to prevent seizures and also may assist in lowering blood pressure by reducing systemic vascular resistance. For details of magnesium therapy in pre-eclampsia and the toxic effects of magnesium see *PRE-ECLAMPSIA AND ECLAMPSIA*.

2 *Torsade de pointes.* See entry. Give 2 g IV over 10 min followed by an infusion of 0.5–0.75 g/h for 12–24 h.

3 *Magnesium deficiency.*

4 *Ventricular dysrhythmias associated with digoxin toxicity.*

5 To control *preterm labour*, although its usefulness is questionable.[4]

6 May reduce *post acute myocardial infarction mortality*, especially in the elderly and high risk patients.[1] 2 g IV over 5–15 min, then 18 g over 24 h.[1]

7 May be useful for atrial fibrillation with a rapid ventricular rate, supraventricular tachycardia, ventricular dysrhythmias during acute myocardial infarction, refractory ventricular tachycardia or ventricular fibrillation and multifocal atrial tachycardia.[1]

8 Phaeochromocytoma surgery. See *PHAEOCHROMOCYTOMA.*

Administration

Dilute 2.47 g (1 ampoule) in 5% glucose made up to a volume of 20 mL. Give by slow IV bolus over 15 min.

M

Magnetic Resonance Imaging (MRI) Anaesthesia

Basic Principles of the MRI Scanner

MRI scanning involves the use of high strength magnetic fields to provide digitalised, tomographic high resolution images of tissues and organs. The device consists of:

1 a *cryogenic magnet*, formed by a liquid nitrogen cooled superconductor in an environment of liquid helium at a temperature of 4.22 K. This magnet produces a magnetic field of up to 2 Tesla. It takes ≈ 72 h to establish this field. 1 Tesla (T) = 10 000 gauss (G). The earth's magnetic field is 5×10^{-5} T (≈ 0.5 G).

2   *gradient coils.* These are loops of wire that have gradient currents
    induced in them during the production of radiofrequency pulses.
    Torque in these wires results in the audible noise of the scanning
    process.[5]

How an Image is Obtained
1   Atoms with net electrical charges due to an odd number of
    protons and/or neutrons are aligned by the static magnetic
    field.
2   A radiofrequency pulse deflects the orientation of these
    atoms. When the pulses cease the atoms return to their
    (relaxed) aligned state in the static magnetic field, releasing
    energy.
3   These 'relaxation' rates vary between tissues and enable dif-
    ferentiation of structure. The 'energy' released by realignment
    is detected by the receiver coil and used to create the MRI
    image.
4   Hydrogen atoms are the most commonly used for imaging.

Contraindications to MRI Scanning or Close Exposure to MRI Equipment
1   Cardiac pacemakers.
2   Ferromagnetic intracerebral aneurysmal clips.
3   Intra-ocular metallic foreign body.
4   Other ferromagnetic devices that can be displaced by the
    magnetic field such as cochlear implants. If an implanted device
    is not ferromagnetic (e.g. stainless steel, nickel, titanium) then
    it does not present a risk.
5   A metal object in the patient that is well fixed, and the function
    of which is not affected by a magnetic field (e.g. sternal wires), is
    not a risk to the patient. However, such objects may affect image
    quality.

Hazards in the MRI Scanning Room

1 Patients or staff can be injured by ferromagnetic objects becoming missiles.
2 Electronically encoded information on objects such as credit cards may be destroyed by the magnetic field.
3 Patients may experience discomfort due to iron-containing pigments in tattoos or make-up.
4 Asphyxiation may result from 'quenching', in which liquid helium leaks into the MRI room and rapidly expands. Frostbite can also occur due to the coldness of the helium. O_2 sensors must be installed and functional to warn of this hazard.[6]
5 Acoustic noise can be a risk to hearing.

Approach to the Patient Requiring MRI Anaesthesia

Many MRI suites routinely scan anaesthetised patients and have well-established MRI-compatible monitors and anaesthetic machines. For a detailed description of problems with monitors in the MRI suite, see Rosewarne.[7]

M

In addition to the hazards and difficulties described above, other issues are:

1 remoteness from the patient
2 difficulty observing the patient
3 inadequate space in the scanner for resuscitation. Patients may need to be removed from the MRI scanning room if resuscitation is required.

Infusion pumps should not be used unless placed remotely with long infusion lines.

The metal spring in the LMA pilot balloon valve may cause image degradation.[8]

Malignant Hyperthermia (MH)

Topics Covered in this Section

▶ Description and Clinical Features
▶ Triggering Factors for Malignant Hyperthermia
▶ Diagnosis of MH
▶ Patients Susceptible to MH
▶ Treatment of the Acute Phase of MH
▶ Treatment of the Post Acute Phase of MH
▶ Anaesthetic Management of the MH Susceptible Patient
▶ Obstetrics and MH Susceptibility
▶ Investigation of a Suspected MH Reaction

Description and Clinical Features

Malignant hyperthermia is a potentially inherited syndrome in which a triggering agent results in a markedly accelerated metabolic state. The triggering agent causes release of calcium ions from skeletal muscle sarcoplasmic reticulum, causing hyperactive muscle fibre shortening. The genetic mutation is on the RYR1 gene on chromosome 19 and relates to the ryanodine calcium gate on skeletal muscle fibres. Two types of clinical reaction are recognised: in one there is muscle rigidity (75% of cases) and in the other there is absence of muscle rigidity.[9] Mortality without specific treatment is 70%. With appropriate treatment the current mortality is about 1%.[10]

The main signs are:

1 rigidity in skeletal muscle (but see above). Masseter spasm may occur (see *MASSETER SPASM*).

2 fever, profuse sweating. Above 43°C proteins begin to denature and irreversible cerebral damage may occur.[10]

3   tachypnoea and cyanosis

4   increased O_2 consumption and CO_2 production

5   tachycardia, unstable blood pressure, arrhythmias

6   hyperkalaemia, acidosis

7   dysfunction in many other organ systems.

Renal failure and DIC may occur.

Triggering Factors for Malignant Hyperthermia

This syndrome is known to be triggered by certain drugs including:

1   all volatile anaesthetic agents

2   suxamethonium, decamethonium and carbachol. Curare is probably also a trigger.

3   caffeine, xanthines, cocaine, phenothiazines.

4   possibly sympathomimetics—it is not clear whether they are unsafe. Ephedrine appears to be safe.[11]

Diagnosis of MH

This diagnosis of MH is based on clinical presentation. In cases of suspected MH elevated serum creatine kinase, myoglobinaemia and myoglobinuria are biochemical evidence of an MH reaction.

Patients Susceptible to MH

1   Patients diagnosed as MH susceptible from muscle biopsy testing.

2   A positive family history of MH or a suspicious episode of reaction to an anaesthetic in a family member. In one report 75% of cases did not have a known positive family history.[12]

3   Patients with musculoskeletal disorders such as strabismus, kyphoscoliosis, and clubfoot.

4   Central-core disease is almost certainly related to MH. Patients with osteogenesis imperfecta, King-Denborough syndrome and other myopathies may also be susceptible. There is probably *no* association between MH and neuroleptic malignant syndrome.

5   A previous exposure to a triggering anaesthetic does not guarantee a lack of susceptibility to MH. About 33% of cases of

MH occur in patients who have been previously exposed to a triggering agent.

Treatment of Acute Phase of MH[13]

1   Alert the surgeon and immediately cease all possible triggering agents such as inhalational anaesthetic drugs. Hyperventilate with 100% O_2 at a gas flow of at least 10 L/min. Do not turn off the CO_2 absorber as production of CO_2 is greatly increased. Summon skilled help. Keep the patient anaesthetised with a propofol infusion until the surgery is (urgently) completed.

2   Administer *dantrolene sodium* 2–3 mg/kg IV boluses until signs of MH are controlled or up to 10 mg/kg is given. Occasionally a total dose > 10 mg/kg will be required. Each vial of dantrolene contains 20 mg of drug and 3 g of mannitol and needs to be mixed with 60 mL of sterile H_2O. This task alone will entirely occupy one of the resuscitating staff.

3   Administer sodium bicarbonate 1–2 mEq/kg or as guided by arterial blood gas analysis.

4   Actively cool the hyperthermic patient with IV iced saline 15 mL/kg over 15 min × 3. Also surface-cool patient with ice and consider lavage of stomach, bladder, rectum and open cavities with iced saline. Stop cooling when the patient's temperature falls below 38°C. *Do not induce hypothermia.*

5   Hyperkalaemia is common. Treat with hyperventilation, sodium bicarbonate, actrapid 10 units + 50 mL of 50% glucose. Calcium chloride 2–5 mg/kg may also be useful. See *POTASSIUM, Hyperkalaemia.*

6   Treat cardiac dysrhythmias with reversal of hyperkalaemia and acidosis + anti-arrhythmic drugs appropriate for the particular dysrhythmia *with the exception of calcium channel blockers.* These can cause hyperkalaemia and cardiovascular collapse in a patient with MH.

7   Monitor serum K^+, Ca^{2+}, clotting studies and urine output, aim for at least 2 mL/kg/h urine output.

8   Do not transfer patient to the intensive care unit (ICU) until a satisfactory response to treatment has occurred, as worsening of the condition may occur if the patient is transferred prematurely.

Treatment of Post Acute Phase of MH

1   Observe the patient in the ICU for a minimum of 24 h. Give dantrolene 1 mg/kg IV 6 h for 24–48 h, then oral dantrolene 1 mg/kg 6 h for another 3 days.

2   Counsel the patient and family regarding MH and ensure that the patient understands the implications of their condition. Arrange for follow-up muscle biopsy testing of the patient and relevant family members.

Anaesthetic Management of the MH Susceptible Patient

M

1   Prepare the anaesthetic machine by removing all vaporisers. Also replace the CO_2-absorbent, anaesthetic tubing and fresh gas outlet tubing with fresh equipment. Flush the anaesthetic machine and breathing system with O_2 at 10 L/min for at least 10 min (20 min if the fresh gas outlet tubing cannot be replaced). A 'volatile anaesthetic free' anaesthetic machine can also be used but this is probably not necessary.

2   Use a 'non-triggering' anaesthetic technique. Non-triggering drugs include:

   (a) intravenous anaesthetic drugs such as barbiturates, propofol, ketamine and benzodiazepines

   (b) opioids, N_2O, all local anaesthetic drugs

   (c) non-depolarising neuromuscular blocking drugs including rocuronium, vecuronium, atracurium and pancuronium

(d) atropine and neostigmine

(e) droperidol.

Amide LA agents may be used but *do not use local anaesthetics with adrenaline.* ·

3 Dantrolene must be immediately available. Do not give prophylactic dantrolene unless the patient has a history of awake stress-induced MH or is a poor anaesthetic risk. The dose of dantrolene in this situation is 2.5 mg/kg IV at induction or 1.25 mg/kg 6 h PO for 2–3 days pre-operatively.[14]

4 In addition to routine monitoring,[15] monitor the patient's temperature carefully intra-operatively and for 4 h postoperatively.

Obstetrics and MH Susceptibility

1 Monitor temperature and heart rate during labour.

2 An epidural or spinal anaesthetic is preferred for Caesarean section, but *do not use LA agents with adrenaline.* If GA is required, use a non-triggering technique as described above.

3 Be aware of the possibility of a MH-susceptible foetus in a non-MH-susceptible mother, if the father is MH-susceptible.

4 Ephedrine is probably safe, as is syntocinon.

Investigation of a Suspected MH Reaction

MH is initially a clinical diagnosis. Elevated serum creatinine kinase, myoglobinaemia and myoglobinuria are biochemical evidence of a possible MH reaction.

Muscle biopsy testing is the only definitive diagnostic test. Quadriceps muscle fibres removed from the patient are exposed to caffeine ± halothane and contractions are measured. A DNA test is available for detection of 1 of the 15 known abnormalities of the RYR1 gene but is only helpful if positive (25% of families).[11]

Mallampati Score

See *DIFFICULT AIRWAY MANAGEMENT.*

Mannitol

An alcohol used for osmotic diuresis, mannitol is useful in:

1   the treatment of raised intracranial pressure. See *INTRACRANIAL PRESSURE (ICP) AND TREATMENT OF RAISED ICP.*
2   preservation of renal function during procedures such as repair of abdominal aortic aneurysm. See *ABDOMINAL AORTIC ANEURYSM REPAIR.*
3   short-term management of acute glaucoma.

Dose

Depends on the indication; see relevant cross-references listed above.

Masseter Spasm

Masseter spasm is defined as jaw tightness that interferes with intubation after a dose of suxamethonium. This reaction is most common in children but is occasionally noted in adults. The incidence of this reaction in children is about 0.1–0.5%.[16] It may be so severe as to prevent jaw opening. It is hypothesised that a percentage of these patients are susceptible to malignant hyperthermia (up to 50%).[16] Masseter spasm may also be the first sign of MH. Some patients who develop masseter spasm have an underlying muscle abnormality.

Treatment

1   Maintain oxygenation. Relaxation of the jaw usually occurs after a few minutes at most.
2   Abandon elective surgery if the masseter spasm is marked and allow the patient to awaken. Follow-up as discussed below.
3   If surgery is urgent and the masseter spasm is isolated continue anaesthesia with a technique that is non triggering for MH. See *MALIGNANT HYPERTHERMIA.*

4   In all cases observe for the development of MH, check serum creatine kinase, myoglobin and urine myoglobin concentration and consider referral for muscle biopsy.

Massive Blood Transfusion

See *BLOOD TRANSFUSION*.

Mediastinal Mass and Anaesthesia

Introduction

Mediastinal masses can occur in any age group and have a wide variety of aetiologies including lymphoma, thymomas, thyroid masses, oesophageal cysts, neurofibromas and vascular tumours. These masses may compress the:

1   superior vena cava. These are usually malignant masses on the right side. See *SUPERIOR VENA CAVA SYNDROME*.
2   heart and pericardium. The heart may be directly involved by tumours and cause effects such as dysrhythmias.[17]
3   trachea and bronchi
4   pulmonary arteries.

The major concerns therefore are that a mediastinal mass can cause catastrophic obstruction to major airways or the heart, SVC or pulmonary arteries under anaesthesia.

Anaesthetic Assessment, Investigation and Preparation

1   Look for any evidence of superior vena cava syndrome (see entry).
2   Evaluate for signs of pericardial tamponade such as pulsus paradoxus and consider echocardiography.
3   Look for pulmonary artery obstruction, which can result in right ventricular outflow obstruction and greatly diminished pulmonary venous return to the left side of the heart. One

simple test is to ask the patient to perform a Valsalva manoeuvre, which may produce syncope or presyncope.[18] Pre-operative CT and MRI scans should be carefully scrutinised for this complication.

4 Look for any evidence of bronchial or tracheal obstruction. Symptoms and signs include:
   (a) wheezing, stridor, decreased breath sounds
   (b) recurrent infections
5 Appropriate investigations include:
   (a) CXR
   (b) CT/MRI of chest
   (c) upright and supine pulmonary function tests looking at peak expiratory flow rate, flow volume loops.
6 Mass effects on major vessels can be elucidated by echocardiography in the erect and supine position.[19]
7 If practical and appropriate, consider pre-operative radiotherapy and/or chemotherapy to shrink the mediastinal mass.

Anaesthesia for Patients with Mediastinal Mass

GA may unmask compression that is not obvious in the awake patient. The specific anaesthetic approach depends on many factors such as the site and size of the mass and the age of the patient and the type of surgery. Options to consider include:

1 local and regional anaesthesia
2 maintenance of spontaneous respiration during anaesthesia if appropriate for the type of surgery
3 awake fibre-optic examination and intubation, with careful positioning of the ET tube beyond an obstruction prior to induction of anaesthesia[20]
4 postural repositioning to reduce compression such as lateral, upright or prone[21]
5 rigid bronchoscopy to splint the airway
6 jet ventilation past a proximal obstruction

7   tracheal stenting
8   cardiopulmonary bypass either planned or immediately available.

Unanticipated Airway Obstruction in the Patient with Mediastinal Mass

In this scenario tracheal intubation is successful but ventilation is ineffective. Try:

1   repositioning the patient (lateral, prone) to shift the mass off the trachea/bronchus
2   rigid bronchoscopy and placement of the tube beyond the obstruction
3   cricothyrotomy and placement of a long ET tube beyond the obstruction
4   median sternotomy to decompress the mediastinum.

Mental Nerve Block

Anatomy

The mental nerve arises in the mandibular canal from the inferior alveolar nerve. It exits the mandible through the mental foramen to supply sensation to the skin of the lower lip and chin and mucous membrane lining the lower lip.

Technique

1   Anaesthetise the mucous membrane of lower lip adjacent to the 2nd premolar tooth (in line with the pupil, with the eyes in the neutral position) using gauze soaked in 4% topical lignocaine.
2   Insert a 25 G needle about 1 cm deep towards the mental foramen and inject 2 mL of LA (e.g. 2% lignocaine).

M-Entropy

See *TIME FREQUENCY BALANCED SPECTRAL ENTROPY.*

Metabolic Cart

See *CARDIAC INVESTIGATIONS*.

Metabolic Equivalent

See *CARDIOVASCULAR PERI-OPERATIVE RISK PREDICTION FOR NON-CARDIAC SURGERY*.

Metaraminol (Aramine)

Synthetic sympathomimetic amine used as a vasoconstrictor agent for the treatment of hypotension. Acts by a direct agonist effect on α receptors with lesser stimulation of β receptors. There is some uptake of metaraminol into adrenergic nerve endings from where it is released as a weak neurotransmitter.

Dose

Adult: Give 0.5–1 mg IV, titrate to desired effect. Effects begin within 1–2 min with a maximum effect in 10 min. Effects last 20–60 min.

IV infusion in adult: Load 50 mg into 100 mL N/S and run at 2.5–60 mL/h.

Child: 0.01 mg/kg IV boluses.

IV infusion in child: 0.1–1 µg/kg/min, titrate against blood pressure.

Methadone

Synthetic opioid agonist with efficient oral absorption and long duration of action. Less sedating than morphine. Used for:

1 analgesia
2 treatment of heroin addiction
3 cough suppression in terminal disease.

M

Dose

For *heroin addiction* give methadone in a dosage that is about 25% of the heroin dosage in mg.

For *analgesia* 5–10 mg PO or subcutaneously or IM every 6–8 h as required.

Methaemoglobin

Methaemoglobin (MetHb) is haemoglobin in which ferrous iron in the molecule has been oxidised to the ferric state. Methaemoglobin-aemia occurs when MetHb exceeds 1% of total Hb. This can occur due to drugs such as:

1 prilocaine in doses > 600 mg, due to the metabolite o-toluidine
2 nitrates, nitrites and sodium nitroprusside.

Effects of Methaemoglobin

1 Oxyhaemoglobin dissociation curve is shifted to the left.
2 As MetHb level increases, pulse oximetry will read 80–85% regardless of the true saturation.
3 Diminished O_2 carrying capacity of the blood.
4 MetHb is brownish in colour and produces a slate grey colour in the patient. Cyanosis is seen at 10–15% MetHb, weakness and dizziness at 30–40% and death at > 70% MetHb concentration.

Treatment

Give methylene blue 1 mg/kg IV (use the 1% solution) over 5 min or ascorbic acid.

Methohexitone

Intravenous methylated oxybarbiturate anaesthetic agent.

Advantages

1 Faster recovery from anaesthesia than thiopentone, so this drug is favoured for ultra-short procedures, e.g. electroconvulsive therapy.

2 It is less irritant than thiopentone if extravasation occurs.
3 Methohexitone may be preferable for use in the asthmatic patient compared with thiopentone.[22]

Disadvantages

1 There is an increased incidence of excitatory effects compared with thiopentone. Methohexitone may also cause an epileptiform pattern on the EEG.
2 Pain on injection may occur.
3 Like thiopentone, it is contraindicated in some types of porphyria. See *PORPHYRIA*.

Dose

1–1.5 mg/kg IV, 6.6 mg/kg IM or 15–20 mg/kg PR.

Methoxamine

Synthetic sympathomimetic amine drug, acts as a selective α1 receptor agonist, producing vasoconstriction. It is used for the treatment of hypotension.

Dose

Adult: 1 mg IV boluses to a maximum of 5–10 mg. Acts within 1–2 min and effects last for 1 h or 5–20 mg IM.

Methoxyflurane

Halogenated ethyl methyl ether volatile inhalational anaesthetic agent.

Physical Properties and MAC

Blood:gas solubility coefficient	13
Oil:gas solubility coefficient	970
Saturated vapour pressure at 20°C	24 mmHg (3.19 kPa)
Boiling point	105°C
MAC	0.16%

Advantages

The most potent inhalational anaesthetic agent in former and current use. It has good analgesic properties at subanaesthetic concentrations.

Disadvantages

1 The high blood gas solubility coefficient results in slow induction of anaesthesia and slow recovery.
2 30–50% of the administered dose of methoxyflurane is metabolised. This can result in renal toxicity due to increased blood inorganic fluoride levels. The toxic level of fluoride is 50 µmol/L and this level may be reached after 2.5 MAC h.[23]
3 Methoxyflurane may result in nephrotoxicity due to intrarenal metabolism of the drug producing elevated intrarenal F⁻ion levels. See SEVOFLURANE.

Methylene Blue

See METHAEMOGLOBIN.

Metoclopramide (Maxolon)

This drug is a chlorinated procainamide derivative used for:
1 the prevention and treatment of nausea and vomiting
2 increasing the rate of gastric emptying.

It acts mainly by antagonising central and peripheral dopaminergic receptors (DA2) and has a direct action on gastrointestinal smooth muscle.

Dose

Adult: 10 mg IV, IM or PO as required up to 8 h.
Child: 0.12 mg/kg/dose to a maximum of 15 mg either IV, IM or PO.

Disadvantages

1 Extrapyramidal side effects may occur. See *DYSTONIC REACTION, ACUTE*.
2 Not suitable for patients with Parkinson's disease.
3 Low efficacy. There is little evidence that metoclopramide is an effective anti-emetic at the usual adult dose of 10 mg.[24]

Metoprolol

β1 selective β adrenergic receptor blocking drug used for the treatment of:
1 supraventricular tachycardia
2 hypertension
3 angina
4 premature ventricular ectopics.

Dose

Adult: 1–2 mg IV boluses minutely to a maximum total dose of 15–20 mg.
Child: 0.1 mg/kg (max. 5 mg) over 5 min, repeat 5 minutely to a max. of 3 doses. Consider infusion 1–5 µg/kg/min.

Midazolam

A water-soluble benzodiazepine with a fast onset and short duration of action. Useful for:
1 premedication, due to its sedating, amnesic and anxiolytic effects
2 sedation for procedures, usually combined with other drugs, e.g. fentanyl ± propofol
3 seizure control
4 intrathecally to potentiate the analgesic effects of local anaesthetic agents.[25]

M

Dose

▶ *Adult*

Sedation for procedures: Inject 1–2 mg IV increments until patient is tolerant of procedure but still able to maintain verbal contact.

Premedication: 0.07–0.08 mg/kg IM 30–60 min prior to the procedure.

Infusion for prolonged sedation: Give LD of 0.1–0.2 mg/kg, then 0.1–0.2 mg/kg/h titrated to clinical effect.

▶ *Child*

Premedication: 0.2 mg/kg up to 5 mg PO mixed with a sweet drink (midazolam is very bitter) 1 h before procedure.

Infusion: 3 mg/kg in 50 mL of N/S run at 2 mL/h.

The Intrathecal Midazolam Controversy

Intrathecal midazolam is being used by an increasing number of anaesthetists to enhance opioid and LA analgesia.[26] This practice has generated much controversy. Several small-animal studies have indicated that neurotoxicity with intrathecal midazolam is common.[27] However, other studies in sheep and pigs do not show intrathecal-midazolam-induced spinal cord damage.[29] Human studies have not resulted in symptoms suggestive of neurological injury or significant adverse side effects.[26,30]

Despite widespread and apparently successful use of intrathecal midazolam in humans Yaksh and others have urged caution because:[31]

1 Neurotoxicity in some animal species is a persistent concern.

2 Midazolam's solubility is pH dependent and midazolam may precipitate in CSF, especially when mixed with other drugs.

3 The midazolam used should be the hydrochloride form and not contain preservatives such as benzoate, and should be at a concentration not exceeding 1 mg/mL.

M

Dose of Intrathecal midazolam

1–2 mg of preservative-free midazolam hydrochloride as a single dose. Use the 1 mg/mL solution. This prolongs analgesia from bupivacaine for about 4.5 h.[32] A continuous infusion of up to 6 mg/day has been given without apparent ill effects, for chronic pain.[33]

Special Notes

Midazolam should be used with caution in patients on efavirenz,an antiviral drug, due to similar metabolic pathways. The anticholesterol drug atorvastatin results in a prolongation of midazolam's drug effects.[34]

Milrinone

Second-generation phosphodiesterase III inhibitor. Effects include positive inotropy and vasodilatation, resulting in increased cardiac output without compromising myocardial O_2 supply–demand ratio. This is due to a reduction of preload and afterload and the lack of a significant tachycardia. Used for the treatment of cardiac failure, e.g. post bypass or as a bridge to transplantation.

M

Dose

Give an IV loading dose of 37.5–50 µg/kg over 10 min, then infusion 0.375–0.75 µg/kg/min.[35]

Advantages

1 Does not cause thrombocytopaenia with chronic use, unlike amrinone.
2 The inotropic effect of milrinone is $20 \times$ that of amrinone.[36]
3 Less prodysrhythmic than β stimulants.

Disadvantages

1 Vasodilation may cause significant hypotension.
2 Dysrhythmias may occur.
3 Dosage should be reduced in renal failure.[35]

Minute Volume

Defined as the volume of gas leaving the lung per minute.
This volume = tidal volume × respiratory rate.
Adult: 85–100 mL/kg
Child: 100–200 mL/kg

Mitral Incompetence (Regurgitation)

Mitral incompetence results in regurgitation of blood into the left atrium. The left ventricle (LV) is thus subjected to an increased work load, leading to hypertrophy. LV failure may occur in chronic cases. Left atrial dilatation develops and atrial fibrillation may occur in mixed lesions (mitral stenosis and mitral incompetence) or chronic mitral incompetence. There is a slow deterioration in exercise tolerance. If mitral incompetence occurs acutely, pulmonary oedema may occur and rapid decompensation and death may follow. Echocardiography will help define the cause and severity of mitral incompetence. A regurgitant fraction > 0.6 indicates severe disease.[37]

Management Aims During Anaesthesia

1   Give antibiotic prophylaxis against bacterial endocarditis. This lesion carries the highest risk of bacterial endocarditis compared with all other valve lesions.[38] See *BACTERIAL ENDOCARDITIS PROPHYLAXIS.*

2   Avoid increasing systemic vascular resistance (SVR), whichwill increase the regurgitant fraction and decrease the cardiac output (CO). Decreasing SVR in a controlled fashion can significantly increase CO.

3   A mild tachycardia can improve CO by preventing overdistension of the LV and mitral valve distortion. Conversely avoid bradycardia.

4 Avoid hypovolaemia so that left atrial filling pressure is maintained. A well-filled left atrium leads to less blood regurgitating back into this chamber and improved left ventricular filling.

5 Be aware of the risk of systemic emboli and/or complications of patient's anticoagulant drugs.

6 Avoid myocardial depressant drugs.

Mitral Regurgitation and Obstetrics

A carefully administered epidural anaesthetic should be well-tolerated as long as:

1 Appropriate monitoring is used, depending on the severity of the patient's condition.

2 Left atrial filling must be maintained with adequate fluid volume loading.

3 Ephedrine is preferable to aramine for treating hypotension.[39]

4 General anaesthesia is usually well-tolerated as long as the above management aims are followed.

Mitral Stenosis (MS)

The normal mitral valve area is 4–6 cm^2. Symptoms occur when the valve area is reduced to 2.5 cm^2 and symptoms become severe at a valve area of < 1 cm^2.[32] The normal atrial–ventricular diastolic pressure gradient across the mitral valve is < 5 mmHg. Severe disease is present if this pressure is > 10 mmHg. When the valve area is < 1 cm^2, the diastolic pressure across the valve may be > 25 mmHg.[37] Symptoms include exertional dyspnoea, orthopnoea and occasionally angina.

To compensate for the stenosed valve, the left atrium contracts more forcefully, leading to left atrial dilatation and hypertrophy. Left atrial pressure is increased and if it exceeds colloid osmotic pressure (25–30 mmHg) pulmonary oedema may occur. Some patients develop irreversible pulmonary hypertension with right ventricular hypertrophy, which may lead to right ventricular failure. See *PUL-MONARY HYPERTENSION*. Pulmonary and tricuspid valve incompetence may also occur secondary to pulmonary hypertension.

Atrial fibrillation (AF) may develop, which can produce sudden cardiac decompensation and emboli.

Aims of Anaesthetic Management

1   Avoid tachycardia/precipitation of AF or fast AF, as this will reduce left ventricular filling time and decrease cardiac output (CO). Therefore avoid atropine, glycopyrronium, ketamine and pancuronium. Control AF pre-operatively. Cardiovert the patient if AF develops intra-operatively.

2   Give prophylactic antibiotics for the prevention of endocarditis. See *BACTERIAL ENDOCARDITIS PROPHYLAXIS*.

3   Avoid large decreases in systemic vascular resistance (SVR) because the left ventricle is restricted in its ability to increase CO, and blood pressure may fall precipitously.

4   Avoid an excess volume load, which may precipitate pulmonary oedema. Also avoid hypovolaemia, which may lead to a reduced CO.

5   Myocardial depressant drugs may cause severe hypotension and must be used cautiously.

6   Be aware of measures that may increase pulmonary hypertension, including N_2O, hypoxia and acidosis. These may be unsafe if pulmonary vascular resistance is already elevated. If pulmonary hypertension is present, the pulmonary capillary wedge pressure may not correlate well with left atrial filling pressure.

7   Avoid Trendelenburg positioning, which may lead to pulmonary oedema.

Mitral Stenosis and Obstetrics

1   Asymptomatic patients without pulmonary oedema are at minimally increased anaesthetic risk.[39]

2 Epidural anaesthesia has been used successfully in patients with mitral stenosis. It is very important to avoid overfilling or underfilling the patient.[40] Avoid adrenaline-containing solutions.

3 Appropriate monitoring, depending on the severity of the lesion, must be instituted.

4 Cardioversion, if required, appears to be relatively safe for the foetus.[41] For AF of sudden onset, start with 25 J. See *CARDIO-VERSION*.

5 If hypotension occurs, metaraminol is preferred to ephedrine.[39]

Mitral Valve Prolapse

Mitral valve prolapse is usually a benign condition and occurs in about 2.4–10% of the population, depending on diagnostic criteria.[37] The condition is due to billowing of the posterior mitral valve leaflet into the left atrium during systole. In a minority of patients, usually with abnormal mitral valves, this lesion can result in strokes, endocarditis, significant or severe mitral valve regurgitation, dysrhythmias such as supraventricular tachycardia and sudden death. Suspect this diagnosis in patients who develop unexpected atrial or ventricular dysrhythmias intra-operatively.[38]

Aims of Anaesthetic Management

1 Increased ventricular emptying can increase the degree of prolapse and lead to acute regurgitation. Therefore, avoid factors that increase contractility, such as increased sympathetic nervous system activity. Also avoid decreasing systemic vascular resistance, and the head up or sitting position.

2 Give antibiotic prophylaxis against bacterial endocarditis. See *BACTERIAL ENDOCARDITIS PROPHYLAXIS*.

3 Avoid hypovolaemia, which can lead to decreased preload and decreased ventricular filling.

4   Avoid tachycardia, which may result in increased LV emptying, which in turn may increase the degree of prolapse.

5   Avoid high airway pressures, which may accentuate prolapse.

Mivacurium

Benzylisoquinolinium diester non-depolarising neuromuscular blocking drug (NDNMBD), with a short duration of action. It is metabolised primarily by plasma cholinesterases. It is cleared from the plasma in about 3 minutes but its effects last much longer than this.[42]

Advantages

1   It has shorter duration of action than other currently available NDNMB drugs (14–16 min),[42] making it useful for brief procedures.

2   It does not require reversal drugs. Routine reversal of mivacurium may not be necessary.[43] Can be given to patients with renal or liver failure.

3   Mivacurium can be given by infusion.

Disadvantages

1   Relatively slow onset of paralysis (3–4 min).[42]

2   Recovery time may be delayed in some individuals possibly due to variations in plasma cholinesterase activity. In patients with atypical plasma cholinesterase, recovery may be delayed > 6 h.[44] Neostigmine may not effectively reverse blockade in these patients.[45]

3   Histamine release can occur, causing flushing and hypotension, especially if the drug is given rapidly (< 10–15 s).[43]

4   Neostigmine reversal of profound mivacurium neuromuscular blockade may cause prolongation of block due to impairment of plasma cholinesterase activity. Edrophonium may be preferable to neostigmine for reversal due to this inhibition effect.[43]

Dose (All IV)

Adult: 0.2–0.25 mg/kg;[45] *top-up dose* 0.1 mg/kg required at ≈ 15 min intervals; *infusion dose* 0.36–0.42 mg/kg/h.

Child: 0.1–0.2 mg/kg; *top-up dose* 0.1 mg/kg; *infusion dose* 0.6–1 mg/kg/h.

Monoamine Oxidase (MAO) Inhibitor Drugs

These drugs are used in the treatment of severe depression when other drugs are unsuccessful, and in the treatment of Parkinson's disease (selegiline).[46] These medications are of two types: non-selective MAO inhibitors and selective drugs for inhibition of MAO B or A.

Non-selective MAOI Drugs

These include phenelzine and tranylcypromine. These non-selective drugs are associated with hypertensive crises if tyramine- or phenylethylamine-containing foods are ingested. Drug interactions include the following:

1 The use of indirectly acting sympathomimetic drugs such as ephedrine, metaraminol and phenylephrine can precipitate a sympathetic discharge, leading to life-threatening hypertension and/or hyperthermia. Direct-acting sympathetic drugs such as adrenaline are not contraindicated.

2 Pethidine administration can lead to severe hypotension, profound respiratory depression, agitation, hypertension, seizures and coma.[47] Fentanyl and morphine can be used.

3 Reserpine, methyldopa and guanethidine may also precipitate hypertension.[48]

4 Levodopa and imipramine are also contraindicated.

5 Cocaine should also be avoided as it inhibits reuptake of nor-adrenaline, leading to a build-up.

If elective surgery is planned, consider stopping MAOI drugs 2 weeks prior to anaesthesia.[48]

However, some authors suggest that the risk of suicide is greater than the risk of avoidable drug reactions and recommend continuance.[47]

Treatment of Hypertensive Crisis

Give phentolamine 2.5–5 mg IV boluses and titrate to blood pressure.

Selective MAOI Drugs

These drugs include selective MAO B inhibitors such as selegiline, and MAO A inhibitors such as moclobemide. Selegiline and moclobemide are associated with much less potential for hypertensive crisis after exposure to tyramine or phenylethylamine orally.

Moclobemide has a half-life of only 4 h. *Use with pethidine is contraindicated.* Indirectly acting sympathomimetic drugs such as ephedrine should not be used with moclobemide.[49]

Morphine

Alkaloid of opium used for:
1 analgesia (agonist at mu 1, delta and kappa opioid receptors). See *OPIOID RECEPTORS.*
2 cough suppression and control of diarrhoea
3 treatment of pulmonary oedema.

Dose

▶ *Adult*

IM: 0.1–0.2 mg/kg up to 4 h as required.

IV: 2–2.5 mg 5 min (up to 10–15 mg) until pain is controlled.

IV infusion: 1 mg/kg morphine in 500 mL N/S. Run the infusion at 10–40 mL/h (10–40 µg/kg/h).

Epidural: 1–5 mg injected into epidural space provides analgesia for prolonged periods, e.g. 5 mg epidural morphine can provide analgesia for 18 h.[50] However, it takes about 1 h for the pain relief to be effective.[50] *Note that there is a risk of delayed respiratory depression with epidural morphine.*

Intrathecal: 0.1–0.5 mg of morphine can provide analgesia for > 24 h.[51] *Note that there is a risk of delayed respiratory depression with intrathecal morphine.* The optimum dose of intrathecal morphine for patients undergoing hip arthroplasty for postoperative pain relief was found in one study to be 100 µg.[52]

Oral: For every 20 mg morphine given IM, give 60 mg of oral morphine. Morphine mixture is given 4 h, MS Contin tablets are given 12 h. To convert the dose of morphine mixture to MS Contin, divide the total daily dose of morphine mixture by 2. Give this dose of MS Contin every 12 h (e.g. if taking morphine mixture 200 mg/day, give MS Contin 100 mg 12 h).

▶ *Child*

IM or subcutaneously: 0.1–0.15 mg/kg via a subcutaneous cannula (preferably placed intra-operatively) or the same dose IM. The IM route is less well-tolerated in children because of the fear of needles.

IV: Load 0.15 mg/kg morphine in 10 mL N/S in a syringe. Give incrementally 1 mL per 5 min to control pain.

IV infusion: Load 1 mg/kg morphine in 50 mL of 5% glucose. Run the infusion at 0.5–2.5 mL/h = 10–50 µg/kg/h.

Important Side Effects of Morphine

1 Drowsiness, sedation and euphoria. These are thought to be kappa receptor agonist effects. There is a risk of dependence due to these effects.

2 Respiratory depression (mu 2 agonist). This can be delayed in the case of intrathecal/epidural morphine.

3   Pruritus, nausea and vomiting.

4   Spasm of the sphincter of Oddi may occur, increasing bile duct pressure.

5   Urinary retention.

6   Epidural morphine may reactivate herpes simplex labialis virus in obstetric patients.[53]

7   Morphine causes histamine release and is traditionally avoided in asthmatic patients. See *ASTHMA*.

Treatment of Side Effects

1   For life-threatening respiratory depression in adults give naloxone 100 µg increments. For children give naloxone 2 µg/kg/dose repeated every 2 min. See *NALOXONE*.

2   For pruritus consider the following strategies:

   (a) *Naloxone*: Small incremental doses, e.g. 50 µg bolus IV, then add 350 µg to patient's next litre bag of IV fluid. Alternatively, give naloxone 40 µg IV 5 minutely prn up to 5 doses.

   (b) *Diphenhydramine*: 10–50 mg IV. Antihistamines are often not effective.[54]

   (c) *Propofol*: 10 mg IV. This is effective in about 80% of cases and the effects last about 1 h.[55] Propofol can also be given by a continuous infusion of 0.5–1 mg/kg/h in severe cases.[55]

   (d) *Droperidol*: 2.5 mg IV.

   (e) *Ondansetron* is effective for the treatment of pruritus due to intrathecal or epidural morphine. Give 8 mg IV for adults.[56] Prophylactic IV ondansetron may also decrease the incidence of pruritus associated with intrathecal morphine.[57]

   (f) For patients with treatment resistant pruritus on PCA morphine, consider changing the patient to *fentanyl* PCA.

3   For nausea and vomiting from morphine PCA, consider *droperidol* 2.5 mg added to morphine 100 mg.[58]

Morphine and Renal/Liver Failure

Use morphine cautiously in renal failure due to the accumulation of the metabolite morphine-6-glucuronide, which can cause severe respiratory depression and decreased level of consciousness. Also use morphine cautiously in liver failure as hepatic encephalopathy may be precipitated.

Multifocal Atrial Tachycardia

See *SUPRAVENTRICULAR TACHYCARDIAS*.

Muscarinic Receptors

See *CHOLINERGIC RECEPTORS*.

Myasthenia Gravis

This is a relatively rare condition with an incidence of 1 per 30 000.[59] About two-thirds of sufferers are female.[59] Myasthenia gravis (MG) is a progressive autoimmune disease in which acetylcholine receptors at the neuromuscular junction are inactivated or destroyed by anti-acetylcholine receptor antibodies and T-cells. This results in weakness and rapid fatigue of the affected skeletal muscle. The disease is associated with thymus gland abnormalities, and thymectomy is frequently beneficial. Types of MG (as described by Osserman and Genkins)[60] are:

1 type I: extraocular muscles only involved.
2 type IIA: slowly progressive mild muscle weakness; muscles of respiration spared
3 type IIB: severe and rapidly progressive muscle weakness; muscles of respiration may be involved
4 type III: fulminant form of MG with rapid progression and high mortality

5   type IV: severe disease resulting from a progression of type I
or II.

The disease may be exacerbated by conditions such as pregnancy, surgery and viral illness.[62]

Conditions Associated with Myasthenia Gravis

1   Cardiomyopathy and cardiac dysrhythmias.
2   Other autoimmune conditions such as rheumatoid arthritis and SLE.
3   Thymoma. This neoplasm can cause airway or vascular obstruction.

Treatment of MG

1   Anticholinesterase inhibitor drugs such as pyridostigmine.
2   Corticosteroids.
3   Plasmapheresis.
4   IV immunoglobulin.
5   Immunosuppressive drugs such as azathioprine and cyclophosphamide.
6   Thymectomy.
7   Patients may take propantheline to block the muscarinic effects of anticholinesterase drugs.

Cholinergic Crisis and Myasthenic Crisis

An overdosage of anticholinesterase drugs can result in a cholinergic crisis. Effects include:

1   muscle fasciculations and severe weakness
2   sweating and salivation
3   pallor
4   bradycardia
5   constricted pupils.

Myasthenic crisis is the development of severe weakness due to an exacerbation of MG. These conditions can be distinguished by injection of edrophonium 2 mg IV. In cholinergic crisis the muscle weakness will get worse and in a myasthenic crisis the weakness should improve. Treat cholinergic crisis with antimuscarinic drugs (atropine) and respiratory support.

Anaesthetic Considerations

1 Patients on immunosuppressive drugs and/or steroids should be considered for prophylactic antibiotic therapy.

2 In poorly controlled patients consider pre-operative plasmapheresis.

3 In patients with significant weakness requiring muscle relaxants, continue pyridostigmine up to the time of surgery. A reduced dose of pyridostigmine can be considered in milder disease; however, management of individual cases will depend on the experience and beliefs of the attending anaesthetist.

4 Provide increased corticosteroid dosage to patients on long-term steroid therapy to cover the stress of surgery. See *STEROID 'COVER'*.

5 Be prepared for the potential need to ventilate patients post-operatively. It is suggested that the need for postoperative ventilation is more likely in patients with:[62]

- duration of disease > 6 years.
- history of coexisting respiratory disease.
- daily dose of of pyridostigmine > 750 mg/day.
- vital capacity < 2.9 L.

Although initially stable, patients with MG may suffer respiratory impairment some hours after surgery. Monitor the patients in a high dependency area. Use opioids with caution due to their inhibitory effects on ventilation.

The patient's anticholinesterase inhibitor drugs may have to be given IV postoperatively until oral intake is re-established.

Myasthenia Gravis and Neuromuscular Blocking Drugs

1 Patients with MG may require an increased dose of suxamethonium (1.5–2 mg/kg) but the effects of suxamethonium may last longer than in normals.

2 MG patients may be exquisitely sensitive to non-depolarising neuromuscular blocking drugs (NDNMBD). Consider titrating small doses of an intermediate duration NDNMBD to assess its effect. Do not use long-acting NDNMBDs such as pancuronium.

3 A NDNMBD may not be necessary for intubation and ventilation in these patients when anaesthetised. Modern volatile agents such as sevoflurane and desflurane can depress neuromuscular transmission in myasthenics.[59]

4 Cisatracurium may produce more predictable results than vecuronium.[61]

5 Mivacurium may have a prolonged action in patients taking pyridostigmine.

6 Reversal of NDNMBDs with anticholinesterase inhibitor drugs can precipitate a cholinergic crisis (see above). This is a controversial and unresolved issue. It may be preferable to await spontaneous recovery.

Myasthenia Gravis and Nonanaesthetic Drugs

1 Aminoglycoside antibiotics may exacerbate weakness in myasthenics.

2 β adrenergic blocking drugs can also caused increased weakness.

Myocardial Infarction (MI)

Topics Covered in this Section
▶ Effects of Recent MI on Peri-operative Risk
▶ Diagnosis of Peri-operative MI
▶ Management of Peri-operative MI

Effects of Recent MI on Peri-operative Risk

Patients with a past history of MI are 5–10 × more likely to suffer a peri-operative MI than patients with no history of MI.[63] The mortality of peri-operative MI is about 30%.[64] Important risk factors are:

1 elapsed time since MI. Less than 6 weeks is associated with high risk and 6 weeks to 3 months is considered to be an intermediate risk factor.[65]
2 nature of surgery
3 degree of myocardial damage.

The risk of peri-operative infarction can be reduced in patients with a history of recent MI with aggressive management including extensive use of ICU resources, invasive monitoring and prolonged postoperative monitoring and care. The results of aggressive management are illustrated in Table M1.

Table M1 Risk of peri-operative MI (non-cardiac surgery) in patients with recent MI

Time elapsed since MI (months)	Periop infarct. rate	
	Non-specific manag. (Steen)[66]	Aggressive manag. (Rao)[67]
0–3	27%	5.8%
4–6	11%	2.3%
>6	4.1%	1.5%

M

Elective surgery should be delayed for 3–6 months after MI, although the evidence for this recommendation is lacking.[64]

Diagnosis of Peri-operative MI

1 Chest pain/diaphoresis in awake patients.
2 ECG changes. For 12 lead ECG changes see *ELECTROCARDIO-GRAPHY*. May see ST segment elevation > 1 mm measured

0.04 s after the J point, T wave inversion, new onset LBBB. With posterior MI may see ST depression in leads V1–V4.

3   Biochemical evidence of peri-operative MI includes elevated troponin levels. A troponin level of 0.05–0.1 µg/L suggests minor cardiac damage, while a reading of > 0.1 µg/L indicates significant cardiac damage/infarction.

Management of Peri-operative MI

▶ Aims of Treatment

1   Optimise oxygen delivery to the myocardium.
2   Reduce myocardial oxygen demand.
3   Reperfusion of the ischaemic myocardium. Options include urgent stenting of coronary artery bypass grafts. Thrombolytic therapy should be considered but will usually be contraindicated after significant surgery.
4   Adequate analgesia in the awake patient. Obtain urgent cardiological opinion. Ideally, stenting should be undertaken within 90 min of myocardial infarction.[68]
5   Continuous ECG monitoring to detect dysrhythmias, particularly VF.

Optimising myocardial oxygenation and reducing myocardial oxygen demand are discussed below in the section on *MYOCARDIAL ISCHAEMIA, PERI-OPERATIVE.*

Myocardial Ischaemia, Peri-operative

Topics Covered in this Section
▶ Factors Determining Myocardial O_2 Supply and Demand
▶ Prevention of Myocardial Ischaemia
▶ Detection of Myocardial Ischaemia
▶ Treatment of Myocardial Ischaemia

Factors Determining Myocardial O_2 Supply and Demand

Myocardial ischaemia occurs when O_2 supply to the myocardium fails to meet O_2 demand. The main determinants of O_2 supply are coronary blood flow and O_2 content of arterial blood. Coronary blood flow is determined by heart rate (80% of total flow occurs during diastole), coronary artery calibre, cardiac output and blood viscosity. Myocardial O_2 demand is determined by heart rate, wall tension and basal metabolic requirements. O_2 demand is thus increased if afterload and/or preload increases or contractility increases or heart rate increases. Myocardial O_2 demand is nearly proportional to the *tension time index* (= tension in heart muscle during contraction $\times$ duration of contraction).

Prevention of Myocardial Ischaemia

The underlying principles in preventing myocardial ischaemia are to optimise factors which improve myocardial O_2 supply and reduce O_2 demand.

1 Continue the patient's anti-anginal drugs throughout the peri-operative period.

2 Of the anti-anginal drugs, β blockers are thought to be the most effective in preventing peri-operative myocardial ischaemia. This is thought to be due to their ability to suppress peri-operative tachycardia.[69] Well-conducted clinical studies have consistently shown that peri-operative β blockers reduce the risk of death due to ischaemic heart disease for as long as 2 years after surgery.[70,71] Prophylactic IV nitroglycerin is probably not effective for the prevention of myocardial ischaemia.[72]

3 Correct anaemia. Aim for a Hb of 10 g/100 mL.

4 Prevent/correct hypothermia which is associated with postoperative myocardial ischaemia.

5 Continue supplementary O_2 therapy well into the postoperative period.

M

Detection of Myocardial Ischaemia

1 Chest pain/diaphoresis in awake patients.

2 ECG and ST segment analysis. See *ST SEGMENT ANALYSIS* for a description of the ECG changes associated with ischaemia. For lead positions to optimise detection of ischaemia see *ELECTRO-CARDIOGRAPHY.*

▶ *Pulmonary Artery Catheter Findings*

Pulmonary capillary wedge pressure typically rises significantly with myocardial ischaemia to > 15 mmHg. In addition, V waves > 20 mmHg may occur.

▶ *Transoesophageal Echocardiography*

May show wall motion abnormalities and wall thickening.

Treatment of Myocardial Ischaemia

1 Ensure that the patient is adequately anaesthetised and/or analgesed.

2 Notify the surgeon and request that surgery be cancelled or expedited.

3 Optimise O_2 delivery to the myocardium by the following:
   - Ventilate with 100% O_2
   - Correct anaemia. Transfuse to a haemoglobin of 10 g/100 mL.
   - Correct hypovolaemia/hypotension with fluid loading ± vaso-constrictors such as *metaraminol.*

4 Treat severe bradycardia. Type of treatment depends on cause, e.g. *atropine* for sinus bradycardia, *isoprenaline* for complete heart block. Treat other dysrhythmias as appropriate.

5 Insertion of an intra-aortic balloon pump will improve myocardial perfusion during diastole.

6 Reduce myocardial O_2 demand by the following:
   (a) Reduce preload using a venodilator such as *glyceryl trinitrate* (GTN). (*Note*: Inadequate preload must be excluded as the cause of ischaemia.)

(b) Sublingual nitroglycerine 0.3 mg can be used while a nitro-glycerine infusion is being organised. Start GTN at 10 µg/min and increase dose by 10 µg/min every 3–5 min until myocardial ischaemia is controlled, or significant hypotension occurs (< 95 mmHg systolic) or a maximum dose of 400 µg/min is reached.

(c) Reduce afterload by the use of an arterial vasodilator such as *sodium nitroprusside.*

(d) Reduce/control heart rate. Consider using β blocker therapy for this purpose. Aim for a heart rate of between 50 and 60 bpm.

(e) Plan for urgent cardiologist review and possible ICU admission.

See *MYOCARDIAL INFARCTION (MI)* above.

M

Nn

Naloxone

Opioid receptor antagonist used to reverse the effects of opioid drugs, especially respiratory depression, nausea and vomiting and pruritus.

Dose

▶ *Adult*

IV bolus dose: 50–100 µg. Acts within 2 min and effects last for 20 min. Additional doses may therefore be required.

IV infusion dose: 4 µg/kg/h

▶ *Child*

2 µg/kg/dose, repeat every 2 min.

Nasal Anaesthesia

See *AWAKE FIBRE-OPTIC INTUBATION*.

Nasal Mucosa Vasoconstrictors

These include the following:

* cocaine (see *AWAKE FIBRE-OPTIC INTUBATION*)
* cophenylcaine forte spray
* drixine drops (oxymetazoline HCl).

Nausea And Vomiting Prevention, Postoperative

The overall incidence of postoperative nausea and vomiting (PONV) is about 20–30%.[1] Factors strongly associated with PONV include female gender, laparoscopic and other abdominal surgery, childhood, obesity, history of PONV or motion sickness, postoperative pain and movement, and non-smokers. For drug dosages, see the individual entries for each drug.

Prevention Strategies for PONV

1 Prophylactic anti-emetic therapy with a 5 hydroxytryptamine 3 (5-HT$_3$) receptor antagonist drug such as ondansetron combined with dexamethasone. These drugs are superior to the more traditional anti-nausea drugs such as metoclopramide.
2 Generous IV hydration.
3 Aggressive pain control with non-opioid analgesic drugs.
4 Avoidance of N$_2$O.[2]
5 Total IV anaesthesia with propofol with avoidance of volatile anaesthetic drugs.[3]
6 Postoperative O$_2$ therapy.[4]

Neck Haematoma

Seen most commonly after thyroid surgery and carotid endarterectomy. Neck haematoma can result in fatal airway compression and make direct laryngoscopy impossible.

N

Management

1 Notify the surgeon and arrange for an operating theatre urgently.
2 If the airway is threatened by significant haematoma, attempt to release the haematoma under LA infiltration (open up the incision). This can be life saving.[5]
3 If the above measure is not successful, spray the tongue and pharynx with LA and attempt awake direct laryngoscopy. If able to see the vocal cords easily, administer GA and muscle relaxants and intubate.
4 If not able to see the vocal cords decide whether the cause for this is likely to be reversible, i.e. the patient is uncooperative. If the cause is reversible, conduct a gaseous induction of general

anaesthesia and perform laryngoscopy when the patient is 'deep'. The surgeon should be scrubbed and ready for urgent tracheostomy. If able to see the vocal cords, paralyse and intubate. If unable to see vocal cords but the patient is easy to ventilate, proceed with surgery.

5   If airway difficulties occur during gaseous induction or the decision is made that direct laryngoscopy is likely to fail, perform an awake intubation using either:
    (a) fibre-optic technique. See *AWAKE FIBRE-OPTIC INTUBATION*.
    (b) retrograde technique. See *DIFFICULT AIRWAY MANAGEMENT*.

6   Alternatively, direct the surgeon to perform a tracheostomy under LA infiltration.

Needle-stick Injury

General Measures after Needle-stick Injury

1   Promote active bleeding from the wound.
2   Cleanse the wound thoroughly with soap and water.
3   Notify appropriate 'staff health' personnel if available for documentation of injury, management of infection prevention and counselling.

Human Immunodeficiency Virus Infection

Overall the risk of HIV infection from a single needle-stick injury is ≈ 3 per 1000.[6] Apart from blood, high-risk fluids include CSF, pleural, peritoneal, synovial fluid and breast milk. Low-risk fluids are vomit, urine, faeces and saliva.[7]

HIV Infection Prophylaxis

Post-exposure prophylactic therapy should ideally commence within 1 h of injury and be continued for 4 weeks. Triple therapy with zidovudine, lamivudine and indinavir is recommended.[7] HIV infection risk may be reduced by > 80% with this regimen.[8]

Hepatitis B

The risk of seroconversion after a needle-stick injury in a non-immunised individual is ≈ 30%. The non-immunised individual can be given a rapid hep B vaccination course plus hep B immunoglobulin after needle-stick injury.

A chronic carrier state occurs in 10% of patients infected with hep B. Of this group about 20% will die from complications of hep B such as cirrhosis and hepatocellular carcinoma.[9] Hep B immunisation has greatly reduced the risk of this illness to health care workers.

Hepatitis C

The risk of hep C transmission from a needle-stick injury is 3–4%. There is no effective infection prophylaxis at the time of writing. About 50% of people infected with hep C develop chronic hepatitis and an estimated 20% of these will progress to cirrhosis.[10] Some of these patients will progress to hepatocellular carcinoma.

Negative Pressure Pulmonary Oedema

Negative pressure pulmonary oedema is defined as transudation of fluid into the alveoli due to intense negative pressure produced by vigorous inspiratory effort in the presence of upper airway obstruction, e.g. laryngospasm, biting the endotracheal tube. Maximum inspiratory effort against upper airway obstruction can produce an intrathoracic pressure of 50–100 cmH_2O.[11] This condition can occur with a single breath and can cause significant hypoxia.

Treatment

1 Relieve the upper airway obstruction.
2 High concentration oxygen therapy.
3 CPAP in spontaneously breathing patients.
4 Diuretic therapy with lasix.

5 In severe cases mechanical ventilation with IPPV ± PEEP may be required.

The pulmonary oedema normally resolves after 12–24 h with supportive therapy.[11]

Neonatal Resuscitation

See Table N1 for Apgar scoring. Apgar scores are measured at 1 and 5 min. The 5 min score correlates with the degree of neonatal depression, and aids in predicting neonatal mortality.[12]

Table N1 Apgar scoring		
Characteristic	Description	Score
Colour	Cyanosed generally	0
	Body pink, limbs blue	1
	Pink 'all over'	2
Pulse	Nil	0
	<100	1
	>100	2
Grimace due to catheter in nose	Nil	0
	Grimacing	1
	Cough	2
Muscle tone	Limp	0
	Some flexion	1
	Active motion	2
Respiratory effort	Nil	0
	Weak cry	1
	Strong cry	2

N

Approach to Neonatal Resuscitation

If the newborn has absent or depressed respirations or a HR < 100 bpm, resuscitation is required. The anaesthetist's primary responsibility is to care for the mother, so ideally the neonatal resuscitator should be someone else.

The steps in neonatatal resuscitation are the following:

1. It is imperative to minimise heat loss. Utilise an overhead radiant heater and dry the baby off with a towel immediately. Ensure that the umbilical cord is securely clamped. Suck out the oropharynx and nose with an 8–10 Fr catheter. The maximum suction pressure that should be used is 100 mmHg.[13] These measures will also stimulate the baby.

2. Optimise the airway. Consider a towel under the shoulders to compensate for the large occiput. Jaw thrust may be required.

3. If meconium-stained liquor is present and the baby is not vigorous, suck out the oropharynx, then the nose. Perform direct laryngoscopy and suck away the meconium under direct vision. If the meconium is thin and the infant is vigorous, then tracheal suctioning is probably not required. However if the meconium is thick or particulate, intubate the trachea with the suction catheter to remove the meconium from below the cords. Alternatively, apply suction directly to an endotracheal tube placed in the trachea and then replace this with a fresh tube. Additionally, aspirate meconium from stomach.[12]

4. If the baby is not breathing or gasping after 15 s from birth, ventilate with 100% O_2 using a self-inflating bag and an appropriately sized face mask. The appropriate sizes of mask are:

   preterm   0
   term   1
   large newborn   2

   Give 5 ventilation breaths at an initial pressure of 30–40 cmH$_2$O over 2–3 s. These breaths are needed to provide initial lung

N

expansion (i.e. 'inflation breaths').[14] Note that the 'pop off' valve on the neonatal Laerdal bag is usually set at 30–35 mmHg.[13] As ventilation continues a lower ventilation pressure is sufficient i.e. 15–20 cmH_2O at a rate of 30–40 breaths/min. The normal tidal volume for a newborn is 6 mL/kg (20 mL for the average term infant).

5   If the heart rate (HR) is absent or < 60 and not increasing and 15–30 s of positive pressure ventilation has elapsed, begin external cardiac compression (ECC).This can be done by placing two fingers at right angles to the chest with the other hand supporting at the back, or the two thumbs on the sternum with hand encirclement technique. Depress the lower third of the sternum 1.5–2 cm or one-third the anterior posterior diameter of the chest. Use a chest compression rate of 90 per min and a ventilation rate of 30 breaths/min (a 3:1 ratio). Stop ECC if HR > 60.

6   If there is a poor response to the above resuscitation, intubate with the appropriate-sized endotracheal tube. The appropriate sizes are:

preterm infant	2.5
term infant	3.0
large term infant	3.5

Listen to the chest to detect correct placement of the endotracheal tube and exclude endobronchial intubation. The distance in cm from the tube tip to the patient's lips should be ≈ 6 cm + patient's weight in kg. If unable to intubate the neonate consider insertion of a size 1 LMA.

7   If the above resuscitative efforts do not result in an adequate spontaneous circulation, establish IV access. To establish IV access consider a peripheral vein or umbilical vein cannulation using a 3.5–5.0 Fr umbilical vein catheter with a single end hole.

Technique for Umbilical Vein Catheterisation

(a) Fill the umbilical vein catheter with saline via a 3-way tap prior to insertion to reduce the possibility of air embolus.

(b Insert the catheter into the umbilical vein. Note that the umbilical vein turns sharply in a cephalad direction just below the skin. Insert the catheter ≈ 4 cm.[12] If the catheter is inserted too far it may enter a hepatic vein. The liver can be damaged by direct infusion of vasoactive drugs or bicarbonate. Attempt to enter the ductus venosus by having the tip of the catheter turned anteriorly (the ductus venosus comes off the anterior wall of the umbilical vein). Free flow of blood should be present.

(c) Place a purse-string silk suture around the base of the cord to prevent subsequent haemorrhage.

If the spontaneous heart rate remains below 60 bpm, give adrenaline 10 μg/kg (0.1 mL/kg of adrenaline 1:10 000). If the response to the initial dose is inadequate, repeat this dose of adrenaline every 3–5 min. If unable to establish IV access, give adrenaline via the endotracheal tube using the same dose as the IV route.

8 Suspect hypovolaemia in any infant who fails to respond to resuscitation. If the infant appears pale with poor perfusion and thready, weak pulse, significant blood loss from the neonate may have occurred. Give volume expansion with 10 mL/kg of N/S or Hartmann's solution over 5–10 min. If blood loss is suspected give O –ve blood 10 mL/kg and assess the response.

9 Consider sodium bicarbonate 1–2 mmol/kg. Dilute the 1 mmol/L solution to 0.5 mmol/L by mixing with 10% glucose. Inject sodium bicarbonate over at least 2 min to decrease the risk of intraventricular haemorrhage.[13] The neonate must be receiving effective ventilation if sodium bicarbonate is given.

10 If low cardiac output persists despite adrenaline, start a dopamine infusion at 5 µg/kg/min initially.

11 If the mother has received an opioid within 4 h of delivery, consider giving naloxone 100 µg/kg IV or via the ET tube.

12 *Do not give naloxone to the baby if the mother is an opioid addict.* This is because of the risk of a severe withdrawal response, such as neonatal seizures.[13]

13 Treat hypoglycaemia (blood sugar level < 2.2 mmol/L) with an IV bolus of 10% glucose 5 mL/kg.

Cessation of Resuscitation Attempts[12]

If no response to resuscitation has occurred after 20 min and after consultation with the neonatal intensivist, consider the discontinuation of resuscitative efforts. If there has been no 'gasp' after 20 min (excluding drug effects), then the outlook is usually extremely poor, i.e. death or severe morbidity.

Neostigmine

This quaternary amine functions as a reversible, acid-transferring cholinesterase inhibitor. Acts by binding to acetylcholinesterase, thus competing with acetylcholine binding. Used for the reversal of the effects of non-depolarising neuromuscular blocking drugs (NDNMBD) and in the treatment of myasthenia gravis.

Dose (for the Reversal of NDNMBD)

50 µg/kg IV given with an appropriate dose of anticholinergic drug. The maximum dose of neostigmine that can be used is 60–80 µg/kg. See *ATROPINE* and *GLYCOPYRRONIUM (GLYCOPYRROLATE)*.

Neostigmine has been used intrathecally in a dose of 25–100 µg. It is an effective analgesic agent but intrathecal neostigmine is associated with a high incidence of nausea and vomiting.[15]

Nerve Stimulator Positions

Common Peroneal Nerve
Attach the negative electrode (black) to the skin just behind the most lateral portion of the head of fibula and positive electrode (red) over the patella.

Facial Nerve Branches
Place the negative electrode just above and lateral to the orbit, and the positive electrode just lateral and below the orbit.

Ulnar Nerve
Place the negative electrode over the volar surface of the distal wrist on the ulnar side and the positive electrode just proximal to this. Stimulates adductor pollicis muscle.

Posterior Tibial Nerve
Place the negative electrode just posterior and distal to the medial malleolus and the positive electrode just posterior and proximal to medial malleolus. With stimulation, plantar flexion of the toes is seen.

Neuroanaesthesia

(See also *CEREBRAL ANEURYSM SURGERY*.)

Aims
1 Prevent/treat elevation of intracranial pressure (ICP) and blood pressure.
2 Provide optimal operating conditions for surgery, e.g. ensure patient does not move during surgery.

Monitoring and Pre-operative Preparation
For major intracranial procedures such as removal of tumours:
1 large bore IV access e.g. 16 G cannula
2 peripherally placed central venous access

3 arterial line

4 precordial Doppler probe, if the risk of air embolus is high, such as when the sitting position is used. The Doppler probe should be placed over the right side of the heart (to the right of the sternum) between the 3rd and 6th intercostal spaces.

5 urinary catheter, temperature probe, nerve stimulator.

Induction and Maintenance

1 Fentanyl $\approx$ 3 µg/kg

2 Thiopentone: appropriate induction dose.

3 Lignocaine 1–2 mg/kg at least 2 min before intubation.

4 Non-depolarising muscle relaxant of choice.

5 Prior to intubation, spray the vocal cords and larynx with 3 mL of 4% topical lignocaine.

6 Secure the endotracheal tube carefully. An armoured tube is required if the patient is placed prone, in the sitting position or supine if the head is not in the neutral position. This is to prevent kinking of the endotracheal tube.

7 Maintain anaesthesia with isoflurane, sevoflurane and/or a propofol infusion. Desflurane, halothane and enflurane are not recommended for neuroanaesthesia (see individual entries). The use of nitrous oxide in neurosurgical anaesthesia is a debated issue. N_2O can cause an increase in intracranial pressure due to cerebrovasodilation.[16] N_2O can also potentially expand air that has been trapped after dural closure, resulting in raised intracranial pressure.[17] However, the significance of the potential deleterious effects of N_2O is questioned by several researchers.[18]

8 Maintain paralysis with a cisatracurium infusion 0.06–0.1 mg/kg/h.

9 Boluses of fentanyl as required. A remifentanil infusion can also be used.

10 The surgeon will frequently request the following:

  (a) Mannitol 20% solution 0.25–1 g/kg IV

    (b) Phenytoin 15 mg/kg in N/S (*not glucose*). Max. rate of administration 50 mg/min IV

    (c) Dexamethasone up to 20 mg IV

11 Antibiotic cover such as cephazolin 1 g.

12 Ventilate, aiming for optimal oxygenation and moderate hypocapnia of $\approx$ 30 mmHg CO_2. A lower $PaCO_2$ may cause cerebral ischaemia.[19] Check $PaCO_2$ formally on arterial blood gas sample.[19] It is preferable not to use positive end-expiratory pressure (PEEP) as it may cause increased intracranial pressure and a reduction in mean arterial pressure. PEEP does not protect against venous air embolism during neurosurgery in the sitting position.[20]

13 Do not infuse glucose containing solutions as elevated blood glucose levels can worsen cerebral ischaemic injury. Use N/S, which has a higher osmolarity than Hartmann's solution (300 mOsm/L vs 274 mOsm/L) and may therefore result in less brain swelling.[21]

14 If the patient is or becomes hypertensive, antihypertensive drugs to consider include the following:

    (a) *Thiopentone* boluses are effective for treating sudden hypertension, e.g. at intubation.[22]

    (b) *Clonidine* 50 µg increments to a max of 300 µg.

    (c) β *blocker*, e.g. atenolol or esmolol.

    (d) *Trimetaphan* is a rapidly acting therapy with a similar onset time to sodium nitroprusside but causing less cerebral vasodilatation. However, trimetaphan use is associated with a high incidence of bladder and bowel dysfunction and tachyphylaxis develops rapidly.

    (e) Sodium nitroprusside or glyceryl trinitrate may be used for hypertension unresponsive to the above drugs or when controlled hypotension is required. However, both agents can cause increased intracranial pressure.[23]

N

15 Mild intra-operative hypothermia provides significant cerebral protection against ischaemia. The patient can be allowed to passively cool to ≈ 35°C until surgery is completed and closure begins. Active rewarming should then commence, aiming for normothermia on emergence.[23]

Emergence

Give 1–2 mg/kg lignocaine IV at least 2 min before extubation and consider extubating the patient 'deep' in order to minimise coughing.

Neuroleptic Malignant Syndrome (NMS)

This syndrome can be severe and potentially life-threatening. It is triggered by drugs such as butyrophenones (haloperidol, droperidol), phenothiazines and thioxanthenes. NMS can also occur with the withdrawal of levodopa in Parkinson's disease.[24] The syndrome resembles, but is in no way related to, malignant hyperthermia. NMS is thought to be due to dopamine receptor blockade in the basal ganglia and the hypothalamus.[24] NMS has a high mortality rate, ranging from 14% with oral drugs to 38% with parenteral drugs.[24]

Factors Predisposing to the Development of NMS

These include:

1   acute hyponatraemia[25]
2   pre-existing fever
3   stress/exhaustion
4   dehydration
5   pre-existing brain damage or dysfunction.

Clinical Presentation

NMS is characterised by:

1   hyperpyrexia

2   muscle rigidity with excessive heat production. May see 'lead pipe' rigidity. The rigidity is a central effect, whereas in malignant hyperthermia the muscle rigidity is a direct peripheral effect.

3   autonomic dysfunction

4   altered mental state

5   renal failure due to rhabdomyolysis

6   dyspnoea, respiratory failure

7   myocadial infarct and cardiac arrest

8   evidence of muscle damage (elevated creatinine kinase levels and myoglobinuria)

9   peripheral neuropathy[26]

10 disseminated intravascular coagulopathy.

Treatment

1   Ensure an adequate airway, that ventilation is occurring and the patient is well-oxygenated. Intubate the patient if indicated.

2   Check pulse and blood pressure and ensure circulation is adequate. Support the patient's circulation if required.

3   Cease the causative drug.

4   Give IV fluids and ensure hydration is optimal.

5   Cool the patient (cooling blankets, cooled IV solutions).

6   Dantrolene (see entry). This drug relieves muscle spasms and helps reduce muscle-related heat production.[26]

7   Bromocriptine mesylate is given orally to reduce creatinine kinase levels, reduce confusion and alleviate extra-pyramidal effects.[26] It acts via its dopamine receptor agonist effect. Amantadine is an alternative.

8   Circulatory and respiratory support.

9   Plasmapheresis has been used successfully in an intractable case of NMS.[24]

10 Other drugs to consider include levodopa-carbidopa, anticholinergics and calcium channel blocker drugs.[26]

N

New York Heart Association Functional Classification of Patients with Heart Disease

See Table N2.

Table N2 New York Heart Association functional classification of patients with heart disease

Class	Description
1	Asymptomatic at rest, symptoms with heavy exercise.
2	Symptoms with ordinary activity but comfortable at rest.
3	Symptoms with minimal activity but comfortable at rest.
4	Symptoms at rest.

Nicardipine

Dihydropyridine calcium channel antagonist drug used IV for the treatment of angina and hypertension and for inducing intra-operative hypotension. IV nicardipine has a rapid onset, is short acting and produces only slight myocardial depression.[27]

Dose

For the treatment of hypertension or induction of hypotension, IV bolus 0.017 mg/kg.[27]

Nifedipine

Dihydropyridine calcium channel antagonist used for the treatment of hypertension, angina and coronary artery spasm during coronary angiography or angioplasty. It is a potent arterial vasodilator with minimal venodilating effects.

N

Dose

Adult: 10–40 mg PO 12 h for moderate to severe hypertension. If reduction in blood pressure is urgent, a 10 mg tablet can be chewed, then swallowed.[28]

Nimodipine

Calcium channel antagonist drug, which preferentially causes smooth muscle relaxation of cerebral arteries. It is used for the prevention and treatment of vascular spasm after subarachnoid haemorrhage (SAH). In SAH patients nimodipine decreases the incidence of cerebral infarction by one-third.[29]

Dose

Adult: 60 mg 4 h PO starting within 4 days of SAH and continued for 3 weeks *or* 1 mg/h IV via a central venous line for 2 h, increased to 2 mg/h if the patient's blood pressure is not significantly compromised. Start as soon as possible and continue for 5–14 days (continue for at least for 5 days after surgery). See *CEREBRAL ANEURYSM SURGERY*.

N

Nitrous Oxide

Gas used:

1 for supplementation of general anaesthesia, usually in a concentration of 70%
2 as an analgesic for labour and painful procedures
3 for laparoscopic surgery to provide pneumoperitoneum.

Presented as a liquid in blue cylinders at a pressure of 44 bar at 15°C.

Physical Properties and MAC

Blood:gas solubility coefficient	0.48
Oil:gas solubility coefficient	1.4

Boiling point	–88°C
Critical pressure	71.7 atmospheres
Critical temperature	36.5°C
MAC	105

Advantages

1. Potent analgesic properties equivalent to 10–15 mg of morphine.[30]
2. Effective sedative properties without respiratory depression.[30]
3. Decreases the MAC of volatile anaesthetic agents and accelerates the uptake of these agents. Although N_2O is not without risk, its use may reduce the use of other drugs with possibly increased toxic effects.
4. It appears to be safe in patients with malignant hyperthermia susceptibility.
5. Inexpensive to produce.
6. Rapid onset and offset of action due to its relative insolubility.

Disadvantages

1. N_2O decreases myocardial contractility, although this is offset by a stimulating effect on the sympathetic nervous system, increasing peripheral vascular resistance. It also causes increased pulmonary vascular resistance in patients with pre-existing pulmonary hypertension.[31,32]
2. 35 × more soluble than nitrogen in blood, thus causing a rapid increase in the size of air-filled spaces, e.g. pneumothorax, and in the size of gas emboli. This property also leads to diffusion hypoxia when N_2O administration is ceased. Supplementary O_2 is thus required at this time.
3. Supports combustion and thus can contribute to fires.
4. Contributes to postoperative nausea and vomiting.[31,32]
5. May increase intracranial pressure by increasing cerebral blood flow.[31,32] See *NEUROANAESTHESIA*.

N

6   Inhibits methionine synthetase and mild megaloblastic bone marrow changes can be seen after only 12 h of N_2O exposure in healthy patients.[33] This effect is due to N_2O oxidising cobalamin in vitamin B_{12}. In patients chronically exposed to N_2O, megaloblastic anaemia and subacute combined degeneration of the spinal cord may occur. Routine N_2O anaesthesia has resulted in subacute combined degeneration of the spinal cord after a single exposure in patients with pernicious anaemia and/or vitamin B_{12} deficiency.[33]

7   N_2O has abuse potential and people who are using N_2O recreationally may suffer the complications described above.

8   Contributes to 'greenhouse' gases and the destruction of ozone.[34]

9   Teratogenicity is suspected from animal studies[35,36] but N_2O has never been conclusively shown to be teratogenic in human pregnancy.[37] The Australian Drug Evaluation Committee currently rates N_2O as a Category A drug, i.e. *no proven long-term harmful effects on the human foetus despite extensive use.*

10 N_2O lacks potency and there is a high risk of awareness if it is used as a sole anaesthetic agent.

11 N_2O anaesthesia causes elevated blood homocysteine levels, which may increase the risk and incidence of myocardial ischaemia.[38]

Warning: Nitrous Oxide and Ocular Surgery

Intra-ocular gas such as perfluoropropane (C_3F_8) or sulfurhexa-fluoride (SF_6) may be used therapeutically for the treatment of conditions such as retinal detachment and vitrectomy. Intra-ocular gas bubbles can exist for up to 10 weeks.[39] If N_2O is used for subsequent non-eye surgery during this time, sudden blindness may occur in the treated eye, due to expansion of the intra-ocular gas. N_2O is therefore contraindicated in this situation.

Non-steroidal Anti-inflammatory Drugs (NSAIDs)

General Comments

NSAIDs have analgesic and anti-inflammatory actions due to their ability to inhibit cyclo-oxygenase (COX1 and COX2). Cyclo-oxygenase catalyses the production of prostaglandin and thromboxane and COX inhibition decreases their production. COX1 produces prostaglandins that are involved with platelet aggregation, renal function and gastric mucosa integrity. COX1 inhibition offers no therapeutic benefit and is the cause of the unwanted side effects of NSAIDs. COX2 results in prostaglandins involved with inflammation and nociception and inhibition of COX2 produces the desired therapeutic effects (anti-inflammatory and analgesia). These drugs have peripheral and probable central sites of action.[40] NSAIDs are thus divided into two groups: drugs that are non-selective (inhibit COX1 and COX2) and selective COX2 inhibitors.

Precautions Applicable to Both Selective and Non-selective NSAIDs

1 These drugs are contraindicated in patients with:
   (a) peptic ulcer disease
   (b) gastrointestinal bleeding or bleeding diathesis
   (c) aspirin-sensitive asthma. NSAIDs should be used with caution in other asthmatics.[41]
   (d) allergy to NSAIDs or aspirin.

2 These drugs should be avoided in patients with:
   (a) renal impairment. Acute renal failure can be precipitated by NSAIDs such as *ketorolac*. Patients on an ACE inhibitor and/or diuretic therapy may be at increased risk of renal failure if given NSAIDs.[40]

(b) pregnancy. These drugs may cross the placenta and cause premature closure of the foetal ductus arteriosus.

(c) patients with pre-eclampsia, hypovolaemia or uncontrolled hypertension.[41]

3 Use NSAIDs with caution:

(a) in the elderly

(b) in patients with diabetes or vascular disease

(c) after major vascular surgery or renal, cardiac or hepatobiliary surgery.

(d) in patients with heart failure on diuretics. NSAIDs cause sodium retention and may precipitate heart failure or hypertension in predisposed patients.[42]

(e) patients on cyclosporin or triamterene

(f) patients taking renally cleared drugs with a low therapeutic index such as digoxin or aminoglycoside

(g) asthmatics. If aspirin-sensitive asthma, see contraindications above.

4 NSAIDs can cause severe hepatic toxicity leading to fulminant liver failure and death.[40]

Precautions Specific to Non-selective NSAIDs

These drugs increase bleeding time and blood loss in some studies due to platelet inhibition. For example, they should be avoided in tonsillectomy and plastic surgery patients.

Non-selective NSAIDS vary in their risk profile. High-risk agents include piroxicam and ketoprofen, while lower risk agents include diclofenac and ibuprofen.[43]

See *DICLOFENAC* and *KETOROLAC*.

Precautions Specific to COX2 Selective Inhibitors

1 Do not interfere with platelet function.

2 Lower incidence of gastroduodenal ulcers than non-selective NSAIDs.[44] However, these drugs should be used with caution in

patients with a history of peptic ulcer disease or a history of gastro-intestinal bleeding and patients on steroids.

3   The undesirable effects of NSAIDs on the kidney may be similar for both selective and non-selective agents. There have been reports of renal failure occurring in association with these drugs.[45]

4   Rofecoxib increases INR in patients on warfarin.

5   Celecoxib is contraindicated in patients allergic to sulfonamides.

6   See *CELECOXIB, PARECOXIB (DYNASTAT), ROFECOXIB.*

Noradrenaline

A catecholamine sympathomimetic agent acting mainly on α and β1 adreno-receptors with almost no effect on β2 (vasodilating) adreno-receptors. Used mainly as a vasoconstrictor to treat refractory hypotension, such as occurs in septic shock. Increases both systolic and diastolic blood pressure and diverts blood flow from the skin, liver, kidney and bowel to the brain and heart. There is thus a risk of ischaemia to the organs from which blood is diverted.

Dose

Give by central line only. Add 6 mg to 100 mL N/S or 5% glucose. Run at 0.05–0.30 μg/kg/min (titrate to desired effect). For a 70 kg patient this equals 3–20 mL/h. Start infusion at 5 mL/h.

Note

1   If extravasation occurs, infiltrate the area of extravasation with 5–10 mg of phentolamine in 10–15 mL of N/S. This may reduce the risk of tissue necrosis.[46]

2   Do not administer noradrenaline in IV lines containing alkaline solutions as the noradrenaline may be inactivated.[46]

Normal Saline

Crystalloid intravenous solution with the following properties:

Sodium	150 mmol/L
Chloride	150 mmol/L
Osmolarity	300 mOsm/L
pH	4.0–7.0

Only 25% of infused saline remains in the intravascular space. Massive infusion of normal saline can result in hyperchloraemic acidosis and pulmonary oedema due to decreased colloid osmotic pressure.

NovoSeven

See *RECOMBINANT ACTIVATED FACTOR VII.*

Nupercaine

See *SUBARACHNOID BLOCK (SAB).*

N

Oo

Obesity

See *BODY MASS INDEX (BMI) AND OBESITY*. The problems of morbid obesity and anaesthesia overlap with those of obstructive sleep apnoea (see below).

Obstructive Sleep Apnoea (OSA) Syndrome

This common disorder is characterised by recurrent and often prolonged episodes of apnoea/hypopnoea and hypoxaemia during sleep, which can produce severe and potentially fatal physiological effects.

Clinical Manifestations

These may include:

1 pulmonary and systemic hypertension
2 right and left heart failure
3 dysrhythmias
4 polycythaemia
5 excessive daytime sleepiness
6 respiratory failure

There is often associated obesity.

Diagnosis

The 'gold standard' for diagnosis of OSA is the full overnight polysomnography. A detailed description of sleep study diagnosis of OSA is beyond the scope of this manual. Most patients with OSA are undiagnosed at the time of anaesthesia.[1]

Treatment

1. Avoid sedating drugs such as alcohol, benzodiazepines.
2. Avoid supine sleep posture (i.e. sleep laterally).
3. Reduce weight if obese.
4. Drug therapy (progesterone, protritylline) is helpful in some patients.[2]
5. Surgery to reduce airway obstruction, e.g. uvulopalatopharyngoplasty.
6. Nasal continuous positive airway pressure (CPAP) machine.
7. Tracheostomy may be considered for life-threatening OSA.[2]

Anaesthetic Implications

▶ *Pre-operative Aspects*

1. Consider investigating patients for cardiorespiratory complications of OSA, e.g. CXR, looking for cardiomegaly and evidence of pulmonary hypertension. Echocardiography may be appropriate.
2. Check FBC for polycythaemia. Phlebotomy should be considered if the haematocrit is greater than 55%.
3. Discuss/consider regional analgesia/anaesthesia if appropriate for the procedure.
4. Avoid sedating premedication such as benzodiazepines and opioids.
5. OSA patients may also be difficult to intubate and may be at risk of aspiration due to associated obesity and gastro-oesophageal reflux.[3] Consider the need for awake fibre-optic intubation, pre-operative drying agents and antacid therapy.

Intra-operative Management

See *DIFFICULT AIRWAY MANAGEMENT*.

1. Due to possibly associated aspiration risk, consider rapid sequence induction. Make adequate preparations for failed intubation should this occur.

2 If the patient has pulmonary hypertension, see *PULMONARY HYPERTENSION* for details of management.

3 Minimise intra-operative opioids if possible. Use short-acting opioids preferably.

4 Ensure NMBDs are fully reversed prior to emergence. Extubate the patient when he/she is fully awake/alert.

5 Consider extubation in the semi-upright position.

Postoperative Management

1 This phase may be a particularly 'at risk' period for the OSA patient due to reduced supervision and monitoring. Unsupervised OSA patients on PCA or morphine infusions have suffered death and hypoxic brain damage.[1]

2 Nurse patients sitting up in bed, or laterally, rather than in a supine position.

3 Supplementary oxygen therapy is usually desirable but this is a debated issue.[1,4] Oxygen therapy may be detrimental in patients relying on hypoxic drive to maintain ventilation. Close postoperative observation will help reduce risk.

4 Consider non-opioid analgesia such as NSAIDs.

5 Patients should use their nasal CPAP machines during sleep periods while in hospital.

6 Nusing in a high dependency unit with pulse oximetry monitoring may be prudent. Continue to intensively monitor until opioid requirements are minimal.

Occipital Nerve Block

See *SCALP BLOCK*.

Oculogyric Crisis

See *DYSTONIC REACTION, ACUTE*.

Ondansetron

An antagonist at the 5-HT$_3$ (serotonin) receptor both peripherally and centrally, ondansetron is used for the treatment/prevention of nausea and vomiting. Odansetron may also be useful for preventing morphine induced pruritus (see *MORPHINE*). It lacks the extrapyramidal side effects seen with dopamine receptor antagonist drugs such as metoclopramide.[5]

Dose
Adult: 4–8 mg IV up to 8 h as required.
Child: 0.1–0.2 mg/kg to a max. of 8 mg.

Disadvantages
There is an increased risk of postoperative headache and constipation with ondansetron.[6]

One-lung Ventilation

Topics Covered in this Section
▶ Indications for One-lung Ventilation
▶ Double Lumen Endotracheal Tubes
▶ Bronchial Blockers
▶ Predictors of High Risk for One-lung Ventilation/Pneumonectomy
▶ Physiology of One-lung Ventilation
▶ Optimisation of Oxygenation During One-lung Ventilation

Indications for One-lung Ventilation
The indications for one-lung ventilation include:
1   prevention of spillage of blood or pus from one lung to the other
2   isolation of the lung that is causing leakage of ventilating gases.

Causes of a leak from one lung include bronchopleural fistula and surgical or traumatic opening of a main conducting airway.

3 unilateral bronchopulmonary lavage
4 improving exposure of operative site for surgeon.

Double Lumen Endotracheal Tubes (DLT)

One-lung ventilation is usually achieved by insertion of a DLT. A left-sided tube is easier to place than a right-sided tube and is usually adequate for left- or right-lung ventilation unless there is pathology in the left mainstem bronchus.

DLT Sizes

Vary from 28 to 41 Fr. Adult male 39–41 Fr, adult female 35–37 Fr.

Placement of a Left–sided Mallinckrodt BronchoCath™ DLT

This disposable plastic DLT has two curves: a distal curve for insertion into the left main bronchus and a proximal curve. Ensure the cuffs are well-lubricated prior to insertion.

1 Induce anaesthesia, paralyse and ventilate.
2 Insert the DLT with the distal curve concave anteriorly. Once the distal part of the DLT has passed through the vocal cords, remove the stylet, and rotate the tube 90° so that the proximal curve is now concave anteriorly.
3 Advance the DLT until slight resistance felt, usually at ≈ 29 cm (27–31 cm).[7]
4 Inflate the tracheal cuff with ≈ 5 mL of air and the bronchial (blue) cuff with ≈ 1.5 mL of air.
5 Ventilate the patient and ensure that both lungs are being inflated. If only one lung inflates both tube lumens may be in one bronchus.
6 Clamp the bronchial lumen tube connection, open the bronchial lumen to air, and then assess ventilation. The right lung only should inflate. If both lungs inflate, deflate both cuffs

0

and gently and incrementally insert the DLT further into the trachea. Repeat steps 4, 5 and 6.

7 Clamp tracheal lumen tube connection, open the tracheal lumen to air, and assess ventilation. The left lung only should inflate. If the right lung only inflates the right bronchus has been intubated. Deflate both cuffs, withdraw the DLT and reinsert the DLT with the head turned to the right and DLT rotated to the left.[7]

8 Ensure that the left lung apex is being ventilated, i.e. bronchial lumen may obstruct the left upper lobe bronchus.

9 If there are persistent problems with placement, insert a fibre-optic bronchoscope down the tracheal lumen to check the position of the DLT. A 3.6–4.2 mm external diameter paediatric bronchoscope will fit through all sizes of DLT.[8] A 4.9 mm external diameter will pass through 41–39 DLTs.

10 Repeat steps 6 and 7 when the patient is repositioned.

A Second 'Blind' Technique of DLT Placement[9]

1 Select the DLT that will be long enough to extend from the lips to 1 cm below the carina. This is estimated by placing the DLT with the proximal curve facing posteriorly. The bifurcation point of the tube should lie just below the anterior border of the ear lobe and the bronchial cuff should be 1 cm below the manubrio-sternal junction.

2 Insert the tube as described in steps 1 and 2 above into the trachea just below the cords and inflate the bronchial cuff with 3–5 mL of air. Clamp the tracheal lumen tube connection and open the tracheal lumen to air, so that ventilation is through the bronchial lumen only. Ventilate the patient, ensuring both lungs inflate evenly.

3 Advance the DLT gradually until only one side of the chest is moving (the left side with correct placement). If only the right side inflates, withdraw the tube back into the trachea and rotate

tube 180° anticlockwise, then reinsert. If again unsuccessful repeat the manoeuvre but with the cuff deflated.

4   When the left bronchus is entered, indicated by left-lung inflation only, deflate the cuff and insert the DLT 1 cm further plus the width of cuff. Reinflate the bronchial cuff with sufficient air to make a seal.

5   Test ventilate each lung separately as described above.

Troubleshooting

If unable to deflate the appropriate lung despite several attempts at repositioning the DLT, consider the following steps:

1   Pass the fibre-optic bronchoscope (FOB) down the bronchial lumen while continuing to ventilate the tracheal lumen.

2   Deflate both cuffs and pull the DLT into the trachea until the carina can be visualised.

3   Intubate the left main bronchus with the FOB.

4   Railroad the bronchial part of the DLT into the left main bronchus.

Bronchial Blockers

These devices enable the occlusion of the left or right bronchus to cause collapse of the appropriate lung.

▶ Univent Tubes

An example of such a device is the Univent tube, which consists of a single endotracheal tube with a separate channel for a manoeuvreable bronchial blocker that can be positioned in the left or right bronchus. The Univent has an oval lumen and adult sizes range from 6.0–9.0 mm internal diameter. Oxygen can be supplied to the deflated lung via the lumen of the bronchial blocker tube.

Technique for Placement of the Univent[10]

1   Test the bronchial and tracheal cuffs and ensure that the tube is

well-lubricated. When fully inflated the bronchial cuff requires 6–8 mL of air.

2 Withdraw the blocker into its channel.

3 Intubate the patient in the conventional manner.

4 Use a fibre-optic bronchoscope to ensure accurate placement of the bronchial blocker into the right or left bronchus. In the left bronchus the optimal position is when the inflated cuff (6–8 mL of air) can just be visualised 5 mm distal to the carina. In the right bronchus correct placement is when the cuff is just proximal to the origin of the right upper lobe bronchus.

Advantages of the Univent Tube Compared with the DLT

1 The Univent tube is much more like a conventional endo-tracheal tube.

2 It is able to be used as an effective lobar blocker.

3 The Univent does not need to be replaced at the end of the case if ongoing ventilation is required.

4 The Univent tube is easier to insert in the patient who is difficult to intubate than a DLT. It can also be inserted using an awake fibre-optic intubation technique.

5 A bronchial blocker can be used in a patient who is too small for a DLT.

Disadvantages of the Univent Tube Compared with the DLT

1 Placement requires a fibre-optic bronchoscope due to the risk of trauma to the trachea or bronchus.

2 Inflation of the bronchial cuff can traumatise the trachea or bronchus.

3 During right upper lobe lobectomy the bronchial blocker may be caught in the suture line.

4 Inflation of the bronchial lumen may result in obstruction of the tracheal lumen.

Predictors of High Risk for One-lung Ventilation/Pneumonectomy

For predictors of poor tolerance of one-lung ventilation and/or pneumonectomy see *RESPIRATORY FUNCTION TESTS*.

Physiology of One-lung Ventilation

Blood flow to the dependent lung is ≈ 60% of the total pulmonary blood flow. If both lungs are ventilated, ventilation preferentially goes to the non-dependent lung. If the chest is opened, this increases the mismatch of ventilation and perfusion. When the non-dependent lung is not ventilated, hypoxic vasoconstriction increases the blood flow to the dependent lung to 80% of the total. However, volatile anaesthetic agents decrease hypoxic vasoconstriction. At 1 MAC isoflurane, the dependent lung blood flow is reduced to ≈ 75% of the total pulmonary blood flow.

Optimisation of Oxygenation

Optimisation of oxygenation can be achieved by applying the following measures:

1   Ensure the position of the DLT is optimal, i.e. that left upper lobe is being ventilated. Suck out the lumens to remove secretions, and identify and correct kinking of the tube. If any doubt exists at any stage check the position of the DLT with the fibre-optic bronchoscope.

2   It is difficult to predict the optimal tidal volume and ventilating pressure for the individual patient. Start with tidal volume of 10 mL/kg and limit the plateau airway pressure to 25 cmH$_2$O initially.[11] Increase the tidal volume to a maximum of 15 mL/kg if necessary. If the airway pressure is excessive (> 30 cmH$_2$O) decrease the tidal volume and increase the respiratory rate.

3   Set the respiratory rate so that PaCO$_2$ is maintained at 40 mmHg.[8] It is usually necessary to increase respiratory rate

by about 20%.[8] Consider permissive hypercapnia if barotrauma is a risk.

4   Apply continuous positive airways pressure (CPAP) of 5–10 cmH_2O to the non-dependent lung using a separate anaesthetic circuit.[11] Allow the non-dependent lung to inflate to a size that does not interfere with surgery. CPAP is most effective if commenced before the lung is deflated[11] or after a large tidal volume inflation to overcome critical opening pressures in the collapsed lung.[8] Alternatively, O_2 can be insufflated into the non-dependent lung via tubing such as a suction catheter placed in the correct lumen.

5   Consider applying 5 cm positive end expiratory pressure to the dependent lung if oxygenation is not satisfactory with CPAP. This will reduce atelectasis but may divert blood to non-dependent lung and worsen oxygenation.

6   Increase FiO_2, up to 100%. The use of N_2O can result in increased dependent lung atelectasis. Therefore, air/O_2 mixtures are preferable if less than 100% O_2 is used.

7   Intermittent reinflation of non-dependent lung or return to two-lung ventilation may be required.

8   Clamping of pulmonary artery to the non-dependent lung will cease shunting of blood to that lung.

9   Ensure that cardiac output (CO) remains adequate as a decreased CO will contribute to hypoxaemia.

10 Treat any other reversible causes of hypoxaemia such as bronchospasm.

11 Intravenous anaesthesia with propofol has no effect on hypoxic vasoconstriction and may be of benefit.[12]

12 Adrenaline, noradrenaline, phenylephrine and dopamine all cause vasoconstriction in the dependent lung, worsening ventilation/perfusion mismatch. However, if a vasopressor is required, dopamine maybe the agent of choice as it has the least effect on hypoxic vasoconstriction.[12]

Opioid Receptors

These are classified as:

- Mu1: stimulation causes miosis, euphoria, supraspinal analgesia, abuse potential[13,14]
- Mu2: respiratory depression, inhibition of gut motility and bradycardia[15]
- Kappa: ventilatory depression, sedation and spinal analgesia
- Sigma: dysphoria, hallucinations, mydriasis, respiratory stimulation and tachycardia
- Delta: ventilatory depression and modification of mu receptor activity.[13]

Opioids: Relative Potencies[13,16]

IV Opioids

Morphine 10 mg IV is equivalent to (all doses are IV):

Alfentanil	500 µg
Buprenorphine	300 µg
Carfentanil	40–50 µg
Codeine	120 mg
Fentanyl	80–100 µg
Heroin	5 mg
Hydromorphone	2 mg
Lofentanil	10–20 µg
Methadone	10 mg
Oxycodone	15 mg
Papaveretum	16 mg
Pethidine	75–100 mg
Remifentanil	80–100 µg
Sufentanil	20 µg

Oral Opioids

Morphine PO 30 mg is equivalent to:

Codeine	240 mg
Dextromoramide	15 mg
Dextropropoxyphene	300 mg
Methadone	20 mg
Oxycodone	30 mg
Pethidine	240 mg

Oxycodone

Synthetic opioid analgesic drug.

Dose

Adult: Start with 5 mg 6 h, increase as required, or 30 mg suppositories PR 6–8 h.
Child: 0.1–0.2 mg/kg PO 4–6 h max. 10 mg.

Oxygen

Gaseous element essential for respiration. Stored in cylinders with black bodies and white shoulders in sizes from 170–8800 L (C–J). The pressure in full cylinder of O_2 is 137 bar at 15°C. Liquid O_2 is stored in vacuum insulated evaporator tanks at less than –150°C. One volume of liquid O_2 can yield 840 volumes of gaseous O_2.

Some Physical Properties of Oxygen

Critical temperature	118.4°C
Critical pressure	50.8 atmospheres
Boiling point	–183°C

Oxygen Content of Blood

Calculated from the equation:

O_2 content/100 mL =
$1.34 \times O_2$ saturation $\times$ Hb concentration/ 100 mL + $0.003 \times PaO_2$

Oxymetazoline

Sympathomimetic used to constrict the arteriolar network of the nasal mucosa. Drixine contains a 0.05% solution of oxymetazoline.

Oxytocin

A naturally occurring polypeptide secreted by the hypothalamus and stored in the posterior pituitary gland. The synthesised form (syntocinon) is free of vasopressin, and is used for induction and augmentation of labour, and to cause and maintain uterine contraction postpartum. It is also used to cause uterine contraction in the setting of miscarriage.

Dose

1 *For augmentation of labour* 1.5–12 mUnits/min titrated to response. Do not infuse with glucose because of the risk of water intoxication due to the antidiuretic effects of oxytocin. Infuse with Hartmann's solution or N/S.

2 *For uterine contraction after delivery or evacuation of the uterus after miscarriage* 10 units IV or IM. Effects last for ≈ 1 h.

Note

Do not infuse oxytocin in the same line as blood or plasma because the drug will be inactivated by plasma oxytocinase. Causes vaso-dilatation and if used in large amounts can cause hypotension and tachycardia.

Pp

Pacemakers and Anaesthesia

Topics Covered in this Section
▶ Classification of Permanent Pacemakers
▶ Anaesthetic Management of Patients with Permanent Pacemakers
▶ Temporary Pacemaker Wire Insertion and Pacing
▶ Transcutaneous Cardiac Pacing (TCP)
▶ Transoesophageal Pacing

Classification of Permanent Pacemakers

More than 1500 types of pacemaker have been produced in the USA. Types of pacemakers include:

1 *asynchronous* (VOO): this type contains no sensing circuitry
2 *synchronous*: in this type, in response to the patient's R wave, the device either triggers (VVT) or inhibits (VVI). VVI pacemakers are the most common type.
3 *sequential*: this type maintains the atrio-ventricular contraction sequence. DDD pacemakers sense the patient's P and R waves and pace atria and ventricles.
4 *programmable*: this type can have their functions such as rate, output, sensing changed.

Permanent pacemakers are classified by a three- or five-letter code:

- The *first code letter* indicates the chamber paced, i.e. **V**entricle, **A**trium, **D**ual, or **O** none.
- The *second code letter* indicates the chamber sensed (**O**, **A**, **V**, or **D** as above).

- The *third code letter* stands for the mode of response to sensing, i.e. **T** = triggered, **I** = inhibited, **D** = double (triggered and inhibited), **R** = reverse (pacemaker activated when tachycardia sensed) and **0** none.
- The *fourth code letter* indicates programmability: **R** = rate responsive, **C** = communicating, **M** = multiprogrammability, **P** = simple programmable. Rate responsive pacemakers can respond to such stimuli as respiration (changes in transthoracic impedance), temperature or QT interval. They are able to increase heart rate in response to presumed exercise.
- The *fifth code letter* indicates anti-tachydysrhythmic function: **S** = shock (implantable defibrillator), **P** = pacing and **D** = both P and S.

Anaesthetic Management of Patients with Permanent Pacemakers

▶ *Elective Surgery*

1 Organise for a pacemaker technician to switch off the programmable features of the pacemaker. Consider reprogramming the pacemaker to an asynchronous (VOO) mode at a rate of 60–70.[1] The risk of VOO mode is that competition between paced and spontaneous beats could lead to sustained tachycardia or fibrillation, particularly in the diseased heart. If the patient has a good intrinsic heart rate, consider VVI mode.

2 Check the ECG to see how frequently pacing spikes occur to assess whether the patient is pacemaker-dependent. If the patient is pacemaker-dependent, plan a strategy for emergency pacing if a malfunction of the permanent pacemaker occurs. Disable the 'artifact filter' on the ECG so pacemaker spikes can be detected.

3 Although endocarditis has been reported with pacing wires[2] prophylactic antibiotics are not indicated unless additional risk factors are present.[3]

4 The use of diathermy can interfere with pacemaker function.[3] The risk of diathermy effects can be reduced by the following:

   (a) Use short bursts of diathermy current at the lowest acceptable power output.

   (b) Do not use diathermy within 15 cm of pacemaker or heart.

   (c) Place the indifferent plate as far away from the heart and as close to the cutting blade as possible.

   (d) The direction of the diathermy current (blade to plate) should be at right angles to the pacemaker system.

   (e) Use bipolar diathermy (the current flows through the two points of forceps) rather than unipolar (blade to plate). If unipolar diathermy is used, 'pure cut' is better than 'blend' or 'coag' settings.

5 Defibrillation, if required, should be carried out with the paddles (or electrode pads) at right angles to the pacemaker wire. Do not place a defibrillation paddle over the pacemaker box.

6 'Pacemaker syndrome' may occur in patients with VVI pacemakers and consists of sudden hypotension with the onset of ventricular pacing.[3] It is due to the loss of atrioventricular synchrony and reflex vasodilatation due to atrial stretch-receptor stimulation. It is treated by reducing the pacemaker rate so that sinus rhythm predominates, or increasing the sinus rate with atropine or isoprenaline.

7 The pacemaker should be rechecked postoperatively and reprogrammed by qualified staff.

8 If pacemaker failure occurs during anaesthesia consider the following options to maintain heart rate:

   (a) atropine

   (b) transcutaneous pacing

(c) isoprenaline infusion

(d) adrenaline infusion.

9 Place nerve stimulators well away from the pacemaker.

▶ Emergency Surgery with Inability of Pacemaker Technician to Attend Patient Pre-operatively

The same considerations as above apply. However, it may not be possible to obtain the assistance of a pacemaker technician.

1 A pacemaker magnet should be immediately available. If significant pacemaker malfunction occurs during surgery, application of a magnet to the pacemaker may convert it to a fixed rate mode. However, application of an external magnet to a pacemaker can produce unwanted, unpredictable results. The pacemaker technician, if contactable, may be able to indicate what will happen if a magnet is applied to a particular pacemaker.

2 Contact the cardiologist urgently if life-threatening pacemaker malfunction occurs that is not responsive to application of a magnet. Once a magnet is placed over the pacemaker, it should not be removed until a pacemaker technician is available. If the magnet is removed, a new program may become apparent. If the effects of the new program are deleterious, then reapply the magnet and contact the cardiologist urgently.

3 Suxamethonium is best avoided as muscle fasciculations may result in pacemaker malfunction.[3]

4 The pacemaker should be checked postoperatively by qualified staff.

▶ Automatic Implantable Cardioverter Defibrillator

1 If the patient has an automatic implantable cardioverter defibrillator (AICD) the defibrillating function should be deactivated prior to anaesthesia by appropriate technical staff.[4]

2 External defibrillation pads and connections should be applied before anaesthesia. If external defibrillation is required, place

the pads in an anterior/posterior position. A higher than normal defibrillation energy may be required.

3 If emergency surgery precludes the deactivation of the unit and inappropriate defibrillation occurs, consider placement of an external magnet over the unit. This may deactivate the AICD and audible tones may be heard from the AICD.

4 Removal of the magnet may reactivate the unit.

5 Medical staff are not at risk if in contact with the patient during AICD defibrillation.[4]

▶ *Specific Procedures and Pacemakers*

Magnetic resonance imaging (MRI) is, in general, contraindicated in patients with pacemakers. If MRI is considered essential, discuss implications with the cardiologist.

Lithotripsy can be performed in a patient with a pacemaker unless the pulse generator (or 'can') is abdominally placed. The above precautions should be used and a programmer should be available throughout the procedure. Contralateral lithotripsy can probably be safely performed in patients with AICDs.[4]

Temporary Pacemaker Wire Insertion and Pacing

A typical unit used is a Medtronic 5375 Demand Pulse Generator.

1 Insert a central venous sheath as described for *INTERNAL JUGULAR VEIN CATHETERISATION*.

2 Insert a pacing wire towards the apex of the right ventricle under X-ray guidance or use a flotation-guided cardiac pacing wire.

3 Connect the pacing leads to the corresponding red and black leads and ask an assistant to connect these to the pacing box. The settings to be adjusted are:
    (a) sensitivity: the pacemaker's ability to sense intrinsic rhythm
    (b) output: the pacing current
    (c) rate: the pacing rate.

4   With the generator switched off, set the 'output' to between 1.5 and 3 mA and the 'rate' at 10 > than the intrinsic rate. Turn the generator on. Advance the wire until ventricular 'capture' occurs (paced beats are seen on the ECG monitor).

5   Deflate the balloon and determine the 'threshold', i.e. turn down the voltage gradually until pacing is 'lost'. This should be at < 1.5 mA.

6   Gradually increase the output until capture is regained. Set the 'output' to 2–3 × this level.

7   Turn the 'rate' down to 10 below the patient's rate, then slowly increase the sensitivity until the patient's rhythm is being sensed and the pacemaker stops pacing, i.e. the 'sensitivity threshold'. Set the sensitivity so that it is 2–3 × more sensitive than the sensitivity threshold.

8   Set the pacemaker rate as appropriate for the patient's requirements, depending on the diagnosis.

Transcutaneous Cardiac Pacing (TCP)

1   The optimal transcutaneous pacing electrode pad placement is the anterior/posterior position. Apply the anterior electrode to the left of the sternum over the cardiac apex. Apply the posterior electrode immediately behind the anterior electrode to the left of the spine. Alternatively, the apex/anterior position can be used.

2   The pads are connected to the pacing unit and the desired rate set. The default rate is typically 80 per minute.

3   The strength of the pacing signal is gradually increased until 'capture' occurs, e.g. 50–90 mA in patients with spontaneous circulation, up to 140 mA in cardiac arrest patients.[5] Pace at a current that is 10% above the capture threshold.

4   With effective pacing you should see a wide QRS complex and a T wave after the pacing spike, and be able to feel a pulse.

5   If capture does not occur with maximum output (usually 140 mA) try repositioning the electrodes.

6   As well as treating bradycardia and asystole, transcutaneous pacing can be used to treat ventricular tachycardia and supraventricular tachycardia by either 'underdrive' pacing (pacing at a rate less than the tachycardia) or 'overdrive' pacing (pacing at a rate faster than the tachycardia). Although the latter is more successful, it is not possible to do if the tachycardia rate is > 170 bpm (the maximum pacing rate).[6]

Transoesophageal Pacing

This is another non-invasive form of pacing but it is not as reliable as transcutaneous pacing.[6] Transoesophageal pacing can be used to provide atrial pacing (TAP) which preserves atrial priming pump function,[7] and to provide atrial overdrive pacing in the treatment of torsade de pointes, supraventricular tachycardia and atrial flutter.[6] This technique involves insertion of an oesophageal electrode that can be incorporated into an oesophageal stethoscope and placement of an external grounding electrode on the patient. Typical settings are square wave pulses of 10 ms at a current of 10 mA.

Packed Cells

See *RED CELLS*.

Pancuronium

Bis-quaternary aminosteroid, long-acting non-depolarising neuromuscular blocking drug.

Dose

0.1 mg/kg IV. Effects last 45–60 min. Give top-up doses of 0.03 mg/kg.

Advantages

Its long duration of action is useful for long operations and for patients who are being ventilated postoperatively.

Disadvantages

Pancuronium causes an increased heart rate, mean arterial pressure and cardiac output via a vagolytic action and enhanced sympathetic activity. This may be deleterious in patients in whom an increased heart rate is undesirable, e.g. severe ischaemic heart disease.

It is metabolised in the liver ($\approx$ 40%) and also excreted in the urine as the unchanged drug ($\approx$ 50%). The dose should therefore be reduced in the presence of renal or liver impairment.

Papaveretum (Omnopon)

Contains a mixture of opium alkaloids including:
- morphine $\approx$ 50%
- codeine 2.5–5%
- noscapine $\approx$ 20%
- papaverine.

Papaveretum 20 mg is $\approx$ equivalent to morphine 12.5 mg. Used as an analgesic drug and for pre-operative sedation for major surgery often with scopolamine (hyoscine).

Dose for Analgesia and Premedication

▶ *Adult*

IM/subcutaneous dose: 10–20 mg
IV dose: 5 mg IV increments to a total of 20 mg

▶ *Child*

IM/subcutaneous dose: Up to 1 month 150 µg/kg, 1–12 months 200 µg/kg, 1–12 years 200–300 µg/kg.

Advantages

Papaveretum is a potent analgesic agent with possibly more sedating and anxiolytic effects than morphine.

Disadvantages

1 Less potent than morphine with a 25% shorter duration of action.
2 Not suitable for epidural or intrathecal use due to the presence of hydroxybenzoate preservative.

Paracetamol

Acetanilide-derivative analgesic antipyretic drug with an uncertain mechanism of action. Paracetamol is thought to be a potent inhibitor of prostaglandin E synthesis in the central nervous system and peripherally reduces chemoreceptor function responsible for nociceptive impulse generation.[8]

Dose

Adult: 500–1000 mg 4–6 h PO or PR, max. 4 g per day.
Child: 20 mg/kg PO or PR initially, then 15 mg/kg PO, PR subsequent doses 4–6 h, max. 60 mg/kg per day.[9]

Precautions

Hepatotoxicity is the main risk factor with paracetamol use. Paracetamol should be used cautiously in patients with liver impairment due to such causes as chronic alcoholism and extensive liver resection.

Paravertebral Block

Anatomy

This technique involves the blocking of nerve roots as they leave the spinal canal through the intervertebral foramina. These foramina are positioned midway between adjacent transverse processes, and about 2 cm anterior to the plane of the transverse processes. In the thoracic region the nerve root enters a triangular space (the paravertebral space) bounded by the vertebral body, the plane of the transverse process and the pleura.

P

Technique

▶ *Thoracic Paravertebral Blocks*

These are useful for acute herpes zoster infection of the chest, rib fracture and unilateral operations such as breast surgery.[10]

1 Identify the spinous process one level above the chosen nerve root.

2 Sterilise the area around the entry point which is 3 cm lateral to the superior margin of this spinous process.

3 Anaesthetise the skin and deeper tissues at this point, then insert a 10 cm 22 G spinal needle 90° to the skin. Advance this needle onto the rib or transverse process (which will be at a depth of ≈ 3 cm).

4 Walk the needle in a cephalad direction over the cephalad edge of the transverse process/rib.

5 Attach a 10 mL syringe (filled with saline or air) to the needle and test for loss of resistance as the needle point passes through the costo-transverse ligament into the triangular space described above.

6 Aspirate for blood, air or CSF. If negative, inject 5–10 mL of LA, e.g. bupivacaine 0.25%.

▶ *Lumbar Paravertebral Block*

1 Identify the spinous process at the level of the nerve to be blocked.

2 The needle entry point is 3 cm lateral to the superior edge of the spinous process.

3 Prepare the skin as described above and insert a 10 cm spinal needle 10–30° cephalad. The transverse process should be contacted at a depth of 2.5–5 cm.

4 The needle is repositioned to walk off the lower medial edge of the transverse process (i.e. angled medially and more caudad). Advance the needle 2 cm.

5   After careful aspiration inject 5–10 mL of LA solution. A larger volume, e.g. 20 mL, can be injected at a single-level which will block three or more levels.[11]

▶ *Risks of Paravertebral Block*

The main risks are:

- pneumothorax (at the thoracic levels)
- Horner's syndrome (at the thoracic levels)
- subarachnoid or epidural block
- intravascular injection.

Parecoxib (Dynastat)

Second-generation parenteral COX2 selective NSAID useful for treating acute pain. It is a prodrug for valdecoxib and can be given IV or IM.

Dose

40 mg IV or IM by slow deep injection. It is approved for single use only. Reduce dose to 20 mg for small elderly patients. With IV injection effects start in 7–14 min and last up to 24 h.

Advantages

Like other COX2 selective NSAIDs parecoxib has little or no effect on platelet function or gut mucosa.[12,13]

See *NON-STEROIDAL ANTI-INFLAMMATORY DRUGS*.

Disadvantages

See also *NON-STEROIDAL ANTI-INFLAMMATORY DRUGS*.

1   Parecoxib is contraindicated in patients with aspirin-sensitive asthma.
2   The drug should be avoided in patients with renal impairment.
3   Parecoxib is not approved for use in children.
4   Although a potent analgesic (superior to morphine 4 mg), it is inadequate as the sole analgesic for severe pain.

P

Parkinson's Disease

Definition

Parkinson's disease is due to the loss of dopaminergic neurons in the substantia nigra of the brain. It is characterised by rigidity, tremor and bradykinesis. Patient's may suffer from a variety of other complaints such as orthostatic hypotension and cardiac arrhythmias.

Treatment

Drugs used to treat Parkinson's disease include:[14]

1. dopamine precursors such as levodopa. Levodopa has a short half life of 1–3 h.
2. dopamine agonists, e.g. ropinirole, apomorphine
3. monoamine oxidase B inhibitors, e.g. selegeline
4. atypical agents, e.g. amantadine (the mechanism of action is not understood)[14]
5. peripherally acting dopa decarboxylase inhibitors such as benserazide
6. catechol-o-methyl transferase inhibitors (inhibit dopamine breakdown) such as entacapone.
7. anticholinergic drugs such as benzhexol.

Pre-anaesthetic Management

1. Place the patient first on the operating list to ensure medication timing is optimal.
2. Continue drug therapy pre-operatively up to the time of surgery. Give drugs through a nasogastric tube if necessary.
3. Patients who are having planned surgery and who will be unable to take their medication for a prolonged period after surgery should be considered for apomorphine subcut. As this drug is severely emetogenic consider domperidone 20 mg tds for 3 days PO prior to a subcutaneous infusion dose of apomorphine ≈ 30–40 mg over 16 h.[14] Apomorphine can also cause

P

significant hypotension. Domperidone can be continued PR postoperatively.

4 Diphenhydramine can be useful for sedation in patients requiring premedication.[15]

Intra-operative Management

1 Levodopa can be given intra-operatively by naso/orogastric tube.

2 Use of succinylcholine may precipitate hyperkalaemia.[16] However, this advice has been questioned by Muzzi et al. who found no potassium rise in seven patients with Parkinson's disease given succinylcholine.[17]

3 Patients may be on selegeline, which can interact with pethidine. See *MONOAMINE OXIDASE (MAO) INHIBITOR DRUGS*.

4 Opioids may worsen rigidity.

5 Propofol may have dopamine-like effects, causing improved tremor control or dyskinesia. Do not use propofol if patients are having stereotactic surgery for Parkinson's disease.[18]

6 Antropine may cause central anticholinergic syndrome. Use glycopyrrolate in preference.[14]

7 Keep patients well hydrated peri-operatively.

Postoperative Management

1 NSAIDs and paracetamol can be used with the usual precautions.

2 Postoperative nausea and vomiting should not be treated with centrally acting antidopaminergic drugs such as metoclopramide and prochlorperazine.[14] Also avoid droperidol.

3 Continue oral therapy as soon as possible after surgery, by nasogastric tube if necessary.

4 Patients with Parkinson's disease are more prone to postoperative confusion and hallucinations.[19] Do not use haloperidol to treat postoperative confusion in Parkinson's patients.[14] Benzodiazepine sedation may be useful in this situation.[15]

Partial Pressure of Gases

In Fully Humidified Inspired Air

O_2	149 mmHg (19.8 kPa)
CO_2	0.3 mmHg (0.04 kPa)
H_2O	47 mmHg (6.25 kPa)
N_2	564 mmHg (75 kPa)

Expired Gas

O_2	116 mmHg (15.4 kPa)
CO_2	26.8 mmHg (3.6 kPa)
H_2O	47 mmHg
N_2	569.9 mmHg (75.7 kPa)

Alveolar Gas

O_2	100 mmHg (13.3 kPa)
CO_2	40 mmHg (5.3 kPa)
H_2O	47 mmHg
N_2	573 mmHg (76.2 kPa)

Arterial Blood

O_2	95 mmHg (12.6 kPa)
CO_2	40 mmHg (5.3 kPa)
N_2	570 mmHg (75.8 kPa)

Venous Blood

O_2	40 mmHg (5.3 kPa)
CO_2	46 mmHg (6.1 kPa)

Patient-controlled Analgesia (PCA) and Patient-controlled Epidural Anaesthesia (PCEA)

Adult Dosages

- *Morphine* (120 mg in 60 mL N/S): start with 1–2 mg IV bolus with 5 min lockout + background infusion.
- *Fentanyl* (1200 µg in 60 mL N/S): start with 10–20 µg bolus IV with 5 min lockout + background infusion. PCA intranasal fentanyl has been used in adults with a dose of 25 µg and a 6 minute lockout.[20]
- *Tramadol* (300 mg in 60 mL N/S): start with 10–20 mg IV bolus with a 5 min lockout period.
- *Remifentanil*: recently there has been research into the use of IV PCA remifentanil for patients in labour. Various regimens have been used, e.g. a background infusion of 0.05 µg/kg/min plus 25 µg boluses with a 5 minute lockout. Patients must be observed very closely for excessive respiratory depression and sedation.[21]
- *Pethidine*: used epidurally (300 mg in 60 mL N/S) 50 mg loading dose then 20 mg bolus with a 10 min lockout + 1 mL/h background infusion (may help prevent blockage of epidural catheter).
- *Bupivacaine*: used epidurally in labouring patients. Epidural bupivacaine can be administered with or without a basal infusion rate. For example, use bupivacaine 0.125% 6 mL/h basal rate with a PCEA dose of 5 mL with a 15 min lockout period.

Child Dosages[22]

PCA techniques are not usually suitable for a child < 5 years.
Morphine: 1 mg/kg loaded into 50 mL 5% glucose. Program 1 mL bolus (20 µg/kg) with a 5 min lockout + background infusion of 0.5 mL/h.

P

Fentanyl: 50 µg/kg loaded into 50 mL 5% glucose. Program 0.5 mL bolus (0.5 µg/kg) with a 5 min lockout + background infusion of 1 mL/h.

Penetrating Eye Injury

See *EYE INJURY, PENETRATING*.

Penile Block

Useful for circumcision, hypospadias repair and penile trauma analgesia.

Anatomy

The penis is innervated by the dorsal nerves of the penis and the perineal nerves (both of which are branches of the pudendal nerves). The injection is made into a triangular space bounded by the symphysis pubis above, corpora cavernosa below and Buck's (Scarpa's) fascia anteriorly.

Technique

Do not use adrenaline-containing LA.

1   Sterilise the skin at the dorsal base of the penis. Insert 23 G 32 mm needle at the 10.30 and 01.30 clock positions, just under the symphysis pubis. Direct the needle through the tough Buck's fascia at an angle of 10–15° to the midline. Alternatively, insert the needle in the midline, then redirect the needle to perform a paramedian injection on each side.

2   Aspirate prior to injection. If no blood is aspirated, inject LA on each side.

Child: Inject 1 mL + 0.1 mL/kg *each side*. Use bupivacaine 0.25%.[23]

Adult: Inject 20 mL of LA; use bupivacaine 0.5% 15 mL + lignocaine 2% 5 mL.

Also inject a bleb of LA at the penile scrotal junction extending to each side of the midline to block ventral branches of the *perineal nerves*. This greatly improves the reliability of the block.[24]

Alternative Technique

Simply inject LA subcutaneously around the base of the penile shaft (1–2 mL of bupivacaine 0.5% or 1.5–5 mL of 0.25%).[25] Do not use adrenaline-containing solutions.

Note: The use of ropivacaine for penile block has been associated with ischaemia of the glans.[26]

Complications of Penile Block

1 Haematoma deep to Buck's fascia causing compression of dorsal veins and arteries with penile ischaemia.
2 Arterial vasospasm due to inadvertent injection of adrenaline-containing solutions.
3 Intravascular injection of LA.

Treatment of Penile Ischaemia Due to Penile Block

Penile ischaemia following penile block may be due to the inadvertent use of adrenaline-containing solutions or compression of penile blood vessels by haematoma formation. Treatments that have possibly been effective include:

1 caudal anaesthesia to provide sympathetic blockade[27]
2 iloprost, a prostaglandin I_2 analogue, which can be given by IV infusion.[26] A dose of 0.5–2 µg/h was used to treat penile ischaemia in an adult.[26]

Pericardial Effusion

See *CARDIAC TAMPONADE*.

Pericardial Tamponade/Pericardiocentesis

See *CARDIAC TAMPONADE*.

Peripartum Cardiomyopathy

Diagnosis

Peripartum cardiomyopathy is diagnosed based on the presentation of cardiac failure in the last trimester of pregnancy or within 5 months of delivery.[28] There should be no other identifiable aetiology other than pregnancy, and conditions mimicking cardiac failure, such as pulmonary emboli, must be excluded. It is a rare condition, with an incidence of 1 per 3000–4000 pregnancies.[28] Aetiology is unknown but thought to be related to viral and autoimmune mechanisms.

There is no specific test for peripartum cardiomyopathy and the diagnosis is essentially one of exclusion of other causes of heart failure.

Pre-anaesthetic Management for Caesarean Section

Management of these patients involves optimisation of preload, afterload and contractility as with all other forms of heart failure. See *CONGESTIVE CARDIAC FAILURE*.

Important strategies include:

1 assessment by obstetric, cardiac and anaesthetic specialists
2 appropriate investigations including ECG and cardiac echocardiography
3 supportive measures including bed rest and oxygen supplementation
4 preload optimisation. This may include fluid restriction, diuretics and venodilation agents such as GTN for reducing preload or fluid therapy to increase preload.
5 afterload reduction with arterial vasodilators such as sodium nitroprusside
6 enhancement of cardiac contractility with inotropic agents such as digoxin and/or dobutamine

P

7   appropriate monitoring including arterial line, central line, PA
    catheter and foetal cardiotocograph
8   thromboembolic prophylaxis

Anaesthetic Management

The aims of anaesthetic management are to provide cardiovascularly stable anaesthesia in addition to the requirements outlined
in the section *CAESAREAN SECTION (CS)*. The type of anaesthesia
chosen will depend on the severity of the cardiomyopathy, and the
skill and experience of the anaesthetist involved. As in the pre-
anaesthetic management optimise preload, afterload and cardiac
contractility throughout the peri-operative period as guided by
invasive pressure monitoring.

General Anaesthesia

General anaesthesia for Caesarean section may be preferred in cases
of severe peripartum cardiomyopathy, due to the risk of potential
cardiovascular instability with regional blockade.[29,30] In addition
to the points made in the section *CAESAREAN SECTION (CS)*, the
following should be noted:

1   The IV induction drug used for rapid sequence, e.g. thiopentone
    or propofol, should be used in an appropriately reduced dose to
    decrease the risk of excessive myocardial depression.
2   One case report recommended maintenance of anaesthesia
    with a propofol/remifentanil infusion.[28]

Regional Anaesthesia

Epidural anaesthesia may be of benefit in some patients due to the
reduction in afterload without reduced contractility. However,
epidural anaesthesia must be induced slowly and carefully with
appropriate invasive monitoring, depending on the severity of the
condition. For example, one patient requiring CS had an epidural
block established to a T4 level over 6 hours with an infusion of
bupivacaine and fentanyl.[28] Subarachnoid block anaesthesia is

generally not recommended in these patients although 'low dose' combined spinal epidural anaesthesia has been used successfully.[31]

Postanaesthetic Care

Mortality is high (25–50%)[30] due to cardiac failure, dysrhythmias and thromboembolic complications.

Pethidine

Synthetic phenylpiperidine opioid receptor agonist used for analgesia and the treatment of postoperative shivering. See *SHIVERING POSTOPERATIVELY*.

Dose

Adult: IV/IM 25–150 mg IM as required up to 3 h. For IV analgesia, give 20–25 mg increments 5 min up to 150 mg.

Adult epidural dose: 25–50 mg. See *PATIENT-CONTROLLED ANALGESIA AND PATIENT-CONTROLLED EPIDURAL ANAESTHESIA*.

Child: 1 mg/kg IM or same dose in 10 mL N/S. Give in 1 mL increments IV 5 min.

Advantages

1 Pethidine may cause less nausea than morphine.[32]
2 Pethidine has little effect on coughing.[32]
3 It causes less spasm of the sphincter of Oddi than morphine.[33,34] Latta et al. have argued in a recent article that this difference in effect may not be clinically significant and prescribing pethidine for patients having biliary surgery is not scientifically validated.[35]
4 Pethidine has local anaesthetic effects and has been used as a sole anaesthetic agent epidurally for surgery in critically ill patients.[36]

Disadvantages

1 Pethidine is inferior to morphine for analgesia at equivalent dosages.[35] It is also shorter-acting.

2 Pethidine can produce severe reactions in patients taking monoamine oxidase inhibitor drugs. See *MONOAMINE OXIDASE (MAO) INHIBITOR DRUGS*.

3 It is not suitable for subcutaneous injection due to stinging.

4 Use pethidine with caution in renal failure as accumulation of the metabolite norpethidine may occur. Accumulation of norpethidine may also occur when pethidine is used in high dose over days. Norpethidine is a potent convulsant and may also cause tremors, twitches and myoclonus. Symptoms of norpethidine toxicity can occur below the 600 mg/day recommended safety level.[35]

5 Pethidine causes more euphoria and is much more likely to be abused than morphine.[35]

6 Pethidine is inferior to hydromorphone for the treatment of ureteric colic.[37]

Phaeochromocytoma

Phaeochromocytomas are rare catecholamine-secreting tumours. 90% arise from the adrenal medulla. About 10% are bilateral and about 10% are malignant.[38] They may also secrete other substances such as enkephalins, somatostatin and calcitonin.

Pre-operative Assessment

The main clinical features are due to secretion of noradrenaline, adrenaline and dopamine. They include:

1 paroxysmal hypertension often associated with dysrhythmias, headaches, sweating and tremor

2 postural hypotension due to volume depletion

3 hyperglycaemia due to α_2 adreno-receptor stimulation decreasing insulin release and promoting glycogenolysis

4 catecholamine-induced cardiomyopathy/cardiac failure

5 possible anxiety, psychosis and visual disturbances.

P

Pre-operative Investigation and Preparation

In addition to routine investigations patients must be evaluated for cardiac dysfunction including ECG and echocardiography. Preparation for surgery takes about 2 weeks. The aims of pre-operative preparation are to:

1 control blood pressure, dysrhythmias and heart failure
2 normalise intravascular volume
3 normalise blood glucose levels.

Recommended treatment and preparation strategies are:

1 α adreno-receptor blockade should be initiated with a drug such as phenoxybenzamine (see *PHENOXYBENZAMINE*). Commence with 20 mg PO bd increasing by 10–20 mg/day. The aims of treatment are to prevent blood pressure rises above 165/90 and to have a mild postural hypotension. Doxazocine is an alternative to phenoxybenzamine. Prazosin can be added if α blockade is inadequate with phenoxybenzamine.[38]

2 β adreno-receptor blockade is indicated for tachydysrhythmias, and tachycardia due to phenoxybenzamine. β *adreno-receptor blockade therapy must never be commenced in the absence of α receptor blockade*. This is because of the risk of blocking β adreno-receptor-mediated vasodilatation, resulting in exacerbation of hypertension. Also β blockade without α blockade may result in myocardial depression sufficient to result in cardiac failure in the presence of elevated SVR. See *ADRENERGIC RECEPTORS*.

3 Alpha methylparatyrosine inhibits catecholamine synthesis by up to 80% and can be useful pre-operatively and intra-operatively to help control blood pressure.[38]

4 α blockade results in vasodilatation of the chronically vasoconstricted intravascular space. Ensure normovolaemia is re-established. A fall in haematocrit of 5% is suggestive of intravascular repletion.

5 Control blood glucose levels. Insulin is rarely required.[39]

Pre-anaesthetic Phase

1 Consider a benzodiazepine premedication.

2 Establish large bore IV access and intra-arterial blood pressure measurement. Use LA liberally for line insertion to reduce nociceptive stimulation, which can precipitate hypertension.

3 Insert a CVP line or PA catheter. This can be inserted after induction of GA. Transoesophageal echocardiography should be considered in patients with significant cardiomyopathy.

4 Thoracic epidural anaesthesia to supplement GA is useful to attenuate the adrenergic response to surgery and for post-operative pain control. However, epidural anaesthesia does not block the hypertensive effects of catecholamine release due to tumour handling. Epidural blockade may also complicate interpretation of extremes of hypertension and hypotension during and after surgery.[40]

5 Avoid morphine, which causes histamine release and may therefore induce catecholamine release.[38] Opioids with minimal histamine-releasing properties include fentanyl, alfentanil and buprenorphine.

6 Do not use droperidol pre-operatively or intra-operatively.[38] This drug can block α_2 receptors and inhibit catecholamine reuptake. Droperidol can also interact with dopamine receptors, resulting in increased catecholamine release.

7 Sodium nitroprusside is often required for severe refractory hypertension and should be preprepared and ready for immediate infusion. Brief episodes of hypertension can be treated with IV phentolamine.

Induction and Maintenance Phase

1 Aim for cardiovascular stability and deal with hypertension and hypotension promptly.

2 Induce anaesthesia with appropriate dosages of midazolam, fentanyl, and propofol or thiopentone. Consider measures to

reduce the hypertensive response to intubation. See *HYPERTEN-SIVE RESPONSE TO INTUBATION (ATTENUATION OF)*.

3   Use a muscle relaxant devoid of histamine release, such as rocuronium or vecuronium. Avoid pancuronium due to its tendency to cause tachycardia, and suxamethonium which may release histamine. Also, fasciculations due to suxamethonium may cause abdominal compression and release of tumour catecholamines.[38]

4   Maintain anaesthesia with isoflurane or sevoflurane. Do not use halothane, which sensitises the myocardium to catecholamines. Desflurane may cause sympathetic nervous system stimulation at higher doses and this should be considered if this drug is used.

5   Consider using a magnesium sulphate infusion. A loading dose of 40–60 mg/kg can be used, then an infusion of about 2 g/h.[41]

6   Phentolamine boluses (1–2 mg) or an infusion can be useful for controlling hypertension. For severe hypertension use a sodium nitroprusside infusion.

7   The use of a remifentanil infusion has been associated with significant hypotension and bradycardia in patients who are undergoing phaeochromocytoma surgery and who are α and β adreno-receptor blocked.[42]

8   Consider β blocker drugs such as metoprolol or an esmolol infusion for intra-operative tachydysrhythmias. In one study two patients with persistent tachycardias resistant to β blockers (and adenosine in one case) responded well to a carefully titrated dose of neostigmine.[43] Nicardipine has also been used.[44]

9   Hypertension is particularly likely to occur on intubation, at the time of pneumoperitoneum (in laparoscopic surgery) and when the tumour is manipulated.

10 Hypotension can occur with removal of the tumour. Treat this with liberal IV fluids. Use a noradrenaline infusion for persistant hypotension unresponsive to adequate fluid loading.

11 Blood loss tends to be poorly tolerated by these patients and blood transfusion should be considered early.

12 Monitor blood glucose levels. Commence glucose-containing IV fluids once the tumour is removed.[38]

13 Reverse neuromuscular blockade with neostigmine and glycopyrrolate. Avoid atropine, which may cause an excessive increase in heart rate.[38]

Advantages of Laparoscopic Surgery[43]

Some phaeochromocytomas are resectable laparoscopically. Advantages include:

1 possibly less blood loss
2 shorter hospital stay
3 less postoperative pain and better cosmetic result.

Disadvantages of Laparoscopic Surgery[43]

1 The creation of pneumoperitoneum can be particularly hazardous and precipitate an adrenergic crisis.[44]
2 Longer operation time.
3 Tendency to greater cardiovascular instability with an increased requirement for sodium nitroprusside.

Postanaesthetic Phase

The patient should be monitored in a high dependency or intensive care unit. Problems to anticipate and treat include:

1 hypoglycaemia. Give glucose-containing solutions postoperatively.
2 hypotension. This may require vasopressor/inotropic therapy (but exclude hypovolaemia/haemorrhage).
3 hypertension. This persists postoperatively in up to 50% of patients.[39] Consider residual tumour or renal ischaemia as possible aetiological factors.

Mortality

The peri-operative mortality for well-prepared patients is 0–3%.[45] For undiagnosed or ill-prepared patients with phaeochromocytoma the mortality approaches 50%.[46] Five-year survival for malignant tumours is about 46%.[47]

Phenoxybenzamine

Tertiary amine (a halo-alkylamine) used for the treatment of hypertension, including the management of phaeochromocytoma. Acts by producing irreversible (non-competitive) α receptor blockade. Its actions therefore last 3– 4 days after a single dose.

Dose

Adult: 10–60 mg PO in divided doses or 10–40 mg IV over 1 h. Effects take ≈ 1 h to manifest.

Child: 0.2–1 mg/kg 12–24 h oral or 1 mg/kg over 1 h, then 0.5 mg/kg/dose 6–12 h.

Phentolamine

Antihypertensive imidazoline agent. Acts by competitive α1 adreno-receptor blockade and to a lesser extent α2 adreno-receptor blockade, resulting in arterial vasodilatation with little venodilatation. Used for the treatment of hypertension, including the peri-operative management of patients with phaeochromocytoma.

Dose

Adult: 5–10 mg IM or 1 mg boluses IV. Effects last 10–30 min. Can also be given by IV infusion at a rate of 1–20 µg/kg/min.

Child: 0.1 mg/kg IV, then infusion 5–50 µg/kg/min IV.

Phenylephrine

Powerful synthetic direct-acting α1 adreno-receptor agonist with weak β adreno-receptor activity. It is similar in action to noradrenaline but is less potent and has a longer duration of action.

Indications

Used:
1 for the treatment of hypotension due to its vasoconstrictor action
2 as a nasal decongestant used topically
3 for producing mydriasis without cycloplegia
4 to overcome paroxysmal supraventricular tachycardia.

Dose for Hypotension

Give by IV infusion. Dilute 10 mg in 500 mL 5% glucose (20 µg/mL). Run at 0.15–0.7 µg/kg/min. For a 70 kg patient give 30–150 mL/h. If giving IV boluses use extremely cautiously, e.g. increments of 50–200 µg.

Precautions/contraindications

Phenylephrine is contraindicated in patients with:
1 severe hypotension
2 ventricular tachycardia.
The drug should be used with caution in patients with:
1 hyperthyroidism
2 bradycardia/partial heart block
3 ischaemic heart disease/severe atherosclerosis.

Phenytoin

1 Hydantoin derivative used for prophylaxis and treatment of seizures.
2 Class 1 anti-arrhythmic drug useful for the treatment of dysrhythmias associated with digoxin toxicity.

Dose for Seizure Control and Prevention

Loading dose: 10–15 mg/kg IV loaded into N/S (*not glucose*). Give no faster than 50 mg/min with ECG monitoring. Give 3–4 mg/kg/day for maintenance.

Therapeutic level: 40–80 μmol/L.

Note

Patients treated with phenytoin have increased dose requirements of vecuronium and pancuronium but not cisatracurium or atracurium.

Physostigmine

Alkaloid anticholinesterase drug from the West African calabar bean. It crosses the blood–brain barrier and is useful for the treatment of:

- glaucoma
- atropine intoxication
- trycyclic antidepressant poisoning.
- central anticholinergic syndrome (see *CENTRAL ANTICHOLINERGIC SYNDROME*).

Pick Line

A useful device for long-term peripheral venous access.

Technique for Insertion

1 Using aseptic technique, insert a 20 G cannula into a suitable vein.
2 Insert the guide wire through the cannula, then remove the cannula.
3 Insert the introducer over the guide wire, then remove the introducer.
4 Insert the banana catheter over the guide wire, then remove the guide wire.

5 Insert the catheter through the banana catheter, then remove the banana catheter by splitting it while it is gradually withdrawn.

6 Suture the pick line into place.

Placenta Accreta/Increta/Percreta

These terms refer to the invasion of placental tissue into the myometrium of the uterus:

- *Accreta* is invasion onto the myometrial surface.
- *Increta* is invasion into the myometrium.
- *Percreta* is invasion into the full thickness of the myometrium. Other organs such as the bladder may be involved.

The term 'placenta accreta' is used in this section to cover all the histological types described above.

Placenta accreta has an incidence of about 1 per 2500 deliveries.[48] This condition is associated with placenta praevia (see below), previous CS or repeated uterine curettage. Due to increasing CS rates the incidence of placenta accreta is increasing. A patient with placenta praevia and a history of two or more CS has a 48% risk of placenta accreta.[49]

Diagnosis

This condition is usually diagnosed at the time of delivery or at CS when there is a failure of the placenta to separate from the uterine wall, associated with severe haemorrhage. Uterine eversion may occur. The condition may be diagnosed prior to delivery by transvaginal ultrasound.[50] MRI imaging can be used to identify the extent of trophoblastic invasion.

Management of placenta accreta

1 If the condition is diagnosed pre-operatively, elective CS hysterectomy is required and preparation must be made for massive blood loss. Consider pre-operative autologous blood

donation. Anaesthetic options are general anaesthesia, epidural anaesthesia or CSE. Spinal anaesthesia as a single-shot technique may not last long enough for this procedure.

2 In one case of known placenta accreta an aortic balloon was placed pre CS and used to control severe intra-operative haemorrhage.[51]

3 Management of undiagnosed placenta accreta at the time of delivery or CS follows the same principles as other conditions associated with massive blood loss. See *BLOOD LOSS ASSESSMENT AND INITIAL MANAGEMENT* and *BLOOD TRANSFUSION*.

Placenta Praevia

Description

This condition is defined as implantation of the placenta in the lower uterine segment over or near the internal os of the uterus. Placenta praevia occurs in about 0.5% of deliveries, with a recurrence risk of about 5%. Diagnosis is usually by antenatal ultrasound. Painless PV bleeding may occur. Caesarean section is required for patients with placenta praevia.

Placenta praevia is associated with an increased risk of placenta accreta, being ≈ 5% if no previous CS have occurred. This risk increases in association with the number of previous Caesarean sections rising to 67% with four or more previous CS operations.[52] See *PLACENTA ACCRETA/INCRETA/PERCRETA*.

Anaesthetic Management for Elective Caesarean Section

Traditionally, general anaesthesia was advocated for elective Caesarean section because of concern over the hypotensive effects of regional anaesthesia combined with potentially massive blood loss. In fact, regional anaesthesia has been used in many centres without any increase in adverse outcome rates.[53] Preparations must be made for massive blood loss, including large bore IV access and the immediate availability of cross-matched blood. As noted above, the risk of haemorrhage is increased by a past history of CS due to the increased risk of placenta accreta.

Anaesthetic Management of the Haemodynamically Unstable Patient

1 Ensure adequate airway and breathing.
2 Resuscitate the patient's intravascular volume with appropriate fluid (crystalloid, colloid, blood).
3 See *BLOOD LOSS ASSESSMENT AND INITIAL MANAGEMENT*.
4 See *CAESAREAN SECTION*. General anaesthesia will be required in almost all cases.

Placental Abruption

See *ABRUPTIO PLACENTAE*.

Platelet Adenosine Diphosphate (ADP) Receptor Antagonists

These thienopyridine drugs are potent inhibitors of platelet aggregation. They are used for the prevention of myocardial ischaemia and infarction, and stroke in susceptible patients. Examples include clopidogrel and ticlopidine.

Description and Mechanism of Action

These drugs are a new class of antiplatelet therapy and act on platelet surface glycoproteins to inhibit platelet adhesion and aggregation. The action of these drugs is delayed for 24–48 h and becomes maximal in 3–5 days.[54] The antiplatelet effect of these drugs is synergistic with aspirin.

Indications

These drugs are used to treat patients with ischaemic heart disease, to reduce the incidence of ischaemia and infarction, and other

P

thrombo-embolic disorders. Platelet glycoprotein antagonists are used acutely in patients undergoing percutaneous coronary interventions or in patients with unstable coronary syndromes un responsive to conventional therapy.

Examples

Oral agents of this type include ticlopidine (Ticlid) and clopidogrel (Plavix).

Anaesthesia and Surgery

1 Cease clopidogrel at least 7 days (and ticlopidine at least 10 days) before elective surgery unless the benefits of antiplatelet therapy outweigh the increased bleeding risk.[54]

2 If regional anaesthesia is contemplated a conservative approach is to stop these drugs for 14 days before surgery (but there is little clinical experience with this situation).[54]

3 Ticlopidine can cause neutropaenia and thrombocytopenia. Check FBC. Platelet function studies may be considered.

4 For emergency surgery associated with severe bleeding due to clopidogrel or ticlodipine, platelet transfusion is the only effective treatment.[54]

Platelet Glycoprotein IIb/IIIa Receptor Antagonists

Drug Description and Indications

These drugs act by ihibiting glycoprotein IIb and IIIa receptors on platelets, thus reducing their ability to aggregate and adhere together. Examples include abciximab (RePro), eptifibatide and tirofiban. These drugs are administered intravenously for such indications as:

1 patients undergoing percutaneous coronary artery interventions

2 patients with angina unresponsive to conventional therapy.

The effects of these drugs can be monitored by activated clotting time or more accurately by turbidometric aggregometry or the platelet function analyser.

Adverse Effects

These include bleeding, allergic reactions and thrombocytopenia.

Platelet GP IIb/IIa Antagonists and Emergency Surgery

1 Cease all antiplatelet therapy as soon as possible before surgery.
2 Consider prophylactic platelet transfusion in patients on abciximab if the drug is ceased less than 12–24 h before surgery.[55]
3 Check platelet count and activated coagulation time.
4 Delay surgery in patients on eptifibatide and tirofiban for 4–6 h.[56] Platelet transfusions are not effective in patients who have received eptifibatide or tirofiban.[57]
5 Consider using an antifibrinolytic drug such as aprotinin.

Platelet Therapy

The normal platelet count is 150–400 $\times$ 10^9/L (150 000–400 000/ µL). An increased risk of surgical bleeding occurs if the platelet count is < 50–80 $\times$ 10^9/L, and spontaneous bleeding can occur below a platelet count of about 20 $\times$ 10^9/L.

Storage of Platelets for Transfusion

Platelet concentrates are stored at 20–24°C and last about 5 days. The bags must be agitated gently and continuously during storage. Compatability testing is not necessary routinely for transfusion.

Contents

A platelet bag contains ≥ 55 $\times$ 10^9 platelets in 40–70 mL of plasma and are collected from a single unit of whole blood.[58] The pH at expiry is 6.8–7.4.

Indications

Platelet therapy is required intra-operatively if the measured platelet count < 50 × 10^9/ L and a bleeding problem is evident,[58] or on clinical grounds, e.g. massive blood transfusion or platelet count > 50 × 10^9/L but the surgical wound is 'oozy'. Platelet transfusion may also be required if a platelet abnormality is present, e.g. platelets exposed to aspirin.[59] See BLOOD TRANSFUSION. 1 unit of platelets increases platelet count in the adult by about 5–10 × 10^9/L.[60] In children 10 mL/kg of platelets increases platelet count by about 30–40 × 10^9/L. Do not use a filter with a pore size < 170 μm. A standard blood-giving set filter is acceptable. Transfused platelets have reduced life spans of 1–3 days. Transfusion can proceed as fast as tolerated and should not exceed 4 h.

ABO Comptability and Platelets

Use ABO-Rh type compatible platelets to increase their life spans. ABO incompatible platelets may be used in an emergency but reactions may occur, such as low-grade haemolysis. If Rh +ve platelets are given to a Rh –ve female with childbearing potential, Rh(D) immunoglobulin should be considered (250 IU per platelet treatment dose).

Pooled Platelets

These are contained in a volume of 160 mL with about 240 × 10^9 platelets. Pooled platelets are indicated for patients with recurrent febrile non-haemolytic transfusion reactions and to reduce the risk of HLA alloimmunisation in patients likely to require multiple transfusions.

Pleural Catheter

See CHEST DRAIN.

Pneumothorax

See *CHEST DRAIN*.

Popliteal Fossa Block

Used to block the *common peroneal* and *tibial nerves* via a single injection in the popliteal fossa. This is effectively equivalent to a sciatic nerve block.

Anatomy

The popliteal fossa is diamond-shaped. The upper medial side is formed by semitendinosus, the lateral side by biceps femoris. The lower medial and lateral sides are formed by the medial and lateral heads of gastrocnemius. The *sciatic nerve* lies at the apex of the diamond and at this point it bifurcates into the *common peroneal nerve*, which runs down on the lateral side of the fossa, and the *tibial nerve*, which runs through the popliteal fossa just medial to the midline. See Figure P1 overleaf.

Common Peroneal (Lateral Popliteal) Nerve (L4, L5 and S1)

1 Forms the *sural nerve* with a branch of the *tibial nerve* supplying the posterolateral calf and lateral side of foot to the fifth toe.
2 Supplies skin over the anterolateral and posterolateral calf.
3 Forms the *superficial* and *deep peroneal nerves*. See *ANKLE BLOCKS AND INNERVATION OF THE FOOT*.

Tibial (Medial Popliteal) Nerve (L4, L5, S1, S2 and S3)

1 Forms part of *sural nerve* (see above).
2 Branches into *medial calcaneal* and *medial* and *lateral plantar nerves*. See *ANKLE BLOCKS AND INNERVATION OF THE FOOT*.

Note: The medial side of the leg and foot are supplied by branches of the *femoral nerve*.

P

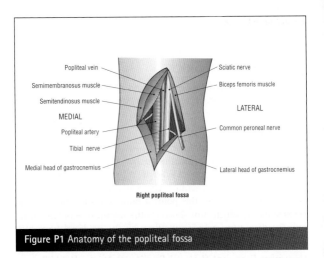

MEDIAL
Popliteal vein
Semimembranosus muscle
Semitendinosus muscle
Popliteal artery
Tibial nerve
Medial head of gastrocnemius

LATERAL
Sciatic nerve
Biceps femoris muscle
Common peroneal nerve
Lateral head of gastrocnemius

Right popliteal fossa

Figure P1 Anatomy of the popliteal fossa

Technique in the Adult[61]

1 Position the patient prone. Draw a triangle formed by semitendinosis, biceps femoris and the skin crease of the popliteal fossa.

2 Bisect the triangle with a perpendicular line from base to apex.

3 Identify the point 5–6 cm cephalad from the skin crease (popliteal fold) along this bisecting line and 1 cm lateral to it. Mark this point with an X. This is the insertion point.

4 Using aseptic technique, insert 7.5 cm 22 G spinal needle through anaesthetised skin at point X at a 45–60° cephalad angle and seek paraesthesia. If a nerve stimulator is available, use an insulated stimulation needle and seek a

P

motor response. Start with a stimulating current of 2 mA with an end-point for injection of muscle reaction just being lost at 0.3 mA.[62] A search pattern perpendicular to the nerve may be required to find it.

5   Inject 30–40 mL of LA (lignocaine 1% or bupivacaine 0.25%).

6   To anaesthetise the medial side of the calf and foot the *femoral* branches can be blocked in by injecting 10 mL of LA over the medial tibial head just below the knee. See also *SAPHENOUS NERVE BLOCK*.

The onset of the block takes 20 min or more.

Technique in the Child[62]

1   In the child the insertion point can be calculated as follows. Again the triangle formed by the popliteal fold and the apex of the popliteal fossa is bisected with a perpendicular line. The distance from the popliteal fold to the point of insertion is 1 cm cephalad per 10 kg of body mass (e.g. in a 25 kg child the distance is 2.5 cm).

2   Insert the insulated stimulation needle at a 45° angle to the skin lateral to the midline.

3   Inject bupivacaine 0.25% using a dose of 0.5 mL/kg.

POR 8

Stands for 8-ornithine vasopressin. Used for skin and tissue vasoconstriction to decrease surgical bleeding. Dilute to 0.1–0.2 units/mL. Do not administer > 0.5 units/kg.

Side Effects

Side effects include hypertension and dysrhythmias. The drug is teratogenic and is therefore contraindicated in pregnancy (POR 8 product information).

P

Porphyria

Topics Covered in this Section
▶ Acute Intermittent Porphyria
▶ Variegate Porphyria
▶ Hereditary Coproporphyria
▶ Types of Porphyria Not Requiring Avoidance of Triggering Drugs

The porphyrias are a group of inherited or acquired enzymatic defects involving heme synthesis.[63] There is an overproduction of porphyrins (required for heme synthesis) and their precursors. These diseases can be classified into hepatic and erythropoietic.

Acute Intermittent Porphyria
▶ *Pathophysiology*
Acute intermittent porphyria is a form of hepatic porphyria more common in females.[63] This illness is associated with attacks of severe abdominal pain and neurotoxity manifesting as psychoses, cranial and peripheral nerve dysfunction and autonomic dysfunction. Hypertensive complications and renal failure are the most frequent causes of death in this group. A significant proportion of pregnant women with porphyria will experience an attack during pregnancy.[63]

▶ *Symptoms and Signs of Acute Attacks*
About 1% of acute attacks are fatal. Clinical manifestations include:
1 severe abdominal pain
2 autonomic instability (tachycardia, hypertension or hypotension)
3 dehydration and electrolyte disturbances

4 neuropsychiatric manifestations, seizures
5 muscle weakness.

▶ *Pharmacological Triggering Agents*

The following drugs can, or are suspected of being able to, precipitate an acute attack as described above:

1 thiopentone and other barbiturates
2 etomidate
3 endogenous steroids and drugs with a steroid structure.[64] Pancuronium and vecuronium are possibly unsafe.
4 enflurane: possibly unsafe. It is contentious but likely that isoflurane and halothane are safe.[64]
5 imipramine and tolbutamide
6 alpha methyl dopa, hydralazine and phenoxybenzamine
7 pentazocine. Other opioids are safe.
8 oral contraceptive pill and griseofulvin: unsafe.
9 phenytoin.[65]

Of the benzodiazepines, nitrazepam and flunitrazepam are considered unsafe and diazepam is possibly unsafe (but see below). Midazolam is considered safe.[63]

Avoid diclofenac, ibuprofen and fenoprofen.

▶ *Pre-anaesthetic Considerations*

1 Avoid prolonged fasting and consider a glucose-saline drip to minimise starvation stress.
2 Acute intermittent porphyria is not an absolute contraindication to regional anaesthesia but consider medico-legal issues including the mental state of the patient and the possibility of neurological deterioration. Bupivacaine is considered safe and lignocaine is probably safe.

▶ *Drugs Considered Safe*

1 Propofol (probably safe),[63] ketamine (probably safe),[64] droperidol (safe). Avoid propofol infusions, which may not be safe.[66]

2 Opioids (except pentazocine) are safe.

3 N_2O is safe. Isoflurane and halothane are probably safe but controversy exists.[63,64]

4 All muscle relaxants are safe, except steroid-based ones, e.g. vecuronium and pancuronium.

5 Anticholinergic and anticholinesterase drugs are safe.

6 Anti-emetics such as droperidol and prochlorperazine are safe but metoclopramide should probably be avoided.

7 Aspirin, naproxen and indomethacin are all safe.

8 Heparin is safe.

▶ *Treatment of an Acute Exacerbation of Porphyria*

1 *Hypertension* and *tachycardia* commonly occur during an acute attack and β blockers are the treatment of choice, especially propranolol.

2 *Seizures*: All commonly used anticonvulsants are porphyrogenic. However, some of the new anti-epileptic drugs such as gabapentin and vigapentin appear to be effective and safe. Diazepam has been used.[67] Check for hyponatraemia as a cause of the seizures. Magnesium sulphate is effective in porphyric patients who are hypomagnasaemic.[63]

3 Keep the patient well-hydrated. If an acute attack occurs, give glucose 20 g/h.

4 Haem arginate (haematin) can produce dramatic clinical improvement during an acute attack by reducing the synthesis of aminolaevulinic acid.[63] The dose of haem arginate is 3 mg/kg/day over 15 min by IV infusion through a central venous line. Give haematin for 4 days. Tin protoporphyrin, an inhibitor of haem oxygenase, may also be useful.

5 Treat severe pain with opioids such as morphine or pethidine.

Variegate Porphyria

Affects both sexes. Avoid triggering drugs as described above. Patients exhibit severe photosensitivity and thin fragile skin.

Hereditary Coproporphyria

Avoid the above triggering agents. This type also exhibits skin manifestations. Acute attacks tend to be less severe than in acute intermittent porphyria.

Types of Porphyria Not Requiring Avoidance of Triggering Drugs:

1 Porphyria cutanea tarda.
2 Erythropoietic uroporphyria.
3 Erythropoietic protoporphyria.

Postanaesthetic Confusion

See *CONFUSION, DECREASED LEVEL OF CONSCIOUSNESS, POSTANAESTHETIC.*

Postdural Puncture Headache

See *EPIDURAL ANAESTHESIA.*

P

Posterior Cutaneous Nerve of Thigh Block (Posterior Femoral Cutaneous Nerve)

Anatomy (S1, S2 and S3)

The posterior cutaneous nerve of the thigh is a branch of the sacral plexus. It supplies skin over the lower lateral part of gluteus maximus, back and medial side of thigh, popliteal fossa and upper part of the back of leg.

Technique

1. With the patient in the lateral position (with the side to be blocked uppermost) identify the greater trochanter and the ischial tuberosity and draw a line between them.

2. Identify the point a quarter the distance along this line from the medial end and mark it with an X.

3. Flex the hip to 90°. The site of entry is just above point X on the gluteal fold.

4. Using aseptic technique, insert a short-bevelled needle and feel for loss of resistance with penetration of the superficial fascia. Attach a saline filled syringe and feel for a second loss of resistance as the needle penetrates the fibrous fatty tissue and gluteus maximus.

5. Inject 4 mL bupivacaine 0.5% for child of 1 year, adding 0.5 mL for each subsequent year up to a maximum of 12 mL.[68]

Postpartum Haemorrhage

Postpartum haemorrhage (PPH) is defined as postpartum loss of greater than 600 mL of blood. Major PPH can be defined as greater than 40% of blood volume or > 2 L.[69] The incidence of PPH is 3–7% of vaginal deliveries.[70] PPH can be due to a variety of causes, including:

1. uterine atony
2. retained placenta
3. trauma to the uterus or birth canal
4. uterine inversion. This may be associated with placenta accreta. See *UTERINE INVERSION* and *PLACENTA ACCRETA/INCRETA/PERCRETA*.

Treatment of PPH

1. Ensuring adequate airway and ventilation of the patient.
2. Obtain large bore IV access.

3 Give appropriate resuscitation fluids (crystalloid/colloid/blood). See *BLOOD LOSS ASSESSMENT AND INITIAL MANAGEMENT* and *BLOOD TRANSFUSION*.

4 Uterine massage and/or bimanual compression of the atonic uterus may reduce blood loss.

5 Appropriate surgical intervention, i.e. ensuring uterus is empty, repair of bleeding tissues.

6 Pharmacotherapy to contract the uterus if uterine atonia is the cause. Appropriate drugs include (see individual entries):

   (a) syntocinon 10 IU IV stat ± infusion of 40 IU in 1000 mL N/S, with the infusion rate titrated to effect.

   (b) ergometrine IV 100–500 µg or IM 200–500 µg. An alternative ergot type drug is methergine in a dose of 200 µg IM or 20 µg IV. *Note that severe hypertension can occur if the patient has received ephedrine or other vasoactive drug in addition to an ergot alkaloid.*

   (c) Prostaglandin F_2 alpha 250 µg IM or intramyometrially. This drug can cause bronchospasm and other adverse effects. See *PROSTIN F_2 ALPHA*.

7 Consider external abdominal aortic compression to temporarily reduce blood loss while more definitive treatment is organised.[70] Compression of the aorta can be achieved because postpartum the abdominal wall is lax and the rectus abdominis muscles diastatic. This technique involves pressing a fist into the abdomen in the midline just above the umbilicus. This results in the abdominal aorta being compressed between the fist and the vertebral column.

8 Consider vaginal/uterine packing or insertion of a Foley catheter balloon into the cervical canal as temporising measures.[71]

9 If the above treatment is unsuccessful, laparotomy is required. Surgical options include uterine artery ligation, internal iliac artery ligation, hypogastric artery ligation or hysterectomy.

10 DIC may occur. See also *DISSEMINATED INTRAVASCULAR COAGULATION (DIC)*.

Potassium

Potassium is the major intracellular cation and is very important in the function of excitable tissue. NR in serum 3.2–5.5 mmol/L.

Hypokalaemia

Hypokalaemia is severe if K^+ level is < 2.5 mmol/L and is associated with:

1 characteristic ECG changes, which include prolongation of the PR interval, T wave inversion and prominent U waves
2 dysrhythmias including atrial and ventricular tachycardias such as torsade de pointes
3 weakness, hypotonicity, ventilatory failure and prolongation of neuromuscular blocking drug effects
4 rhabdomyolysis (if prolonged, severe hypokalaemia).

▶ *Treatment of Hypokalaemia*

1 IV potassium chloride. Do not exceed 40 mmol/h.[72] For rapid correction give 10 mmol in 100 mL 5% glucose over 30 min. Measure K^+ each hour and repeat this dose until serum K^+ reaches 4.0 mmol/L. Rapid correction of hypokalaemia is not without risk ($\approx$ 0.5% morbidity).[73] It should only be done in urgent situations.
2 Treat the cause of the hypokalaemia.

Hyperkalaemia

Hyperkalaemia is severe if serum K^+ is $\geq$ 6.5 mmol/L and very severe at 7 mmol/L or greater. Heperkalaemia may cause:

1 characteristic ECG changes such as flattening of the p wave, tall peaked T waves and widening of the QRS complex and the PR

P

interval. Development of deep S waves, sinus arrest with nodal rhythm, sine wave ECG pattern and asystole may also be seen.

2 cardiac dysrhythmias, including ventricular ectopic beats, atrial arrest, atrioventricular block, ventricular tachycardia and ventricular fibrillation

3 the antagonising of the effects of non-depolarising neuro-muscular blocking drugs

4 tingling, weakness and flaccid paralysis

5 hypotension.

▶ *Treatment of Hyperkalaemia*

Emergency management includes:

1 hyperventilation

2 sodium bicarbonate 50–100 mmol IV

3 calcium chloride 5–10 mL of 10% solution IV

4 IV glucose 25–50 g 50% solution (50–100 mL) with 10–20 units of actrapid insulin

5 dialysis.

Subsequent management (and for less severe hypokalaemia) is:

1 Resonium A or calcium resonium 15 g PO 6 h or 30 g PR 8 h.

2 Treat the cause if possible.

Note: Suxamethonium is contraindicated.

Prazosin

Quinazoline derivative used for the treatment of hypertension, phaeochromocytoma and prostatism. Acts by competitively inhibiting α1 adreno-receptors, resulting in arterial and venous vaso-dilatation.

Dose

Adult: 1 mg 8–12 h, gradually increased to up to 20 mg/day.

Note: Prazosin can cause postural hypotension.

Pre-eclampsia/Eclampsia

Topics Covered in this Section

▶ Pre-eclampsia and Eclampsia Defined
▶ Aetiology of Pre-eclampsia/Eclampsia
▶ Clinical Features
▶ Treatment Aims
▶ Acute Management of Severe Hypertension
▶ Optimising Intravascular Volume and Renal Function
▶ Prophylaxis/Treatment of Seizures
▶ Management of Coagulopathy
▶ Anaesthetic Management
▶ Postpartum Management

Pre-eclampsia and Eclampsia Defined

The Australasian Society for the Study of Hypertension in Pregnancy describes pre-eclampsia as a 'multisystem disorder potentially affecting maternal liver, kidneys, brain and clotting system as well as leading to impaired placental circulation'.[74] This group defines pre-eclampsia as hypertension developing after 20 weeks of pregnancy in the absence of previous hypertension or renal disease and which resolves within 3 months postpartum. Associated with the hypertension are one or more of the clinical features described in the next section. The disease may occur rarely prior to the 20th week of pregnancy, associated with such conditions as a hydatidiform mole.[75]

Pre-eclampsia associated hypertension can be subclassified into:

1 *mild*: systolic blood pressure ≥ 140 mmHg, diastolic blood pressure ≥ 90 mmHg
2 *severe*: systolic blood pressure ≥ 170 mmHg, diastolic blood pressure ≥ 110 mmHg.

If seizures occur eclampsia is diagnosed. The mortality of pre-eclampsia/eclampsia is 2–4%. Up to 7% of pregnant women develop pre-eclampsia[75] and eclamapsia occurs in up to 0.12% of pregnancies.[76]

Aetiology of Pre-eclampsia/Eclampsia

The aetiology of pre-eclampsia is unknown but it is theorised that the fundamental underlying abnormality may relate to the trophoblast leading to placental ischaemia. The abnormality may be a maternal immune maladaption to the trophoblast, inadequate trophoblastic invasion or some other cause. This abnormality results in placental ischaemia with increased release of uterine renin, stimulation of aldosterone secretion and breakdown of placental architecture. This placental breakdown leads to other placental substances being released into the maternal circulation causing:

1 widespread maternal endothelial injury[77]
2 decreased production of vasodilating substances such as prostacyclin and an overproduction of vasoconstrictors such as thromboxane A_2
3 arterial vasospasm, increased platelet aggregation and increased capillary permeability.

Clinical Features

▶ Cardiovascular Effects

An increased systemic vascular resistance, circulatory volume contraction and increased left ventricular work occurs. Cardiac dysfunction may supervene, resulting in cardiogenic pulmonary oedema. Non-cardiogenic pulmonary oedema may also develop due to leaky pulmonary capillaries and decreased plasma oncotic pressure.[75]

▶ Central Nervous System Effects

Headache, visual disturbances, irritability, hyper-reflexia, clonus and seizures may occur. Intracranial haemorrhage may also occur, accounting for 30–40% of deaths from pre-eclampsia.

▶ *Respiratory Effects*

Pulmonary oedema may occur due to low plasma oncotic pressure, increased permeability of alveolar capillaries, ventricular dysfunction and iatrogenic fluid loading.

▶ *Renal Effects*

Proteinuria ($\geq$ 300 mg/day). Oliguria/renal failure may occur with a serum creatinine > 90 µmol/L. Hyperuricaemia $\geq$ 0.35 mmol/L is a marker of potential foetal risk.[74]

▶ *Hepatic Effects*

Hepatocellular damage, swelling and hepatic rupture can occur. Patients may complain of epigastric pain.

▶ *Haematological Effects*

Haemolysis, coagulopathy and increased blood viscosity may occur. The patient may develop disseminated intravascular coagulation.

▶ *Utero/placental/foetal Effects*

Uteroplacental blood flow may be greatly decreased, leading to intra-uterine growth retardation and increased risk of placental abruption.[77]

▶ *HELLP Syndrome*[78]

This is the presence of haemolysis, elevated liver enzymes and low platelet count in the pre-eclamptic or eclamptic patient. HELLP syndrome occurs in 4–12% of pre-eclampsia cases.[79] It is not a separate disease entity but rather a type of presentation of severe pre-eclampsia/eclampsia.

Treatment Aims

1 Control hypertension.
2 Optimise intravascular volume and renal function.
3 Prevent/treat seizures.

4   Maximise perinatal outcome without unduly endangering the mother. Ultimately the safety of the mother is paramount.

Acute Management of Severe Hypertension

1   Treat the hypertension of pre-eclampsia if the diastolic blood pressure > 110 mmHg or systolic blood pressure > 170 mmHg because of the risk of intracerebral haemorrhage.[75] Reduce systolic BP by 20–30 mmHg and diastolic BP by 10–15 mmHg. If the blood pressure is less than 170/110 mmHg, further reduction is controversial. Blood pressure no lower than 140/90 mmHg may or may not be a reasonable treatment aim.[75]

2   Treatment of hypertension must occur at the same time as the optimisation of the patient's intravascular volume. Continuous CTG monitoring should be undertaken to detect foetal compromise due to reduction in blood pressure.[75] Invasive arterial blood pressure measurements should be obtained if continuous IV drug infusions are required. Drug therapies include:

(a) Hydralazine 10 mg IV bolus at 15 min intervals to a maximum of 40 mg.

(b) Nifedipine orally (not sublingually). *Avoid calcium channel blocker drugs if magnesium therapy is to be used because they enhance magnesium toxicity.*

(c) Labetalol. Give incremental doses of 5–10 mg IV. This can be repeated at 5 min intervals up to 1 mg/kg. The total dose required may vary from 20 to 300 mg.[77] Labetalol is not thought to adversely affect the foetal heart rate or uteroplacental blood flow.[77,80]

(d) Diazoxide 30 mg IV minutely to a maximum of 300 mg.

(e) Epidural anaesthesia, if otherwise indicated for labour analgesia or Caesarean section, will further assist in the lowering of blood pressure.

(f) Magnesium therapy (see below).

(g) If patients are on oral clonidine this should be continued during labour and/or peri-operatively because of the risk of rebound hypertension.[75]

(h) Esmolol? There is little information in the literature regarding the use of esmolol in pre-eclampsia. However, in the foetus the duration of effect of esmolol is prolonged with a half-life of 21 min.[77] See the comment on drugs to avoid below.

(i) Sodium nitroprusside (SNP) infusion. Pre-eclamptic patients may be extremely sensitive to SNP.[77] SNP may cause foetal cyanide or thiocyanate toxicity and foetal bradycardia.[77]

(j) Glyceryl trinitrate (GTN) infusion. Note that GTN causes uterine relaxation.

(k) Trimetaphan infusion.

Chronic oral therapy drugs include methyldopa, oxprenolol, labetalol, nifedipine, clonidine and prazosin. Cease these drugs if BP < 120/70 mmHg.[75]

Drugs to *avoid* include atenolol and ACE inhibitors due to potential adverse neonatal effects.[75] β blockers can cause foetal bradycardia and foetal hypoxaemia.

▶ Magnesium Therapy

1 If the above medications are inadequate to control hypertension, commence a magnesium sulphate infusion. Magnesium is a potent anticonvulsant which also reduces systemic vascular resistance, improving uterine blood flow and lowering blood pressure.[77] Give a loading dose of magnesium 4 g (8 mL of a 50% solution of magnesium sulphate in 250 mL N/S) over 20 min via a central line. Magnesium can be given via a peripheral cannula initially in an emergency until central venous access is obtained.

2 Commence a maintenance infusion of 1 g/h following the loading dose. A dose range of 1–3 g/h is suggested.[81] Continue the magnesium infusion for 24 h after the delivery or after the last

seizure. If the initial dose of 4 g does not prevent convulsions, give a second loading dose of 2–4 g over 20 min. Monitor magnesium blood levels every 6 h. The therapeutic level is 2–3.5 mmol/L.[81] Cease the infusion if the blood level of Mg^{2+} > 3.5 mmol/L. Monitor knee jerk reflexes. Stop the infusion and check the Mg^{2+} level if these disappear. Decrease or stop the magnesium infusion if urine output < 30 mL/h (Mg^{2+} is renally excreted).

Table P1 Effects of magnesium therapy

Clinical effect	Mg^{2+} (units in common use)		
	mmol/L	mEq/L	mg/dL
Normal serum level	0.75–1.0	1.5–2.0	1.8–2.4
Therapeutic anticonvulsant level	2–3.5	4–7	4.8–8.4
Loss of patellar reflexes	3.5–5	7–11	8.4–12
Skeletal muscle relaxation	6	12	14.4
SA and AV block/respiratory paralysis	6–7.5	12–15	14.4–18
Cardiac arrest	>12	>25	>30

▶ Magnesium Toxicity

In addition to supportive measures for airway breathing and circulation, treat gross magnesium toxicity with:

1. calcium chloride 1 g slow IV injection
2. fluid loading and diuretic therapy to increase renal excretion
3. glucose and insulin to increase Mg^{2+} entry into cells
4. dialysis.

▶ *Magnesium Therapy and Anaesthesia*

1 Magnesium therapy potentiates the effects of non-depolarising muscle relaxants (NDNMBDs). Dosages of NDNMBDs should be reduced as guided by neuromuscular monitoring. Fasciculations may not be seen with suxamethonium.

2 Magnesium 40 mg/kg given immediately after induction of anaesthesia appears to be effective in reducing the hypertensive response to intubation in pre-eclamptic patients.[82]

Optimising Intravascular Volume and Renal Function

The main causes of death in pre-eclampsia/eclampsia are pulmonary oedema and cerebral haemorrhage. Although these patients tend to be intravascularly depleted (mean value 500–600 mL)[75] volume expansion should be undertaken cautiously. Careful volume expansion is particularly important if vasodilator therapy is to be used or epidural or spinal anaesthesia is to be undertaken. Excess IV fluid therapy can easily precipitate pulmonary oedema in these patients with a high mortality.[83] This is a much more significant threat to the patient than the risk of permanent renal failure, which is rare.

▶ *Steps for Optimising Intravascular Volume*

There is considerable controversy in the literature as to whether crystalloid or colloid is preferable in pre-eclampsia.[83] Each individual obstetric unit must formulate its own protocols. A suggested approach is:

1 Auscultate the lungs for evidence of pulmonary oedema and assess JVP.

2 Measure urine output. Aim for a urine output > 0.5 mL/kg/h.

3 For mild pre-eclampsia give a fluid challenge 500 mL of N/S or Hartmann's solution.

4 If there is no clinical evidence of fluid overload commence N/S or Hartmann's solution at 1–1.5 mL/kg/h.

5 If there is evidence of fluid overload or LV dysfunction, give Hartmann's solution at 0–0.5 mL/kg/h.

6 If urine output falls to < 0.5 mL/kg/h over 4 h and there is no evidence of fluid overload, consider a fluid challenge, i.e. 250 mL bolus of crystalloid over 20 min, and assess the response. If urine output does not improve or there is evidence of fluid overload, consider inserting a central venous line and measuring CVP. If the patient is coagulopathic, consider using an antecubital fossa long line to measure CVP. Cautiously fluid-load the patient to a CVP of 5–6 mmHg. If CVP is already > 6 mmHg or pulmonary oedema develops, consider inserting a PA catheter. Ongoing management may require vasodilator therapy, inotropes and optimal fluid loading as guided by PA catheter readings ± other investigations such as TOE.

Prophylaxis/Treatment of Seizures

Seizures may be preceded by hyperreflexia, clonus, retinal vasospasm and visual disturbances and headache.

1 Magnesium sulphate is the treatment of choice for prevention and treatment of seizures, because of its potent anticonvulsant effects in pre-eclampsia/eclampsia, coupled with its ability to improve uterine blood flow and reduce systemic vascular resistance. Give 4 g over 5–10 min, then infusion. See above.

2 Diazepam (5–20 mg IV given incrementally) can be used to treat seizures acutely.

3 Phenytoin should be added if seizures continue to occur despite magnesium.[75]

4 If prolonged loss of consciousness occurs, intubate and ventilate the patient and organise an urgent cerebral CT scan. Cerebral haemorrhage may have occurred.[76]

Management of Coagulopathy

Give a platelet transfusion if the platelet count < 20 $\times$ 10^9/L (20 000/mm^3). Also give platelets if the count is 20–40 $\times$ 10^9/L and there is active bleeding and/or severe hypertension.[74] Give FFP if coagulopathic.

Anaesthetic Management

▶ *Epidural Anaesthesia*

Pre-eclamptic patients are often hypovolaemic. Adequate circulating volume must be ensured prior to initiation of epidural blockade to avoid sudden hypotension. See comments above regarding optimising intravascular volume. Epidural blockade should be achieved gradually and significant hypotension treated with small doses of ephedrine and IV fluid boluses if appropriate. It is also essential to exclude significant thrombocytopenia and coagulopathy prior to epidural insertion. If the platelet count is > 100 $\times$ 10^9/L (100 000/mm^3) significant coagulopathy is unlikely.[84] If the platelet count is 80–100 $\times$ 10^9/L, the platelet count is not falling precipitously, coagulation studies are normal and the patient does not have clinical evidence of a bleeding tendency, e.g. bruises, it *may* be safe to proceed with epidural placement. Skin bleeding times and thromboelastograghy may or may not be reliable tests of platelet function in this situation[77] and each institution must formulate its own policy. Epidural anaesthesia is contraindicated if the platelet count is < 50 $\times$ 10^9/L. It may be safer *not* to use *adrenaline*-containing LA solutions for epidural blockade but this is debatable.[77]

▶ *Spinal Anaesthesia*

This is usually avoided because of concerns about causing profound maternal hypotension.[77] However, Hood and Curry concluded in their retrospective study that blood pressure decreases were similar for spinal and epidural anaesthesia in severely eclamptic women.[85] As pointed out by Santos in the situation of urgent caesarean section the risks of spinal anaesthesia induced hypotension must be 'weighed against the risk of an airway catastrophe with general anaesthesia'.[86]

▶ *General Anaesthesia*

1   Airway oedema may make intubation difficult and preparations for failed intubation must be made.

2   It is imperative to prevent/control the hypertensive response to intubation pharmacologically. However, no drug protocol available at present is totally reliable. Suggested drug strategies include:

  (a) lignocaine 1 mg/kg IV

  (b) hydralazine 5–10 mg IV at least 10 min before induction

  (c) trimetaphan infusion commenced at 3–4 mg/min and titrated to effect. See *TRIMETAPHAN*.

  (d) sodium nitroprusside infusion titrated to effect

  (e) fentanyl 8 µg/kg, noting that some respiratory depression of the newborn may occur[87]

  (f) magnesium sulphate bolus 40 mg/kg[82]

  (g) remifentanil. Consider an infusion of 0.25 µg/kg/min 1 minute before induction of general anaesthesia (unpublished personal experience).

  (h) esmolol? Esmolol has been used to blunt the pressor effects of tracheal intubation but there are no studies yet proving its efficacy in treating hypertension in pre-eclamptic patients.[77] Esmolol persists in the foetus with a 21 minute half-life and may cause foetal bradycardia and hypoxaemia.[77]

3   Magnesium therapy may affect the patient's response to neuromuscular blocking drugs. See magnesium therapy comments above.

4   If patients have marked airway oedema on intubation consider a period of elective ventilation postoperatively to prevent airway compromise in the early postoperative period.

P

> ### All Types of Anaesthetic

Do not give ergometrine in the presence of eclampsia/pre-eclampsia, due to the risk of precipitating a hypertensive crisis.[75] Oxytocin is acceptable.

Postpartum Management

1 If epidural anaesthesia has been used pre-delivery consider continuing the epidural post-delivery with an infusion of bupivacaine or ropivacaine (plus fentanyl) to maintain peripheral vasodilation.

2 Patients should be monitored in a high dependency area or the intensive care unit.

3 Pre-eclampsia may become more severe in the postpartum period and ongoing vigilance is required. Of the patients who suffer convulsions, about 40% of these begin in the postpartum period.

4 For ongoing oral treatment for hypertension, consider oral therapy with oxprenolol, methyldopa, nifedipine, clonidine or prazosin.

Pregnancy and Non–Obstetric Surgery— Anaesthetic Considerations

There is a slightly increased risk of spontaneous abortion associated with anaesthesia and surgery in the first and second trimester of pregnancy.[88] Preterm labour in the postoperative period is also more likely. It is not possible to separate anaesthesia, the disease requiring surgery, or the surgery itself, as the main causative factor. There does not appear to be an increased risk of foetal abnormality in these patients. Elective surgery should be avoided if possible during pregnancy.

Anaesthetic Drugs and Pregnancy

1 Ketamine in doses > 1.1 mg/kg can significantly increase uterine tone.

2 Avoid giving inhalational agents above 2 MAC as this can decrease cardiac output and adversely affect foetal perfusion.

Cardiovascular Issues

▶ *Supine Hypotensive Syndrome*

Aorto-caval compression, resulting in hypotension when supine, can occur after the first trimester. At term, when supine, 10% of patients have symptoms but 90% have complete aorto-caval compression by the gravid uterus.[89] The compression is relieved by left lateral displacement of the uterus, i.e. place a wedge under the right hip producing left lateral tilt. Avoid hypotension from any cause as this can result in foetal hypoxia.

▶ *Increased Thrombo-embolism Risk*

1 Mobilise the pregnant patient early after surgery and use other precautions against deep venous thrombosis. See *DEEP VENOUS THROMBOSIS (DVT) PROPHYLAXIS*.

2 Maintain adequate blood pressure, as maternal hypotension may lead to foetal asphyxia due to decreased uterine blood flow.

3 Vasoactive drugs such as phenylephrine and dopamine may significantly reduce uterine blood flow.

Respiratory Issues

1 *Aspiration risk*: Patients are at increased risk for aspiration from as early as ≈ 12th week and especially from the 20th week,[90] up until 2–3 days postpartum. See *ASPIRATION, PREVENTION AND TREATMENT*. Patients at risk of aspiration should receive antacid medication and a rapid sequence induction if a general anaesthetic is used. See *RAPID SEQUENCE INDUCTION (RSI)*.

2 *Functional residual capacity is decreased* from about the second trimester while *closing capacity and oxygen consumption are increased*. Thus pregnant patients undergo rapid O_2 desaturation if apnoea or airway obstruction occurs.

P

3 *Increased vascularity and oedema of airway mucosa* may result in the need for a smaller than expected endotracheal tube size, and bleeding with instrumentation of the airway, e.g. nasal intubation.

4 *Hyperventilation should be avoided* in the pregnant patient as this can result in foetal hypoxia and acidosis.

Regional Anaesthesia

Pregnant patients tend to be more sensitive to local anaesthetic agents than non-pregnant patients. It is recommended to reduce the dose of LA used by 25–30%. Ensure there is adequate IV fluid loading and treat hypotension promptly.

Teratogenicity of Anaesthetic Drugs

Major birth defects occur in about 3% of the population. The foetus is most vulnerable to teratogenic drugs during the period of organogenesis (2nd to the 12th week). Agents of concern include the following:

1 Nitrous oxide has been shown to decrease uterine blood flow in animal studies but has never been conclusively shown to cause adverse effects in human pregnancy. See *NITROUS OXIDE*.

2 Benzodiazepine drugs have been anecdotally associated with cleft lip anomalies.[91]

3 Cocaine use has been associated with microcephaly and other congenital abnormalities.

4 Propofol has, in animal studies, resulted in delayed ossification and abnormal cranial ossification in the foetus and an increased incidence of subdural haematomas (Propofol Product Information). Although the manufacturer advises against the use of propofol in pregnancy there is no evidence of terato-genicity in humans.

Foetal Monitoring and Welfare

The most important factors in maintaining foetal wellbeing during anaesthesia are avoiding maternal hypotension, hypovolaemia, hypocapnia and hypoxia. Consider intermittent or continuous foetal monitoring after ≈ 20th week intra-operatively. If monitoring indicates a non-reassuring foetal heart trace consider measures such as:

1 increasing maternal oxygenation
2 increasing maternal blood pressure
3 changing the site of surgical traction
4 increasing uterine displacement.

If intra-operative X-rays are taken, use foetal shielding.

Pressure Units

1 mmHg = 0.133 kPa = 1.36 cmH$_2$O = 100 Pa
1 bar = 100 kPa
1 kPa = 1% of an Atmosphere
1 kPa = 7.50 mmHg
1 torr = 133 Pa
1 lb/square inch (PSI) = 6.89 kPa
1 Atmosphere = 760 mmHg = 14.7 PSI = 1.013 bar
1 Atmosphere = 760 torr = 101.3 kPa

Procainamide

Class Ia anti-arrythmic drug useful for the treatment of:

1 atrial flutter, atrial fibrillation, supraventricular tachycardia
2 unsustained ventricular tachycardia
3 Wolff-Parkinson-White associated atrial fibrillation.

Dose in the Adult

IV: 50 mg/min until the dysrhythmia is controlled or the QRS widens or SBP falls below 85 mmHg up to a maximum dose of 1000–1500 mg. Then provide an infusion of 2–4 mg/min.

Precautions

1 Procainamide is contraindicated in prolonged Q-T syndrome.
2 Procainamide can worsen muscle weakness in myasthenia gravis.
3 Non-depolarising muscle relaxant drugs have a prolonged effect in the presence of procainamide.

Prochlorperazine

A phenothiazine of the piperazine subclass, this drug is useful for the treatment of:
1 nausea and vomiting
2 vertigo.
Prochlorperazine acts by a central antidopaminergic receptor effect.

Dose

Adult PO: 5–20 mg 8–12 h.
Adult IM: 12.5 mg IM up to 6 h. Although not recommended by the manufacturer prochlorperazine can be given IV safely at a rate not exceeding 5 mg/min.[92]

Disadvantages

1 This drug is unsuitable for patients with Parkinson's disease.
2 Prochlorperazine can cause dystonic reactions (see *DYSTONIC REACTION, ACUTE*).
3 This drug can precipitate the neuroleptic malignant syndrome (see entry).

Promethazine

This is a phenothiazine antihistamine drug with sedative and anti-emetic properties. It acts mainly by blocking H1 histaminergic receptors and also has some anticholinergic, antidopaminergic and anti-serotoninergic properties. Promethazine is used for the treatment of:
1 allergic reactions

2   pruritus
3   emesis.

Dose

Adult: 25–50 mg IV or 25–75 mg PO daily in divided doses.
Child: 0.2–0.5 mg/kg/dose 6–8 h IV, IM or PO.
Sedation dose: 0.5–1.5 mg/kg, maximum 100 mg.

Propacetamol

Intravenous form of paracetamol. 1 g of propacetamol IV is equivalent to 500 mg of paracetamol PO.

Propofol

2,6–diisopropyl phenol (a hindered phenol) used as an intravenous anaesthetic agent for induction ± maintenance of anaesthesia and also for sedation. Propofol has also been used to treat pruritus.[93] Presented as a white emulsion of soya bean oil and egg phosphatide containing 1% propofol.

Dose

Adult: 2–2.5 mg/kg.
Child: 3–3.5 mg/kg.

Dose for Total Intravenous Anaesthesia

For unpremedicated patient: 12 mg/kg/h for 10 min, then 10 mg/kg/h for 10 min, then 8 mg/kg/h for 10 min, then 6 mg/kg/h.
For premedicated patient: as above but start at 10 mg/kg/h. Titrate the infusion rate to the patient's physiological response. The usual maintenance dose for anaesthesia is 6–12 mg/kg/h.

Total Intravenous Anaesthesia Using the Diprifusor Technique (Target-controlled Infusion)[94]

This technique involves the use of a computer-controlled propofol infusion pump called a Diprifusor. The computer program includes

P

mathematical modelling of pharmacokinetic parameters, enabling estimation of actual patient blood concentrations of propofol. The patient's weight and age are entered into the pump's computer and the desired blood concentrations are 'dialled up' on the Diprifusor, which is able to adjust infusion rates appropriately to achieve this level. The Diprifusor is not as yet recommended for use in children. The age range available on the Diprifusor is 16–100 years and the weight range 30–150 kg.

Table P2 Suggested blood propofol concentrations for various stages of anaesthesia (Zeneca *Guide for Anaesthetists* Product Information 1999)

Stage of anaesthesia	Blood concentration (µg/mL)
Induction with midazolam 2 mg and fentanyl 100 µg	(Initial target concentration) *Young healthy adult patient*: Unpremedicated 6 µg/mL Premedicated 4 µg/mL (Range 4–8 µg/mL) *For older, sicker patient* use a target concentration of 3–4 µg/mL
Maintenance of anaesthesia (with O$_2$ and N$_2$O)	*Young, healthy patient*: 3.5–5.3 µg/mL *Older, sicker patient*: 2.8–3.5 µg/mL

Notes: 1 Induction times for the initial target blood concentrations outlined above are ≈ 60–120 s; 2 For a gradual induction of anaesthesia in patients who are elderly or unwell begin with 3 µg/mL, then increase concentration gradually in steps of 0.5–1 µg/mL 1 minutely; 3 The target concentration to maintain anaesthesia is 3.0–6.0 µg/mL, depending on factors such as the amount of surgical stimulation and what other drugs are used; 4 Patients will wake up at a propofol concentration of ≈ 1–2 µg/mL.

Dose for Sedation

For adult, give boluses of 20–50 mg or an infusion at a rate of 1–4 mg/kg/h titrated to clinical effect.

Dose for Antipruritic Effect (for Pruritus Due to Opioids or Liver Disease)

Adult: 10 mg IV bolus or infusion 0.5–1 mg/kg/h.[93]

Advantages

1 Propofol can be used for total IV anaesthesia.
2 Less hangover effect and less nausea and vomiting compared with thiopentone.[95]
3 Rapid redistribution and elimination results in a short duration of action even after prolonged periods.
4 Propofol has anticonvulsant properties and has been used to treat status epilepticus in humans successfully [94] (but see below).
5 Propofol has an antipruritic action and anxiolysis effects.[94]
6 Allergic reactions are extremely rare.
7 Safe to use in patients with malignant hyperpyrexia susceptibility.
8 Propofol is probably safe as a single dose for patients with porphyria but may not be safe if given as an infusion. See *PORPHYRIA*.

Disadvantages

1 Pain on injection.
2 Seizure-like movements and seizures have occurred with propofol administration. Seizure incidence has been estimated to be 1 in 47 000 administrations.[96]
3 Causes a 20% drop in mean arterial pressure and a 20% decrease in systemic vascular resistance.[94] This effect is more pronounced in the elderly[97] and hypovolaemic. Propofol must be used with extreme caution in the elderly.
4 Abuse potential.

5 Five × more expensive than thiopentone (for an induction dose).

6 Some deaths have occurred in children in ICU on propofol infusions.[98]

Propranolol

This is an aromatic amine non-selective β receptor blocker without intrinsic sympathomimetic activity. It is used for the treatment of:

1 angina, hypertension and tachydysrhythmias
2 hypertrophic obstructive cardiomyopathy
3 phaeochromocytoma, thyrotoxicosis, migraine and acute exacerbations of porphyria.

Dose

Adult: 1–10 mg IV titrated to desired clinical response.

ProSeal Laryngeal Mask Airway

See *LARYNGEAL MASK AIRWAY (INCLUDING PROSEAL AND FASTRACH)*.

Prostate Surgery

See *TRANSURETHRAL RESECTION OF PROSTATE (TURP)*.

Prostin F$_2$ Alpha

Prostin F$_2$ alpha is the methylated analogue of prostaglandin F$_2$ alpha. It is used to cause uterine contraction for therapeutic abortion and the treatment of postpartum haemorrhage (PPH) due to uterine atony. See *POSTPARTUM HAEMORRHAGE*.

Dose for Uterine Atony with PPH

Give 250 μg IM or intramyometrially for refractory uterine atony. Repeat dose every 15–30 min up to a total dose not exceeding 2 mg.

Note

Prostaglandin F_2 alpha increases airway resistance and is relatively contraindicated in asthma.[99] Overdose of this drug may cause cardiovascular collapse.[100]

Protamine

Obtained from fish sperm, protamine is a mixture of cationic proteins used to neutralise the anticoagulant effect of heparin. It is also ≈ 60% effective in reversing the effects of low molecular weight heparin.

Dose for Reversing Heparin

1 mg of protamine neutralises 100 units of heparin. Give slowly (over minutes), as it can cause acute hypotension, bradycardia and anaphylactoid/anaphylactic reactions. Can also cause pulmonary vasoconstriction/hypertension acutely.

Dose for Reversing Low Molecular Weight Heparin

1 Dalteparin (Fragmin): give protamine 1 mg/100 U of dalteparin.
2 Enoxaparin (Clexane): give protamine 1 mg/1 mg of enoxaparin.

Adverse Effects of Protamine

1 Protamine can cause anaphylactic or anaphylactoid reaction with hypotension, bronchospasm and pulmonary oedema. Patients who have fish allergy, vasectomy, insulin exposure or previous protamine exposure may have an allergic reaction to protamine.[101]
2 Protamine can also cause pulmonary hypertension, possibly through the release of complement.
3 In patients in whom protamine is contraindicated alternative drugs to reverse heparin include fresh frozen plasma, recombinant platelet factor 4, heparinase –I and other experimental drugs.[101]

P

Prothrombin Time

See *INTERNATIONAL NORMALISED RATIO (INR)*.

Pruritus, Due to Opioids

See *MORPHINE*.

Pseudocholinesterase Deficiency

See *SUX APNOEA*.

In patients with pseudocholinesterase deficiency the effects of the following drugs may be prolonged:

1   Suxamethonium
2   Mivacurium.

Pulmonary Artery (PA) Catheter

Topics Covered in this Section

▶ Pulmonary Artery Catheter Measurements and Normal Values
▶ Technique of PA Catheter Placement
▶ Diagnostic Patterns
▶ Cardiac Output Studies
▶ Factors Affecting the Accuracy of PCWP and Cardiac Output Studies

Pulmonary Artery Catheter Measurements and Normal Values

Central venous pressure (CVP)	0–6 mmHg
Mean pulmonary artery pressure (MPAP)	9–16 mmHg
Pulmonary capillary wedge pressure (PCWP)	8–12 mmHg
Cardiac output (CO)	4–8 L/min
Cardiac index (CI)	2.5–4 $L.min^{-1}.m^{-2}$
Stroke volume (SV)	60–130 mL

Right ventricular stroke work (RVSW)	$4-8$ g.m.m^{-2}.beat^{-1}
Left ventricular stroke work (LVSW)	$44-68$ g.m.m^{-2}.beat^{-1}
Stroke volume index (SVI)	$35-70$ mL.beat^{-1}.m^{-2}
Systemic vascular resistance (SVR)	1000 dynes.s.cm^{-5}
Systemic vascular resistance index (SVRI)	$1760-2600$ dyne.s.cm^{-5}.m^{-2}
Pulmonary vascular resistance (PVR)	100 dyne.s.cm^{-5}
Pulmonary vascular resistance index (PVRI)	$44-225$ dyne.s.cm^{-5}.m^{-2}

Technique for PA Catheter Placement

1 Insertion measurements quoted are for the right internal jugular approach. For a much more detailed description of insertion technique refer to Kong and Singer's article listed in the references.[102]

2 Insert the pulmonary artery (PA) catheter sheath (8.5 F) as for an internal jugular or subclavian vein central line insertion (see page 533).

3 After flushing all the lumens and testing the flotation balloon, attach the proximal end of the distal (balloon) lumen to the pressure transducer and calibrate ('zero'). Ensure none of the lumens are open to air at their proximal ends. Insert the PA catheter through the sheath haemostasis valve and transduce the pressure measured at tip of balloon lumen. Once the tip of the PA catheter is in the vein (at $\approx$ 20 cm insertion distance), inflate the balloon with 1.5 mL of air and measure the pressure as the catheter is advanced. With correct placement four types of pressure wave are seen:

(a) SVC and right atrial (0–4 mmHg)

(b) right ventricle, at $\approx$ 30 cm (25/0 mmHg)

(c) pulmonary artery (PA), entered at about 40–50 cm (25/9 mmHg). A dicrotic notch appears on the waveform. The PA diastolic pressure can be falsely elevated if the heart rate exceeds 120 bpm due to insufficient time for the pressure to

P

return to baseline.[103] A mean PA pressure > 20 mmHg is diagnostic of pulmonary hypertension.

(d) Pulmonary artery wedge pressure (8–12 mmHg). Also called pulmonary capillary wedge pressure (PCWP). This pressure is used to approximate left ventricular end diastolic pressure (LVEDP). The PCWP should be equal to, or less than, the PA diastolic pressure.

4 When the balloon is deflated the PA pressure trace should reappear. If it does not, withdraw catheter a few centimetres.

Diagnostic Patterns

See Table P3 for some common diagnostic patterns.

Table P3 Some common diagnostic patterns

Condition	PCWP	CO	SVR
Hypovolaemic shock	Low	Low	High
Cardiogenic shock	High	Low	High
Vasogenic shock	Low	High	Low

> ## *PA Catheter Findings with Some Specific Conditions*

1 *Cardiac tamponade*: There tends to be equalisation of all cardiac diastolic pressures, i.e. RA = RVD = PAD = PCWP.

2 *Myocardial ischaemia*: See elevation in PCWP typically to > 15 mmHg and V waves > 20 mmHg.

3 *Right ventricular infarction*: Typically see high RA pressure, poor RVSW and normal or low PCWP.

4 *Mitral incompetence*: V waves on recording of the pulmonary artery occlusion pressure. The size of the V wave correlates with the degree of regurgitant flow.

▶ *Conditions Causing Elevation of the PCWP*

1   Left ventricular failure.
2   Mitral stenosis and mitral incompetence.
3   Cardiac tamponade and constrictive pericarditis.
4   Volume overload.

Cardiac Output Studies

1   Enter the patient's weight and height into the cardiac output studies program.
2   Enter the patient's CVP and PCWP.
3   Inject cold saline into the right atrial port of the PA catheter at the end-expiration point of the patient's ventilatory cycle. Repeat 4–6 times, aiming for a consistent cardiac output result.
4   Enter the averaged cardiac output value and initiate the calculations function.

Factors Affecting the Accuracy of PCWP and Cardiac Output Studies

1. Thermodilution CO may be inaccurate in patients with tricuspid incompetence, intracardiac shunts and atrial fibrillation.
2   PCWP will be greater than LVEDP in patients with conditions such as mitral stenosis and prolapsing left atrial tumours.[104] PCWP will be less than LVEDP in conditions such as decreased left ventricular compliance and LVEDP > 25 mmHg.[104]
3   In the presence of pathologically large 'a' waves (as occurs with mitral stenosis, complete heart block, atrial myxoma and early acute heart failure), use the end-exhalation diastolic PCWP measurement.
4   If there are pathological large 'v' waves (as can occur with mitral regurgitation, left atrial enlargement and VSD), again use the diastolic end-expiration PCWP measurement.
5   The tip of the PA catheter should lie in West Zone 3 of the lung (where venous and arterial pressure exceed alveolar pressure 95% of the time).[105]

P

6 Peak end-expiratory pressure (PEEP), by increasing pleural pressure, will artificially elevate the measured PCWP value. To correct for PEEP > 10 cmH$_2$O subtract half the PEEP pressure from the measured PCWP or use the formula:[104]

$$\text{actual PCWP (mmHg)} = \text{measured PCWP (mmHg)} - \frac{\text{PEEP} \times 0.75}{3}$$

Pulmonary Embolus

Diagnostic Features

1 Dyspnoea, pleuritic chest pain.
2 Tachycardia.
3 Confusion.
4 Cyanosis.
5 Friction rub, wheezing.
6 Pleural effusion.
7 Evidence of elevated pulmonary artery pressure, i.e. accentuation of pulmonary valve closure sound, widened splitting of the second heart sound, palpable right ventricular heave, raised CVP.
8 Hypotension and cardiovascular collapse and death may occur. Overall mortality is about 10%.[106]

Investigations

1 ECG changes may occur, such as ST depression and T wave inversion in anterior leads, deep S wave in lead I and a Q wave and inverted T wave in lead III.
2 CXR may show an enhanced pulmonary artery shadow, lung oligaemia in the area affected by the embolus and a wedge-shaped area on the pleural surface, suggesting infarction.
3 Echocardiography may indicate RV dilatation and hypokinesis with apical sparing, suggesting PE.[107] Thrombus may be seen in the cardiac chambers and echocardiography enables

measurement of pulmonary artery pressure. A negative echo-cardiogram is not helpful.

4   Arterial blood gases may show hypoxaemia and hypocapnia.
5   Serum D-dimer may be elevated.
6   Ventilation/perfusion scan.
7   Pulmonary angiography may provide a definitive diagnosis.

Treatment

Management of PE is determined by the patient's clinical conditions and available resources.

▶ *Cardiovascularly Unstable Patient*

1   Resuscitate the patient, i.e. ensure adequate airway and ventilation, provide 100% O_2. Ensure adequate cardiac rhythm and blood pressure and support the circulation as required. See *CARDIAC ARREST*. Intravascular volume expansion and inotropic support may be required.

2   Consider thrombolytic therapy with e.g. *streptokinase* 250 000 units IV over 30 min, then 10 000 units/h for 24–72 h or *tissue plasminogen activator* 15 mg IV bolus, then 45 mg/h for 2 h.

  Alternatively, consider surgical embolectomy ± immediate femoral–femoral bypass and pump oxygenation until conventional cardiopulmonary bypass can be established. Percutaneous embolectomy is performed in some specialist centres.

3   Use noradrenaline if a vasopressor is required. Intra-aortic balloon counterpulsation may be required.

4   Inhaled selective pulmonary vasodilators such as nitric oxide or prostacyclin may be of benefit in addition to the other measures discussed.[108,109]

▶ *Cardiovascularly Stable Patient*

1   For less critical situations heparinise the patient using either unfractionated or low molecular weight heparin:

- *Heparin*: Give a loading dose 5000 IU, then infuse heparin at 18 units/kg/h. Maintain the activated partial thromboplastin time (APTT) at 1.5–2.5 × control, i.e. at 50–90 s. The NR for APTT is 25–30 s.
- *Low molecular weight heparin*:
  - Dalteparin 100 U/kg/12 h subcutaneously or 200 U/kg/day.
  - Enoxaparin 1 mg/kg/12 h subcutaneously or 1.5 mg/kg/day.

Therapy with unfractionated heparin or LMW heparin should be continued for at least 5 days overlapping with oral warfarin therapy from day 1. The international normalised ratio (INR) must be in the therapeutic range (2.0–3.0) for at least 2 days before ceasing heparin therapy.

2 If patients cannot be heparinised, e.g. due to ongoing bleeding, consider insertion of an inferior vena caval filter.

Pulmonary Hypertension

Only a very brief outline of this extremely complicated condition is provided. Pulmonary hypertension is diagnosed when mean pulmonary artery pressure > 25 mmHg.[110] Pulmonary hypertension is considered moderately severe when mean pulmonary artery pressure (PAP) > 35 mmHg, and right ventricular (RV) failure is unusual, unless mean PAP > 50 mmHg.[111] It may be primary or secondary to such causes as pulmonary emboli, congenital cardiac disease with left to right shunts, mitral stenosis, morbid obesity and sickle cell anaemia.

Pathophysiology

Pulmonary hypertension results in:

1 right ventricular (RV) hypertrophy and dilatation with eventual RV failure. There is increased RV end-diastolic pressure with subsequent elevated central venous pressure (CVP).

2 pulmonary valve regurgitation

3 right atrial enlargement and tricuspid regurgitation

4 dyspnoea, haemoptysis and chest pain.

Further increases in pulmonary vascular resistance (PVR) result in increased RV failure and/or decreased venous return to the left ventricle with systemic hypotension. Cardiac output is low and fixed.

Acute rises in PAP can cause RV failure, bulging of the intraventricular septum with reduced LV filling and decreased LV output. This can lead to a vicious cycle of reduced coronary blood flow, further reduction in right and left ventricular function, bradycardia due to myocardial hypoxia and cardiac arrest.[112]

General Considerations

1 Factors which (in the presence of pulmonary hypertension) *increase* PVR must be avoided. These include:

   (a) N_2O

   (b) adrenaline, dopamine and other α adreno-receptor agonists

   (c) protamine, serotonin, thromboxane A_2 and prostaglandins such as PGF_2 alpha and PGE_2

   (d) hypoxia, hypercapnia

   (e) acidosis

   (f) positive end expiratory pressure and lung hyperinflation

   (g) cold, anxiety and stress

2 PVR, when elevated, can be *decreased* by:

   (a) hyperventilation to produce hypocapnia

   (b) correction of hypoxia

   (c) drugs such as nitric oxide, morphine, glyceryl trinitrate, sodium nitroprusside, tolazoline and inhaled or IV prostacycline (PGE_2). Also isoprenaline and other β adreno-receptor agonists, aminophylline and ganglion-blocking drugs.

3 To maintain cardiovascular stability:

   (a) Avoid marked decreases in venous return. This will cause

P

decreased RV filling, leading to decreased RV output. Correct fluid and blood loss rapidly.

(b) Avoid marked decreases in systemic vascular resistance. Cardiac output is restricted by a fixed RV output. If SVR falls the patient may not be able to maintain blood pressure by increasing cardiac output.

(c) Avoid drugs that cause myocardial depression.

(d) Maintain heart rate. Bradycardia may result in reduced cardiac output with hypotension and right ventricular failure.

4   These patients are at high risk of thrombo-embolic phenomenon and require pre- and post-operative anticoagulant therapy.

Specific Anaesthetic Management

1   *Monitoring*: Invasive arterial blood pressure and CVP monitoring will usually be required for anaesthetised patients with pulmonary hypertension. The use of pulmonary artery catheter monitoring is controversial due to the risk of pulmonary artery rupture, dysrhythmias and difficulty interpreting the data obtained, especially in the presence of anatomical shunts.[110] If a PA catheter is used, it may provide a useful warning of a sudden rise in PAP. If this occurs, attempt to reduce PAP and aim to decrease PVR more than SVR. This should lead to an increase in cardiac output.[112] Consider evaluating the effects of planned drug strategies prior to anaesthesia.

2   *Intra-operative exacerbation of pulmonary hypertension*: This may result in acute RV failure with progressive elevation in CVP, falling LV output and hypotension. In addition to strategies described above, different drugs have been used in various case reports, successfully reducing pulmonary artery pressure. These include:

(a) sodium nitroprusside[113]

(b) isoprenaline[114]

(c) isoflurane.[115] This may be the preferred inhalational anaesthetic drug in this condition.

(d) inhaled prostacycline 20 μg 4 h

(e) IV prostacycline 4 ng/kg/min[112]

Noradrenaline may be the most appropriate inotrope in this condition due to its ability to increase SVR without causing a tachycardia. PVR has been shown to decrease in animals given noradrenaline.[116]

Antibiotic prophylaxis for bacterial endocarditis is required for patients with associated heart valve or other structural abnormalities.

Obstetric Implications

Pulmonary hypertension and pregnancy is associated with a high incidence of death.[110] Women who have primary pulmonary hypertension and who deliver vaginally have a mortality rate of 50–60%.[110] Ideally, these patients require a multidisciplinary approach with early involvement of the cardiologist, haematologist, neonatologist, obstetrician and anaesthetist.

▶ Vaginal Delivery

1 Epidural blockade for labour can be used but must be carefully titrated with small increments of LA and opioids and carefully monitored, including invasive arterial and central venous blood pressure measurement.[117] Patients should receive continuous oxygen therapy. Use ephedrine for hypotension. Consider intrathecal morphine as an alternative to epidural anaesthesia for labour.

2 It is important to prevent pushing/Valsalva manoeuvre at the time of delivery. Forceps or vacuum extraction should be used.

3 Oxytocin used for induction and/or augmentation of labour was considered safe in the Smedstad et al. patient series.[118] However, syntocinon may cause an acute rise in PVR, leading to

reduced cardiac output, and some clinicians advise avoiding the drug or giving it very cautiously.[119,120]

▶ *Caesarean Section*

Regional anaesthesia can be used for Caesarean section and may be preferable to GA, but there is insufficient experience to recommend one technique over another.[110] If GA is selected or is mandatory, an opioid-based anaesthetic may be appropriate by providing cardiovascular stability.

Pulmonary Oedema

Simultaneously with resuscitation, identify the cause of pulmonary oedema and treat if possible. Causes of pulmonary oedema include:

1 fluid overload (e.g. IV fluids, glycine)
2 acute myocardial dysfunction
3 neurogenic pulmonary oedema
4 postobstruction pulmonary oedema (forced inspiration against a closed upper airway). See *NEGATIVE PRESSURE PULMONARY OEDEMA*.
5 increased pulmonary capillary permeability as occurs with adult respiratory distress syndrome.

Treatment Strategies

1 Ensure adequate airway. Intubate the patient if necessary.
2 Ensure adequate ventilation. Administer 100% O_2. Continuous positive airways pressure (CPAP), bi-level positive airway pressure (BiPAP), intermittent positive pressure ventilation (IPPV) ± positive end-expiratory pressure (PEEP) may be required depending on the severity of respiratory distress. These treatment modalities are of benefit by reducing the work of breathing and by decreasing left ventricular afterload due to

decreased transmural pressure as a consequence of increased positive intra-thoracic pressure.[121] Extravascular lung water is not decreased by these treatments.[122]

3   Ensure circulation is adequate. See *CARDIAC ARREST*. Reduce cardiac preload by sitting patient upright or reverse Trendelenburg.

4   Drug therapy includes:
   (a) frusemide 40–120 mg
   (b) morphine 2 mg increments at 2 min intervals to a total of 10 mg (relieves agitation and probably causes venodilation decreasing preload)
   (c) if the cause of pulmonary oedema is LV failure commence glyceryl trinitrate (GTN) infusion. See *CONGESTIVE CARDIAC FAILURE*. Consider sublingual nitroglycerine 600 μg while preparing the GTN infusion. GTN will reduce LV filling pressure, decreasing LV wall tension and O_2 consumption.

5   Consider inotropic support, e.g. dobutamine may be appropriate due to its effects on β adreno-receptors, causing reduced afterload and a greater effect on inotropy than chronotropy. See *DOBUTAMINE*.

6   Consider using a phosphodiesterase III inhibitor. See *AMRINONE* and *MILRINONE* entries.

7   Consider the use of a mechanical circulatory assist device such as an intra-aortic balloon pump. See *CONGESTIVE CARDIAC FAILURE*.

8   Establish invasive monitoring, i.e. arterial line, central venous line, and consider siting a pulmonary artery catheter.

9   Initial investigations include ECG, CXR, arterial blood gases. A transoesophageal echocardiogram may be readily available in some institutions and helpful in diagnosis. Obtain urgent cardiology consultation.

Pulmonary Valve and Subvalvular Stenosis

Pulmonary valve stenosis is considered severe if the pressure gradient across the pulmonary valve is > 50 mmHg with a normal cardiac output.[123] The stenosed valve eventually causes right atrial and right ventricular (RV) hypertrophy. RV output is maintained until the pressure gradient across the valve exceeds about 80 mmHg. The RV will begin to fail and RV output decreases. This decreases LV preload and thus cardiac output, leading to fatigue, syncopy and angina. SVR increases in an attempt to compensate for low cardiac output. LV stroke volume is low and fixed and dependent on HR.

Secondary infundibular hypertrophy can occur with dynamic right ventricular outflow obstruction as occurs in hypertrophic obstructive cardiomyopathy.[124]

Management Aims

1 Avoid factors that increase right ventricular O_2 requirements such as tachycardia and increased myocardial contractility.
2 Avoid factors decreasing right ventricular O_2 supply, such as hypotension. Treat hypotension promptly with a vasoconstrictor.
3 Venous return must be maintained. Restore fluid and blood loss promptly.
4 Avoid marked decreases in systemic vascular resistance.
5 Marked increases in RV filling pressure are not well-tolerated. Do not overfill the patient's intravascular space.
6 Avoid bradycardia and drugs that decrease myocardial contractility.
7 Consider balloon valvuloplasty of the stenosed pulmonic valve pre-operatively.
8 Provide antibiotic prophylaxis for bacterial endocarditis. See *BACTERIAL ENDOCARDITIS PROPHYLAXIS*.

Anaesthesia and Pulmonary Valve Stenosis

Asymptomatic patients without decompensation tolerate anaesthesia well. In decompensated patients the following is required:

1 Invasive monitoring (arterial blood pressure and CVP). CVP prior to anaesthesia will indicate the patient's usual RV filling pressure. Maintain this filling pressure throughout the perioperative period.

2 Maintain systemic vascular resistance, preload, contractility and a reasonable heart rate (90–110 bpm).[117]

Obstetrics and Pulmonary Valve Stenosis

▶ *Vaginal Delivery*

In decompensated patients, epidural anaesthesia must be provided with extreme caution. Invasive monitoring is required to maintain a 'normal' CVP for the particular patient. Consider intrathecal morphine or other opioid as a possible alternative to epidural blockade. Ransom and Leicht reported on the management of a pregnant patient with severe pulmonary stenosis for labour and delivery. They used an intrathecal sufentanil infusion with LD 10 µg, then an infusion of 5 µg/h as effective for labour pain, supplemented by 1.5mL of 1% lignocaine at the time of delivery.[124]

▶ *Caesarean Section*

There is little information from the literature to guide management. Mangano recommends GA following the principles outlined above.[117]

P

Rr

Raised Intracranial Pressure

See *INTRACRANIAL PRESSURE (ICP) AND TREATMENT OF RAISED ICP.*

Rapid Infusion Catheter Exchanger Set

Used to obtain large bore peripheral IV access. The set contains either a 7 Fr 5 cm catheter or an 8.5 Fr 6.4 cm catheter with a dilator, a 0.64 mm diameter spring-wire guide and a scalpel.

Technique

1   Asepticaly insert a cannula (at least a 20 G) into a suitable large peripheral vein. Anaesthetise the insertion site if the patient is awake.

2   Release the tourniquet and insert the guide wire through the cannula, then remove the cannula.

3   At the site of wire entry, use the scalpel to incise the skin sufficiently to enable the dilator and catheter to pass easily into the vein.

4   Insert the catheter with dilator using a twisting motion. When the catheter is in place, remove the dilator and the guide wire. *Never lose visual contact with wire.*

5   Suture the catheter to the skin.

Rapid Sequence Induction (RSI)

This is a technique for the induction of anaesthesia designed to reduce the possibility of aspiration prior to intubation. A skilled assistant is mandatory for this technique.

The steps are:

1 Check the anaesthetic machine and breathing circuit, and ensure suction is available and within easy reach. Ensure aids to intubation are within easy reach, such as a Teflon introducer.

2 Always have a prepared plan if intubation fails. See *DIFFICULT AIRWAY MANAGEMENT*.

3 Have all the required anaesthetic and emergency drugs drawn up. Decide on drug dosages *before* the anaesthetic begins.

4 Attach all appropriate monitoring to the patient and position the patient for intubation (head extended on a firm pillow, neck flexed).

5 Preoxygenate the patient for at least 5 min.

6 Induce anaesthesia with thiopentone 3–5 mg/kg IV, followed immediately by suxamethonium 1.5 mg/kg. Ask the patient to keep his/her eyes open. Cricoid pressure is applied by the assistant as the patient begins to lose consciousness (eyes begin to close). Cricoid pressure involves the assistant pressing on the cricoid cartilage with the thumb and index finger. To identify the cricoid cartilage see *CRICOTHYROID PUNCTURE AND CRICOTHYROTOMY*. The force of cricoid pressure should be about 30 N.[1]

7 If a nasogastric tube is in situ, it should be left in place. This is because the nasogastric (NG) tube increases the efficiency of cricoid pressure and allows 'venting' of gastric gases and fluids.[1] Remember to apply suction to the NG tube prior to performing RSI to empty the stomach.

8 The patient will be paralysed after fasciculations occur or in 50–60 s if no fasciculations are seen.

9 If suxamethonium is contraindicated use rocuronium 0.6–0.9 mg/kg. Good intubating conditions will be provided by rocuronium in 60 s but this drug is not the equal of suxamethonium for reliability of intubating conditions.

R

10 Intubate the trachea. Cricoid pressure is removed when the intubation is confirmed by end tidal CO_2 monitoring, the tracheal tube cuff is inflated and when the assistant is instructed to by the anaesthetist.

Recombinant Activated Factor VII

Also referred to as Activated Factor VII, NovoSeven, eptacog alfa (activated) and rFVIIa.

Description and Indications

rFVIIa is manufactured from baby hamster kidney cells, which express cloned human factor VII. First used in patients in 1988, this drug is useful for the prevention or control of bleeding during surgery or trauma in haemophiliac patients with inhibitors to factors VIII or IX. It has since been used to successfully treat non-haemophiliacs with massive haemorrhage from various causes (trauma, surgical, DIC, sepsis), unresponsive to all other available coagulation factors. This drug represents a major breakthrough in the management of blood loss as a universal haemostatic agent.

Mechanism of Action

rFVIIa enhances the process of haemostasis at the site of bleeding without systemic activation of coagulation.[2] This is because rFVIIa requires tissue factor (TF) to become active. TF is exposed at the site of injury and the TF-rFVIIa combination activates the coagulation cascade on activated platelet membranes adhering to the site of injury.

Efficacy of rFVIIa

rFVIIa has been typically used in situations where there is:
1 severe blood loss
2 transfusion of blood, platelets, FFP, cryoprecipitate and other clotting factors

R

3 coagulopathy (often dilutional) that may or may not correct with the above treatment

4 ongoing life threatening haemorrhage.

In reports from the literature, administration of rFVIIa produces a dramatic and life-saving resolution of the bleeding problem. A typical example of the efficacy of rFVIIa is reported by Svartholm et al.[3] A 50-year-old female with necrotising pancreatitis continued to bleed after 27 L of packed cells, 4.5 L of FFP, platelets, prothrombin complex concentrate, desmopressin, antithrombin III, fibrinogen, tranexamic acid and aprotinin. A dose of 120 µg/kg rFVIIa was given and repeated 5 h later, with bleeding decreasing after the first dose and ceasing after the second dose.

Dose for Acute Bleeding

1 35–120 µg/kg IV every 2–3 h until control is achieved. Give 35–120 µg/kg every 3–12 h if continued treatment is needed.

2 rFVIIa is presented in vials of 1.2–4.8 mg and a diluent (sterile water) is provided. Give by IV bolus over 2–5 min.

Dose for Surgical Prophylaxis

35–120 µg/kg IV every 2–3 h for 1–2 days, then every 2–6 h if ongoing treatment is required.

Advantages

1 rFVIIa appears to have an excellent safety profile in both therapeutic dosages and overdose. The rate of fatal thrombo-embolic complications is low (0.07% in one report of 5522 patients).[2]

2 There is no infection risk.

3 Drug volume is not an issue compared with potentially large fluid loads with platelets, FFP and other clotting factors.

4 The drug can be given rapidly.

5 rFVIIa may improve platelet function.[4]

Disadvantages

1 rVIIa is extremely expensive.

2 There are rare reports of anaphylactoid reactions. rFVIIa is contraindicated in patients with hypersensitivity to mouse, hamster or bovine proteins.

Red Cells

(Based on the *Australian Red Cross Circular of Information 2003*, with permission.) 'Red cells' (or 'packed cells') means the red cell component of a unit of whole blood when most of the plasma has been removed. Packed cells for transfusion have the following characteristics.

Storage

Packed cells are stored at 2–6°C for up to 42 days. If removed from refrigeration, the blood should be returned to refrigeration or transfusion begun within 30 minutes. Once the packed-cell container has been opened, the contents are considered expired in 4 h.

Contents

Depending on the manufacturer, packed cells contain varying amounts of glucose, mannitol, adenine, sodium chloride, sodium citrate and phosphate. The volume of a unit of red cells is > 240 mL and the haematocrit is 0.5–0.75. Haemolysis at expiry is less than 0.8%. As stored blood ages, the electrolyte and pH values change. See Table R1.

2, 3 diphosphoglycerate, which is one of the regulators of oxygen unloading from haemoglobin, is almost completely dissipated after 3 weeks of storage.[5] However, levels regenerate quickly after transfusion.

Red Cells with Buffy Coat Removed

These are suspended red cells after centrifuging whole blood and removing plasma and the 'buffy coat layer', which contains platelets

Table R1 Physiochemical properties of stored blood[5]		
Physiochemical property	2 weeks' storage	5 weeks' storage
pH	7.2	6.6
Sodium (mmol/L)	168	156
Potassium (mmol/L)	30	48

and white cells. Indications for this type of blood are the same as for leukocyte depleted whole blood. See *WHOLE BLOOD*. This technique is less effective than leukodepletion filters.

Red Cells Leukocyte Depleted

Blood is centrifuged, plasma is removed, and white cells are removed by a filter. Indications are the same as for leukocyte-depleted whole blood. See *WHOLE BLOOD*.

Red Cells Washed

Red cells are washed with normal saline to remove plasma proteins, antibodies and electrolytes. Red cells washed are indicated for patients with IgA deficiency with anti-IgA antibodies. Such patients may suffer allergic transfusion reactions, including anaphylaxis, after multiple transfusions of non-washed red cells.

Risks of Red Cell Transfusion

(See also *BLOOD TRANSFUSION, Massive Blood Transfusion Management*.)

These can be divided into acute and longer term risks.

▶ *Acute Risks*

1 Acute haemolytic reactions due to such causes as ABO incompatability or antibodies to more minor red cell antigens.

2 Allergic reactions.

R

3 Acute sepsis due to bacterial contamination.
4 Transfusion-related acute lung injury.

▶ *Longer Term Risks*

1 Infections—these may be bacterial, parasitic or viral. The risk of HIV infection in Canada from a unit of transfused blood is about 1 per million and for hep C is about 1 per 100 000.[6]
2 Transfusion-associated graft versus host disease.
3 Immunosuppressive effects.

Reflexes

Table R2 Limb reflex nerve roots	
Reflex	Nerve roots involved
Plantar	S1
Ankle	S1, 2
Knee	L3, 4
Biceps	C5, 6
Triceps	C7, 8

R

Remifentanil

This 4 anilidopiperidine is a selective mu receptor agonist opioid drug with extremely fast onset and offset times and a similar potency to fentanyl. Remifentanil is a derivative of fentanyl with an ester linkage that is rapidly metabolised by non-specific plasma esterases, resulting in a context-sensitive half-life of $\approx$ 3 min.[7]

Dose During Induction of Anaesthesia

Run a remifentanil infusion at 0.75–1 µg/kg/min together with a sleep dose of propofol or thiopentone. Remifentanil can be used to attenuate or block the cardiovascular response to intubation.[8] However, remifentanil can also cause severe bradycardia and hypotension in some patients.[9]

Dose During Maintenance of Anaesthesia

After intubation, run the remifentanil infusion at a rate of 0.25–0.5 µg/kg/min. This rate can be increased for periods of extreme stimulation, such as rigid bronchoscopy, to a maximum of 2 µg/kg/min.

Remifentanil and Patient-controlled Analgesia

See *PATIENT-CONTROLLED ANALGESIA (PCA) AND PATIENT-CONTROLLED EPIDURAL ANAESTHESIA (PCEA).*

▶ *Advantages*

1 MAC of volatile agents and the effective anaesthetic infusion dose of propofol are reduced by 50–75% in the presence of a remifentanil infusion.

2 Clearance of remifentanil is independent of renal/hepatic function.

3 Rapidly titratable to desired clinical effect, providing excellent cardiovascular stability.

▶ *Disadvantages*

1 Formulated in glycine, an inhibitory neurotransmitter. *Remifentanil is not recommended for spinal or epidural administration.*[7]

2 The offset of remifentanil is so rapid that patients will be without analgesia within about 10 min of infusion cessation (unless regional anaesthesia or longer-acting opioids are utilised). Similarly, if the infusion of remifentanil stops unintentionally intra-operatively all opioid effects will rapidly disappear.

R

3 Postoperative analgesia should be commenced well before the remifentanil infusion is stopped.

4 Blood pressure is reduced by 15–20% and a mild bradycardia is usual. Severe cardiovascular depression may occur in some patients.

5 When remifentanil is used for sedation there is a higher incidence of nausea and respiratory depression than with propofol.[10]

Renal Protection

See *ABDOMINAL AORTIC ANEURYSM REPAIR*.

Renal Transplant Surgery

Pre-operative Phase

1 Ensure the patient has received pre-operative immunosuppressive therapy including prednisone 20 mg PO, cyclosporin and azothioprine.

2 Pre-operative dialysis is usually provided. Dialysis to within 0.5 kg of ideal body weight is desirable.[11] Aim for $K^+ < 6$ mmol/L and pH > 7.25. Treat pH < 7.25 preferably with dialysis; otherwise give 50 mmol of sodium bicarbonate. For treatment of hyperkalaemia see *POTASSIUM*.

3 Ensure arterio-venous fistulas are identified and protected with soft padding and kept warm. Place IV cannulas and blood pressure cuff on the other limb. Palpate the fistula at intervals to check patency.

4 Obtain large bore peripheral IV access. *Do not use the cephalic vein if possible* (see *VEINS OF THE UPPER LIMB*). Central venous access is essential, but this can be obtained after induction. Invasive arterial blood pressure monitoring is not required unless indicated by the patient's co-morbid conditions.

5 Give antibiotic cover prior to surgery using a broad spectrum antibiotic, e.g. cephazolin 1 g.

Intra-operative Phase

1   Consider a rapid sequence induction if delayed gastric emptying is suspected. Do not use suxamethonium in the presence of hyperkalaemia. Propofol or thiopentone can be used for induction. The most appropriate muscle relaxant is cisatracurium, although a single dose of rocuronium can be given. Maintain anaesthesia with O_2, N_2O and isoflurane. Sevoflurane should probably not be used, at least on theoretical grounds. See *SEVOFLURANE*.

2   Monitor temperature and keep the patient normothermic.

3   Fentanyl at normal doses is the opioid of choice. Pethidine and morphine are unsuitable due the accumulation of active metabolites (norpethidine and morphine-6-glucuronide).

4   Keep patients reasonably well-filled intravascularly. This may require large volumes of fluid (60–100 mL/kg).[11] The target CVP is around 10–12 mmHg.[11]

5   If hypotension occurs during surgery discuss the management with the surgeon, but in general treat with intravascular volume expansion. If volume expansion is ineffective give a vasopressor. Consider inotropic support with dobutamine or dopexamine if hypotension persists.[11]

6   The surgeon may request drugs to optimise renal graft perfusion, such as mannitol 20–50 g ± frusemide 80 mg IV. Dopamine may also be considered (200 mg in 100 mL 5% glucose) although there is little evidence of efficacy.[11] Start the dopamine infusion at 5 mL/h.

7   Prior to arterial unclamping of the graft kidney, aim for a central venous pressure of ≈ 10–12 mmHg.[11] Optimal intravascular fluid volume is essential for graft survival. N/S is the crystalloid of choice (no potassium or lactate).[12]

8   If a blood transfusion is required use a Sepacell leucocyte reduction filter.

R

Postoperative Phase

Use fentanyl IV via a PCA infusion pump for postoperative analgesia. Do not use morphine or pethidine due to the possible accumulation of harmful metabolites.[12]

Respiratory Function Tests

The most useful tests of respiratory function are:

1 *exercise tolerance*
2 *spirometry*. The most useful measurements are:
   (a) *FEV_1*, forced expiratory volume in the first second. An FEV_1 of < 1 L or < 30% predicted is indicative of severe disease. A $\geq$ 10–15% increase in FEV_1 after a bronchodilator such as ventolin indicates a significant response to that drug.[13]
   (b) *FVC*, forced vital capacity
   (c) *ratio of FEV_1 to FVC*. This ratio should normally be greater than 80% of predicted. A ratio < 70% is indicative of *obstructive* lung disease, e.g. asthma, chronic bronchitis and emphysema. 60–70% ratio indicates mild disease, while a ratio of < 50% indicates severe disease. An FEV_1:FVC ratio of > 70%, with a FVC < 80% of predicted, is indicative of *restrictive* lung disease, as occurs with fibrosing alveolitis and chest wall abnormalities.
   (d) *vital capacity*. A vital capacity < 50% predicted or < 2 L indicates increased risk of pulmonary complications.
   (e) *arterial blood gases*. A PaO_2 < 60 mmHg and/or a $PaCO_2$ > 50 mmHg indicates respiratory failure.
   (f) *carbon monoxide (CO) diffusion capacity*. This test measures the transfer of CO into the blood from the lungs (DLCO). The result is given as a percentage of predicted normal. CO transfer is reduced in patients with alveolar disease and pulmonary vascular obstruction such as pulmonary emboli. CO transfer is increased in such conditions as pulmonary

haemorrhage and congestive cardiac failure. A DLCO < 50% predicted is indicative of increased anaesthetic risk.

(g) *measurement of TLC, RV and VC*

(h) *maximum breathing capacity (MBC)*. MBC normally > 100 L/min. If MBC < 50% predicted or less than 50 L/min, there is an increased anaesthetic risk for major surgery.

(i) *flow volume dynamics*. A discussion of this area is beyond the scope of this manual.

Respiratory Factors Predicting Increased Risk for Abdominal Surgery[14]

1 FEV_1 and FVC < 70% predicted.
2 FEV_1/FVC < 65% predicted.
3 MBC and DLCO < 50% predicted.

Respiratory Factors Predicting Increased Risk for Pulmonary Lobectomy[15]

1 FEV_1 < 1 L or < 40–50% of predicted.
2 MBC < 40–70 L/min or < 40% of predicted.

Lung Function Tests Indicating Increased Operative Risk for Pneumonectomy[15]

1 Postoperative predicted FEV_1 < 0.85 L or pre-operative FEV_1 < 2 L ± FEV_1 < 50% of FVC.
2 MBC < 70 L/min or < 55% of predicted.
3 Hypercapnia on room air ($PaCO_2$ > 45 mmHg).
4 Temporary pulmonary occlusion of pulmonary artery on the planned operative side (with PA catheter) can be considered. Increased risk exists if $PaCO_2$ > 60 mmHg, PaO_2 < 40 mmHg or pulmonary artery pressure rises to greater than 40 mmHg.

R

Resuscitation of the Newborn

See *NEONATAL RESUSCITATION*.

Retained Placenta

See *UTERINE RELAXATION FOR RETAINED PLACENTA*.

Retinal Detachment Surgery

During retinal repair surgery the surgeon may inject sulphur hexafluoride (SF_6) intravitreally. If N_2O is being used as part of the anaesthetic, it should be discontinued 15–20 min before injection of gas. This is because the N_2O can diffuse into the gas bubble and greatly increase intra-ocular pressure. N_2O should not be used in subsequent anaesthetics while the intravitreal gas is present.

Retrograde Intubation

Several retrograde intubation kits are available. A basic technique for retrograde intubation, and variations of this technique, are described below:

1 Puncture the cricothyroid membrane with a cannula or needle suitable for insertion of a guide wire or epidural catheter. If an epidural catheter is used it is easier to pass an 18 G cannula through the cricothyroid membrane than a Tuohy needle.[16]

2 The wire or catheter is then retrieved from the oropharynx. If there is a large amount of fluid in the oropharynx (e.g. blood or secretions) air can be injected through the epidural catheter (if this is used), creating bubbles, thus making the tip easier to find.[17]

3 The endotracheal tube is placed over the guide wire/catheter and while both ends are held taut, the ET tube is passed into the laryngeal inlet. Tension on the wire/catheter is then relaxed, enabling the ET tube to be passed into the trachea.

4 Once the trachea has been intubated the wire/catheter is removed through the mouth.

Variations of the Above Retrograde Intubation Technique

▶ Variation 1

The ET tube is passed over the wire/catheter until it is positioned just below the cords at the level of the cricothyroid membrane. A Teflon bougie is then passed through the ET tube into the trachea. The wire/catheter is removed and the ET tube then railroaded over the bougie into the trachea.

▶ Variation 2

Tie a strong silk suture to the proximal end of the catheter and pull this through the cricothyroid membrane and out through the mouth. The suture is then tied to the Murphey eye of the ET tube, which is pulled into the laryngeal inlet by the suture. The trachea is intubated and the suture left in place. When the patient is extubated the tube can be pulled back into the trachea if re-intubation is required.

Rocuronium

Quaternary aminosteroid non-depolarising neuromuscular blocking drug (analogue of vecuronium).

Dose

0.6 mg/kg IV. Rocuronium has a duration of action of 30–40 min. Maintenance bolus doses of 0.15 mg/kg can be given.

Infusion dose: 3–5 µg/kg/min can be given, titrated to the measured twitch response.

Rapid Reversal of Rocuronium

Org 25969 is a drug currently under investigation and has been shown to bind to rocuronium and completely reverse its effects. This drug may enable rocuronium to be used as an ultra-short-acting, non-depolarising neuromuscular blocking drug. Org 25969 may also enable the rapid reversal of rocuronium in situations where this may be desirable, e.g. failed intubation, partially paralysed patients in recovery.[18]

Advantages

1 Rapid onset of action with adequate intubating conditions achieved in 60 s.
2 Minimal cardiovascular side effects. Rocuronium can cause some increase in heart rate.[19] It does not cause histamine release.
3 Suitable for use by continuous infusion.
4 Presented as a ready-to-use solution, unlike vecuronium which is presented as a powder.

Disadvantages

1 Rocuronium is cleared principally by uptake in the liver and secretion in the bile.[20] A small proportion is excreted in the urine. Effects of rocuronium may be prolonged in the presence of hepatic disease and, to a lesser extent, renal disease.[20]
2 Intubating conditions are often not ideal after 60 s; this drug is therefore less reliable than suxamethonium for this purpose.[21]
3 Rocuronium precipitates with thiopentone. This can result in the blockage of IV catheters and bronchospasm.[22] Flush thiopentone from the IV line before giving rocuronium.
4 Requires refrigeration (storage at 2–8°C). If removed from the refrigerator, the rocuronium ampoule should be discarded within 12 weeks.
5 Allergic reactions to rocuronium may be more common than with some other currently used NDNMBDs such as vecuronium.[22,23]

Rofecoxib

COX2 selective NSAID useful for the treatment of acute pain, osteoarthritis and rheumatoid arthritis. The dose in adults is

12.5–25 mg once daily PO. See *NON-STEROIDAL ANTI-INFLAMMA-TORY DRUGS*.

Ropivacaine

Aminoamide local anaesthetic drug. Pure s-enantiomer. Useful for all types of local and regional anaesthetic techniques, except for Bier block.

Dose

Adult: For local or field analgesia 200 mg is the maximum recommended dose, although 250 mg has been used without adverse effect. 200 mg has been given IV accidentally, producing convulsion but no cardiotoxicity.[24]

Lumbar epidural use (adult): 15–25 mL of 0.75% solution for surgical anaesthesia. For postoperative analgesia an infusion of 0.2% can be run at 6–14 mL/h.

Thoracic epidural use (adult): Use 5–15 mL of 0.5% mg/mL solution to establish the block, then an infusion of 4–8 mL/h of 0.2% solution for postoperative analgesia. See *EPIDURAL ANAESTHESIA*.

Subarachnoid block: Use a 0.5% solution. For example, 3.5 mL of 0.5% ropivacaine is effective for hip arthroplasty.[25]

Advantages

1 Less cardiotoxic than bupivacaine.
2 When ropivacaine is used epidurally there is less motor block but similar sensory block compared to bupivacaine, with a faster recovery from motor block.[26]
3 Some vasoconstrictor properties. The addition of adrenaline does prolong the duration of cutaneous analgesia but not the duration of peripheral nerve block.[24]
4 Ropivacaine produces a longer duration of cutaneous block than bupivacaine.[24] For epidural blockade the duration of sensory block is similar for the two drugs. The duration of

R

peripheral nerve block is shorter with ropivacaine than bupivacaine at equal concentrations.[24]

Disadvantages

1 Ropivacaine is more cardiotoxic than lignocaine. Cardiac arrest due to IV ropivacaine with successful resuscitation has been described in several reports.[27,28] In two cases there was progressive bradycardia, hypotension and asystole.

2 Ropivacaine has similar central nervous system toxicity to bupivacaine.

3 Ropivacaine is about 25% less potent than bupivacaine. 7.5 mg/mL ropivacaine is comparable to 6 mg/mL bupivacaine.

4 The vasoconstrictive properties of ropivacaine may potentially result in end organ ischaemia. For example, the use of ropivacaine for penile block has resulted in a report of transitory ischaemia of the penile tip. See *PENILE BLOCK*.

5 Ropivacaine is contraindicated for IV regional anaesthetic technique (Bier block).

R

Ss

'Saddle' Block

See *SUBARACHNOID BLOCK (SAB)*.

Salbutamol

Synthetic sympathomimetic drug used for the treatment of bronchoconstriction and premature labour. Acts by stimulating β2 and, to a lesser extent, β1 adreno-receptors.

Dose for Bronchospasm

▶ *Adult*

Puffer: 200–400 μg inhaled 6–8 h.

Nebuliser: 2.5–5 mg 4 h or more frequently up to every 20 min, depending on the severity of the bronchospasm.

IV: 5 μg/kg bolus over 10 min, then infusion 5–20 μg/min. Mix 15 mg salbutamol with 250 mL N/S. 10 mL/h of this solution = 10 μg/min.

▶ *Child*[1]

Puffer: 100–200 μg 4–6 h.

Nebuliser: 0.03 mL/kg of 0.5% solution of salbutamol 4 h or more frequently, depending on the severity of the bronchospasm.

Alternatively (using 0.5% solution):

Child < 3 years	0.3 mL
Child 3–6 years	0.4 mL
Child 6–12 years	0.5 mL.

Make the volume up to 4 mL with N/S prior to nebulisation.

IV: 5 μg/kg over 10 min, then infusion 1–5 μg/kg/min.

Dose for Uterine Relaxation to Halt Premature Labour

Load 25 mg of salbutamol in 1 L Hartmann's solution and infuse 60–100 mL over 10–20 min.[2] Run the infusion at up to 50 µg/min, although tachycardia usually prevents the infusion rate being safely increased above 20 µg/min. As a general guideline, slow the infusion rate when the maternal pulse rate reaches 120/min, and cease if the pulse rate reaches 140/min.[2]

Potential Side Effects

IV salbutamol therapy can cause:

1 anxiety and tremor
2 widening of pulse pressure, tachycardia and hypotension
3 hyperglycaemia and hypokalaemia
4 pulmonary oedema with prolonged use of salbutamol over days
5 hyperinsulinaemia and hypoglycaemia in the foetus.

Sander's Injector

See *TRANSTRACHEAL JET VENTILATION*.

Saphenous Nerve Block

Anatomy

The *saphenous nerve* is the cutaneous branch of the posterior division of the *femoral nerve* and supplies sensation to the medial side of the leg and foot.

Nerve Stimulator Technique[3]

1 Palpate the point 3.5 cm posterior to the centre of the bony prominence of the medial femoral condyle.
2 Sterilise and anaesthetise the skin at this point. Insert a 5 cm 22 G insulated block needle. Attach a nerve stimulator and set

the stimulating current at 2 mA. Attempt to elicit paraesthesia over the medial malleolus.

3   Reduce the stimulation current and adjust the needle position to maintain paraesthesia, the end-point of nerve localisation being paraesthesia persisting at 0.4 mA. The depth of needle insertion on average is 2.8 cm.

4   Inject 10 mL of LA agent, e.g. lignocaine 2% with adrenaline.

Loss of Resistance (LOR) Technique[3]

1   Identify the sartorius muscle on the medial side of the femur.

2   After sterilising and anaesthetising the skin just above the knee joint insert a 20 G Tuohy needle attached to a 10 mL syringe suitable for a LOR technique. Insert the needle until LOR occurs (identifying the subsartorial fat pad).

3   Inject LA, e.g. 10 mL of lignocaine 2% with adrenaline. There is a 20% failure rate with this technique.

Scalp Block

The posterior scalp is innervated by the:

1   *greater occipital nerve* (C2, 3): supplies the skin over the occiput to the vertex

2   *lesser occipital nerve* (C2): supplies the occipital area immediately above and behind the mastoid, and the skin over the mastoid process. It is derived from the cervical plexus.

3   *third occipital nerve* (C3): supplies the skin of the lower occiput.

The anterior scalp is innervated by the *supra-orbital* and *supra-trochlear nerves*. These are branches of the frontal nerve (in turn a branch of the *ophthalmic division of the V cranial nerve*). There are also contributions from:

(a)   *zygomaticotemporal nerves* (V2)

(b)   *auriculotemporal nerves* (V3)

(c)   *greater auricular nerves* (C2, 3).

S

Technique for Scalp Block[4]

1 Position the patient sitting with the head flexed. Identify the nuchal ridge on the posterior scalp.
2 Identify the point (X) over the occipital protuberance 2.5 cm lateral from the midline.
3 Sterilise the skin and insert a 23 G needle at point X to contact bone. Inject a ridge of 3 mL of LA to anaesthetise the *greater occipital nerve*.
4 To anaesthetise the *lesser occipital nerve*, angle the needle anteriorly and laterally along the back of the skull. Inject subcutaneous anaesthesia from this point to the mastoid process. Use about 8 mL of LA.
5 To anaesthetise the entire scalp, perform the block bilaterally and extend a subcutaneous wheal around the entire scalp circumference. Inject subcutaneously above the ears and continue anteriorly at the same level.

See *FOREHEAD BLOCK*.

Scalp Capillary pH Measurement in the Foetus

Foetal scalp capillary blood pH can help in the diagnosis of foetal hypoxia and acidosis. A pH of < 7.2 may indicate the need for urgent delivery.[5]

Table S1 Foetal scalp pH and significance

pH value	Significance
≥ 7.25	Normal
7.20–7.24	Pre-acidotic
< 7.20	Acidotic

Sciatic Nerve Block

This block is useful for surgery on the foot and lower leg but note that the medial side of the leg, ankle and foot will not be anaesthetised. These areas are supplied by the *saphenous* branch of the *femoral nerve*.

Anatomy

The *sciatic nerve* is formed from the following sacral plexus nerve roots: L4, 5, S1, 2 and 3. The sciatic nerve leaves the pelvis via the greater sciatic foramen and descends beneath the gluteus maximus between the greater trochanter and the ischial tuberosity to enter the thigh behind the adductor magnus. The nerve travels along the postero-medial aspect of the femur and divides at the apex of the popliteal fossa into the *tibial nerve* and *common peroneal nerve*. See *POPLITEAL FOSSA BLOCK*.

▶ Supplies

Motor to the hamstring muscles and all the muscles of the leg and foot. *Sensory*: All the leg and foot below the knee except for the medial side of the leg, over the medial malleolus and posterior thigh.

Techniques of Sciatic Nerve Block

There are many approaches to the sciatic nerve. Four techniques will be described.

▶ Anterior Approach

1 Position the patient supine and identify the anterior superior iliac spine (ASIS) and the pubic tubercle. Draw a line between these two landmarks.

2 Draw a second line parallel to the first, extending from the greater trochanter in a medial caudad direction.

3 At the junction of the medial third and lateral two-thirds of the first line, draw a perpendicular which intersects the second line. This is the entry point.

S

4   Sterilise (and, if the patient is awake, anaesthetise) the skin and insert a 12.5 mm 23 G insulated needle attached to a nerve stimulator.

5   When the lesser trochanter of the femur is contacted walk off the medial border. The nerve will be located ≈ 2.5 cm deeper than this point. Start with a stimulating current of 3 mA at 2 Hz. Reduce the current to 0.2–0.6 mA when the nerve is located (preferably ankle movement is seen).

6   Inject 20 mL of 0.5% bupivacaine (or 30 mL of bupivacaine 0.25% or 30 mL of ropivacaine 5 mg/mL).

▶ Posterior Approach[6]

1   Position the patient in the lateral position with leg to be blocked uppermost and flexed at the hip and knee (Sim's position).

2   Identify the greater trochanter and the posterior superior iliac spine (PSIS) and draw a line between these two landmarks.

3   Draw a second line from the sacral hiatus to the greater trochanter. Drop a perpendicular from the midpoint of the first line and draw an X where it crosses the second line. This is the entry point. Prepare skin as above.

4   The X should overlie the U-shaped sciatic notch at its superior and lateral border. Insert a 10 cm 23 G insulated needle until paraesthesia, a motor response or bone is encountered (usually the lateral border of the notch).

5   Withdraw and advance more medially. The nerve will lie just a little deeper than the bone.

6   Note that the nerve emerges from the upper medial border of the notch, then curves down to lie equidistant from the ischial tuberosity and the greater trochanter; this may help identify the position of the nerve.

7   Inject 20–30 mL of bupivacaine 0.5%.

S

▶ *Lithotomy Approach*

This is a very simple and reliable approach.

1 Position the patient supine, with the leg to be blocked flexed at the hip.
2 Identify the greater trochanter and ischial tuberosity, and the midpoint between these two landmarks. This is the entry point.
3 Insert a 10 cm insulated 23 G needle attached to a nerve stimulator. Start with 4 mA at 2 Hz. Elicit movement in the foot, which should persist when the current is reduced to 0.3 mA.
4 Inject LA, 30 mL of bupivacaine 0.5% or 30 mL of ropivacaine 5 mg/mL.

Lateral Approach

1 Identify the point 2 cm below and 2 cm posterior to the greater trochanter. Prepare the skin as above.
2 Insert a 10 cm 23 G insulated needle attached to a nerve stimulator, contact the femur, then reinsert so that needle passes just behind the femur.
3 When the sciatic nerve is contacted, inject LA as described above.

Sciatic Nerve Sheath Catheter

This is a technique for postoperative analgesia in which the surgeon inserts a catheter into the sciatic nerve sheath during surgery for an above knee amputation. The nerve block is established with 20 mL of bupivacaine 0.25% or ropivacaine 10 mg/mL. This is followed by an infusion of bupivacaine 0.25% run at 10 mL/h.

S

Seizures

See *EPILEPSY, STATUS*.

Serotonin Syndrome

This syndrome is due to excessive serotonin in the central nervous system. It is usually due to an overdose of a single drug or interaction between two different types of drug, e.g. tramadol and sertraline. Examples include:

1 selective serotonin reuptake inhibitors such as sertraline, fluoxetine, paroxetine, venlafaxine
2 monoamine oxidase inhibitors, e.g. moclobemide
3 tramadol
4 prochlorperazine
5 St John's wort.

Symptoms and Signs

1 Mental state changes such as confusion, hypomania, agitation.
2 Motor disturbance such as incoordination.
3 Hyperreflexia.
4 Diaphoresis, tremor, diarrhoea and fever.

Treatment

1 This condition is usually self-limiting (under 24 h) once the causative drugs are ceased, but fatalities have occurred.
2 5-HT antagonists such as methysergide have been used.

Sevoflurane

Volatile inhalational halogenated ether-type anaesthetic agent.

Physical properties and MAC

Blood:gas solubility coefficient	0.69
Oil:gas solubility coefficient	48
Saturated vapour pressure (20°C)	160 mmHg (21.3 kPa)
Boiling point	58.6°C
MAC	2.05%

Advantages

1 The absence of pungency coupled with low blood solubility makes sevoflurane the agent of choice for inhalational induction.

2 Low blood:gas solubility results in sevoflurane providing rapid induction of anaesthesia, and rapid emergence.

3 Cerebralautoregulation is preserved up to an inspired concentration of 1.5 MAC.[7]

4 Sevoflurane causes bronchodilation. Desflurane causes an increase in airway resistance.[8]

5 Ozone-friendly agent.

Disadvantages

1 Concerns have been raised about potential renal toxicity with sevoflurane. About 5% of sevoflurane is metabolised, causing elevation of serum fluoride levels which are known to be nephrotoxic from experience with methoxyflurane. (See *METHOXYFLURANE.*) However, unlike methoxyflurane, sevoflurane does not cause fluoride-induced renal nephropathy.[9] The reason for this is thought to be that sevoflurane does not induce intrarenal F⁻ (through intrarenal metabolism of sevoflurane) as does methoxyflurane.[10]

2 Sevoflurane is degraded by CO_2 absorbers to produce several compounds including compound A, which is toxic to kidney tissue. Compound A production is increased by high sevoflurane concentrations, low gas-flow rates, high soda lime temperature and the use of barium lime.[9] However, there is no evidence of renal injury in humans due to compound A.[9] It is recommended that in the presence of soda lime fresh gas-flow rates should be not less than 2 L/min,[7] and use with barium lime (Baralyme) is contraindicated. In summary therefore, there is no clinical evidence of renal toxicity due to sevoflurane in humans. However, in the United States the FDA and several researchers

S

have cautioned against the use of sevoflurane in patients with pre-existing renal impairment.[11,12]

3 There have been rare reports of smoke/fire, extreme heat and significant carbon monoxide production in anaesthesia machines during sevoflurane anaesthesia while using a desiccated CO_2 absorbent (Abbott Australasia Communication 25 November 2003). This interaction has resulted in airway irritation, difficult ventilation, severe airway oedema and erythema and elevated carboxyhaemoglobin levels. To prevent these events from happening, do not leave gases flowing through the CO_2 absorbent when it is not in use for a prolonged period. Turn off the vaporisers when not in use. It is also recommended to periodically check the temperature of the CO_2 absorbent and to check that the delivered sevoflurane concentration matches the concentration dialled up on the vaporiser. An unusually delayed rise or unexpected decline of inspired sevoflurane concentration compared to the vaporiser setting may indicate significant heating of the CO_2 absorbent.

4 Sevoflurane causes prolongation of the Q-T interval (as does isoflurane and enflurane).[13] Sevoflurane has been implicated in causing torsade de pointes (polymorphic VT).[14] Q-T prolongation due to sevoflurane can be reversed by ceasing sevoflurane and maintaining anaesthesia with a propofol infusion.[15]

5 Less potent than similar halogenated ethers.

6 Postoperative agitation may be more common in children after a sevoflurane anaesthetic compared with halothane.[16]

7 Can rarely cause convulsions at high inhalational doses.[17]

8 Rarely, sevoflurane can degrade in the storage bottle, resulting in a 'hiss' when opening and an acrid odour.[17] Do not use the contents if this occurs.

9 Sevoflurane can induce malignant hyperthermia. Do not use in MH-susceptible patients.

Shivering Postoperatively

Shivering after a general anaesthetic is common (in up to 60% of patients)[18] and usually benign but can lead to undesirable effects such as:[19]

1 increased O_2 consumption
2 raised intra-ocular pressure
3 disruption of delicate surgical repair
4 hypoglycaemia.

Prevention

1 Use warming devices such as warm-air-filled blankets (e.g. Bair Hugger), heating mattress.
2 Minimise the surface area of the patient that is exposed.

Treatment

1 Exclude causes of shivering other than anaesthesia, such as hypoglycaemia, fever and hypothermia.
2 Exogenous heat.
3 Pethidine 0.5 mg/kg IV.[20]
4 Clonidine 1.5 µg/kg IV.[20]
5 Tramadol 1 mg/kg/IV.[21] Tramadol may be more effective than pethidine.[22]

Sickle Cell Disease

Topics Covered in this Section

▶ Spectrum of Sickle Cell Disease
▶ Diagnosis of Sickle Cell Disease
▶ Sickle Cell Anaemia (SCA)
▶ Anaesthetic Considerations for SCA
▶ Obstetric Anaesthesia and SCA
▶ Anaesthetic Considerations for Sickle Cell Trait
▶ Treatment of Sickle Cell Crisis

S

Spectrum of Sickle Cell Disease

Sickle cell disease is a general term for a type of inherited haemo globinopathy involving the production of HbS. In this abnormal variant, valine is substituted for glutamic acid at the sixth amino acid position of the β chain of the globin molecule. Deoxygenation of HbS results in the formation of insoluble globin polymers (long crystals). This gives the red blood cell (RBC) a sickle shape, which results in increased RBC destruction and episodes of obstruction of blood vessels. Repeated cycles of sickling and unsickling eventually result in irreversible sickling. Patients suffer from a chronic haemolytic anaemia and episodes of *sickle cell crisis* in which vaso-occlusion results in tissue ischaemia and infarction with severe pain (see below).

This disease affects mainly blacks and some Mediterranean races. Types of sickle cell disease include:

- *HbSS*, the homozygous form of the disease, associated with severe haemolytic anaemia. This variant is *sickle cell anaemia*. RBC contain 85–95% HbS.[23] Variable increases in HbF occur in patients with sickle cell anaemia, which offers some protection from sickling, reducing the complication rate and increasing survival. Levels of HbF above 20% are particularly effective.[23]

- *HbSC*, sickle cell HbC disease. In this condition, in addition to the HbS gene, a mutant β chain gene causes cellular dehydration and increased intracellular HbS concentration. Most patients will eventually develop symptoms but median survival is longer than for HbSS.

- *HbAS* (sickle cell trait), heterozygote form. Patients are usually not anaemic. The red cell contains 20–45% HbS. Sickling starts at an O_2 saturation of 40% and the critical PaO_2 for irreversible sickling is 20 mmHg. This disease does carry some risk, e.g. splenic infarcts at altitude.[23]

- *Alpha thalassaemia and HbSS* sometimes coexist, resulting in a less severe anaemia than in HbSS alone.[24]

Diagnosis of Sickle Cell Disease

A sickledex test will detect HbS but does not identify the type of sickle cell disease. The genotype can be detected by haemoglobin electrophoresis.

Sickle Cell Anaemia (SCA)

Sickling occurs in response to reduced O_2 tension, acidosis, cold, dehydration and can occur with drug therapy in association with glucose-6-phosphate dehydrogenase deficiency (see *GLUCOSE-6-PHOSPHATE DEHYDROGENASE (G6PD) DEFICIENCY*). At 65% O_2 saturation, 75% of RBC are sickled. The critical PaO_2 for irreversible sickling is 42 mmHg.[23] Patients have a chronic severe haemolytic anaemia, impaired renal concentrating ability and susceptibility to severe bacterial infections. Sickle cell crisis results in hypoxia/infarction of affected tissues. This leads to pain, renal impairment, haemolytic anaemia, fever, tachycardia and a self-perpetuating cycle of acidosis and hypoxia. Patterns of attacks include the following:

1 *Chest syndrome* describes recurrent episodes of chest pain, fever and pulmonary infiltrates.
2 *Sickle cell lung disease* with progressive deterioration in lung function and cor pulmonale occurs.
3 *Sequestration crisis* occurs particularly in young children, due to the pooling of RBCs in the spleen and liver.
4 *Aplastic crisis*, due to sudden severe bone marrow depression, is another potentially fatal complication. This can be precipitated by infection, typically viral.[24]

Anaesthetic Considerations for SCA

▶ *Pre-operative Measures*

1 Pre-operative transfusion therapy to correct anaemia to 10 g/dL is recommended prior to intermediate or high-risk surgery. It is no longer recommended to reduce HbS levels to < 30%.[25]

2   For patients having minor surgery, pre-operative transfusion is
     probably unneccessary.[25]

3   Keep the patient well-hydrated peri-operatively. These patients
     tend to have renal impairment with reduced renal concentrat-
     ing ability.

4   Do not perform elective surgery in the presence of infection as a
     crisis may be precipitated.[23]

▶ *Intra-operative and Postoperative Measures*

1   It is imperative to prevent hypoxia, acidosis, dehydration and
     hypothermia. Maintain a mild respiratory alkalosis with inter-
     mittent positive pressure ventilation. Use higher than usual
     inhaled FiO_2 concentrations.

2   Use prophylactic antibiotic therapy. These patients are prone to
     overwhelming infections, particularly streptococcal infection,
     due to functional hyposplenism.

3   Prevent local circulatory stasis. Vasopressors should not be used,
     if possible.[23]

4   SCA is a relative contraindication to tourniquet use. Tourniquets
     have been used safely in these patients but this technique should
     be undertaken very cautiously.[26] For example, Al-Ghamdi
     reported using exchange transfusion to reduce HbS from 82.6%
     to 47% prior to the sequential application of tourniquets for
     bilateral knee replacement.[27]

5   A cell saver should probably not be used due to the high
     incidence of sickling in the washed cells.[28]

6   Ensure the above management continues post-operatively.

7   Regional anaesthesia is associated with a higher incidence of
     painful crises compared with GA.[29]

Obstetric Anaesthesia and SCA

In addition to the general measures described above:

1   It is especially important to prevent aorto-caval compression in
     this population.

2 The incidence of CS is higher in this group than the normal population.[30]

3 The safety of epidural blood patch for postdural puncture headache (PDPH) is unknown in this group. Chiron et al. used 30 mL of Plasmion (a modified fluid gelatin) heated to 37°C injected into the epidural space in a sickle cell patient with PDPH with good results.[31]

Anaesthetic Considerations for Sickle Cell Trait

1 Extra special precautions should be taken to prevent hypoxia in the peri-operative period in these patients due to an increased risk of complications such as cerebral infarction and superior sagittal sinus thrombosis.[23]

2 A cell saver should probably not be used due to the high incidence of sickling in the washed cells.[28]

Treatment of Sickle Cell Crisis

1 Provide adequate analgesia but observe closely for respiratory depression. Opioids will usually be required, at least initially.

2 Correct/prevent dehydration.

3 Treat infective complications with antibiotics.

4 Keep the patient well-oxygenated.

5 Blood transfusion should only be undertaken if pain is refractory to maximal opioid therapy, or the patient suffers a stroke or acute chest syndrome.[25]

6 *Hydroxyurea therapy*: Hydroxyurea can increase HbF concentration and have other beneficial effects in this condition.[32]

▶ *Treatment of Acute Chest Syndrome*

IV dexamethasone 0.3 mg/kg 12 h × 4 doses may be of benefit.[33]

Sleep Apnoea Syndrome

See *OBSTRUCTIVE SLEEP APNOEA (OSA) SYNDROME.*

Sodium Bicarbonate

Inorganic salt used:

1 in the treatment of severe life-threatening metabolic acidosis
2 in the treatment of cardiac arrest associated with pre-existing metabolic acidosis or after return of spontaneous circulation when there has been a prolonged period of cardiac arrest
3 to reduce the availability of free drug in the serum in situations such as tricyclic overdose. Sodium bicarbonate is also used to alkalinise the urine to increase drug excretion after, for example, barbiturate overdose.
4 in the treatment of severe life-threatening hyponatraemia if hypertonic saline is not available
5 in the treatment of hyperkalaemia (see *POTASSIUM*).

It is presented as an 8.4% solution (1 mmol/mL) with an osmolarity of 2000 mOsm/L.

Dose for Profound Metabolic Acidosis

To restore pH to normal,[34]

$$\text{dose (mmol)} = \frac{\text{base deficit (mEq/L)} \times \text{body weight (kg)}}{3}$$

Give half this dose, then recheck acid–base status.

Note: Sodium bicarbonate inactivates adrenaline and noradrenaline if the two drugs are mixed.

Sodium Nitroprusside (SNP)

Direct-acting vasodilator of resistance and capacitance vessels (arterio- and venodilator). SNP is 44% cyanide by weight. It acts by spontaneously dissociating to form nitric oxide, which causes vasodilatation. SNP is used for the treatment of severe hypertension (in conjunction with invasive blood pressure monitoring) and for the control of blood pressure during surgery such as cerebral aneurysm repair.

Dose

1 Mix 50 mg SNP powder with 100 mL of 5% glucose. The recommended dose range is 0.3–6 µg/kg/min. In order to minimise the risk of cyanide toxicity the lower dose range of 0.3 µg/kg/min–2 µg/kg/min is suggested.[35] The maximum permissible rate of SNP is 10 µg/kg/min and this should not be used for longer than 10 min.

Table S2 Infusion rate for sodium nitroprusside (500 µg/mL) for a 70 kg patient

Dose (µg/kg/min)	Rate of infusion (mL/h)
0.3	2.5
2	17
6	50
10	84

2 If necessary add other hypotensive drugs to reduce SNP dose, such as trimetaphan. SNP can also be given as a bolus of 1–2 µg/kg (in a 70 kg patient this is 0.14–0.28 mL of the above solution).

3 Protect the solution from light by measures such as foil wrapping. In room light 45% will decay in 6 h. If marked degradation does occur the solution changes to a blue colour.

Symptoms/signs of Cyanide (CN⁻) Toxicity

1 Resistance to SNP therapy.
2 Metabolic acidosis/increased serum lactate.
3 Tachycardia, dysrhythmias, sweating and hyperventilation.
4 Cyanide poisoning occurs with CN^- serum levels of ≥ 8 µg/mL.

S

Treatment of CN⁻ Toxicity

1 Cease SNP infusion. Ensure adequate airway, breathing and circulation, and administer 100% O_2. Give sodium bicarbonate to correct acidosis (see *SODIUM BICARBONATE*).

2 Give sodium thiosulphate 150 mg/kg IV over 15 min, then an infusion of 30–60 mg/kg/h (converts CN⁻ to thiocyanate).[35]

3 Sodium nitrite 4–6 mg/kg very slowly IV.[35] This drug results in increased quantities of methaemoglobin to combine with the CN⁻.

4 Other alternative treatments include:
   (a) hydroxycobalamin IV. The dose is not firmly established although 100 µg/kg is suggested.[36]
   (b) dicobalt edetate 300 mg IV over 1 min followed by glucose 50 mL of 50% solution. Give another 300 mg dose if no response.

Sotalol

Non-selective β adrenergic receptor blocker with marked Class 3 anti-arrhythmic properties, useful:[37]

1 for second line treatment of antrioventricular (AV) nodal and AV re-entrant tachycardias. Also used for the prevention of these dysrhythmias.

2 for termination of sustained ventricular tachycardia (VT)[38] and for the prevention of recurrent VT and ventricular fibrillation (VF)

3 for prevention of atrial fibrillation (AF) after cardioversion

4 as an alternative to amiodarone in cardiac arrest due to pulseless VT or VF resistant to defibrillation.

Adult PO Dose

160–640 mg daily in 2–3 divided doses.

Adult IV Dose

0.5–1.5 mg/kg over 5–20 min. In VT/VF associated cardiac arrest give 1 mg/kg over 1 min, then 0.5 mg/kg over 1 min for breakthrough VT.

Problems

1 Sotalol can cause hypotension, bradycardia and AV block.
2 On rare occasions sotalol administration can cause the development of polymorphic VT or torsade de pointes.
3 Sotalol is contraindicated in familial QT syndrome and asthma.
4 Renally excreted. Reduce doseage in patients with renal impairment.
5 Sotalol has a long half-life of 8–15 h.

Spinal Anaesthesia

See *SUBARACHNOID BLOCK (SAB)*.

Spinal Anatomy

There are 33 vertebrae in total: 7 cervical, 12 thoracic, 5 lumbar, 5 sacral (fused) and 4 coccygeal (fused).

Landmarks

A line joining the iliac (Tuffier's line) crests passes through the lower part of L4 vertebra or the L4–5 disc space with some interpatient variation.[39] The C7 spinous process (*vertebra prominens*) is the first prominent spine when running the fingers down the nuchal furrow.

The angle of the scapulae are at the same level as the T7 spinous process.

Spinal Cord

Extends from the medulla to L1–2 disc space in the adult (range T12 vertebra to L2–3 disc).

S

Spinal Nerves

There are 31 pairs of nerves: 8 cervical, 12 thoracic, 5 lumbar, 5 sacral and 1 coccygeal.

Subarachnoid Space

Extends from the foramen magnum to S2 vertebra. At this level the dura continues (without a space) as part of the filum terminale which attaches to the coccyx.

Epidural Space

Extends from the foramen magnum to the sacral hiatus. See *EPIDURAL ANAESTHESIA*.

Spirometry

See *RESPIRATORY FUNCTION TESTS*.

Status Epilepticus

See *EPILEPSY, STATUS*.

Steroid 'Cover'

Need for Supplementary Glucocorticoids for Patients on Long-term Glucocorticoid Therapy

Patients who are on long-term steroid replacement therapy, of more than 10 mg/day of prednisilone, may suffer severe peri-operative cardiovascular collapse due to inadequate endogenous glucocorticoid production in response to the surgical 'stress'. This type of complication is probably extremely rare. However, the administration of steroids to prevent this problem is associated with few if any significant adverse effects. The dose of 'steroid' to be given is unresolved. Chronic steroid therapy can be arbitrarily defined as steroid therapy for more than 1 month during the 6–12 months prior to surgery and/or which has been

S

discontinued for less than 12 months.[40] The maximum endogenous production of steroid in normal patients undergoing severe physiological stress is 75–150 mg/day.[40] Also, in normal patients serum cortisol levels return to normal by 48 h after uncomplicated major surgery.[40]

Several steroid replacement regimes are suggested, including the following.

Regime Suggested by Wall[41]

▶ Dose of Steroid Cover for Major Surgery

Give hydrocortisone 25 mg IV on induction, then 100 mg intraoperatively. Postoperatively give hydrocortisone 50–100 mg IV 8 h for 24 h, then 25–50 mg 8 h for the second 24 h. Then taper the steroid dose gradually to the patient's usual daily dose.

▶ Dose of Steroid for Minor Surgery

Give 50 mg hydrocortisone on induction, then 50 mg intraoperatively. Restart the patient's oral therapy when the patient is able to tolerate oral intake.

Regime Suggested by Nicholson et al.[42]

▶ Dose of Steroid for Major Surgery

Give the patient's usual dose of oral steroid on the day of surgery. On induction give hydrocortisone 25 mg IV, then 100 mg IV by continuous infusion over the next 24 h. Continue with 100 mg IV every 24 h until the patient is able to tolerate his/her usual oral steroid dose.

▶ Dose of Steroid for Minor Surgery

Give the usual dose of oral steroid on the day of surgery. On induction give hydrocortisone 25 mg IV. Resume the patient's usual oral therapy as soon as possible after surgery.

S

Steroid Equivalents

Table S3 Relative potencies of glucocorticoids	
Drug equivalent	Dose (mg)
Hydrocortisone	80
Dexamethasone	3
Methylprednisilone	16
Prednisone	20

ST Segment Analysis

Computerised automated monitoring of ST segments in leads II and V5 will detect about 80% of myocardial ischaemic episodes.[43] Use the *diagnostic* ECG filtering mode. Ischaemia is associated with:

1 transient tall T waves/T wave inversion
2 a non-specific increase in R wave amplitude
3 ST depression denoting endocardial ischaemia, which is significant when > 1 mm from the baseline 60 ms after the J point and which lasts > 60 s. The J point is the end of the QRS complex, where the S wave becomes the ST segment. Down-sloping and horizontal ST segment depression is considered more significant than up-sloping ST segment depression.
4 ST segment elevation denoting transmural ischaemia is significant if ≥ 2 mm.
5 ST segment monitoring may not be helpful if there are intraventricular conduction delays, left bundle branch block, ventricular pacing, no P waves or the patient is taking digoxin.

Subarachnoid Block (SAB)

Topics Covered in this Section

▶ Anatomy Relevant to Subarachnoid Anaesthesia
▶ Contraindications to the Use of SAB
▶ Technique for SAB
▶ Taylor's Approach to SAB
▶ Local Anaesthetic Solutions for SAB
▶ Subarachnoid Opioids
▶ SAB Needles
▶ 'Saddle' Block
▶ Combined Spinal Epidural Anaesthesia
▶ Anticoagulant Therapy and SAB
▶ Continuous Spinal Anaesthesia/Analgesia
▶ Complications of SAB

Anatomy Relevant to Subarachnoid Anaesthesia

In adults the spinal cord extends from the medulla to the L1, 2 interspace, although in some individuals the cord can extend as far as the L2, 3 disc level. A line through the iliac crests passes through the lower part of L4 or the L4, 5 interspace.

Contraindications to the Use of SAB

The absolute contraindications to SAB anaesthesia are:

1 patient refusal
2 significant coagulopathy
3 infection at the site of insertion.

Technique for SAB

1 Obtain large bore adequate IV access and load the patient with 500 mL–1 L of crystalloid IV.

S

2   Position the patient either sitting or laterally with maximum lumbar flexion.

3   Sterilise the skin over the lumbar spine and anaesthetise the site of insertion. Use the L3, 4 or the L4, 5 interspace. A midline or paramedian approach can also be used. See *Taylor's Approach to SAB* below.

4   Insert the spinal needle into the subarachnoid space, as evidenced by the return of cerebrospinal fluid (CSF).

5   Inject the LA solution (see below for drug types and dosages), then place the patient in the supine position, unless intending to produce 'saddle' analgesia (see *Saddle Block* below). Anticipate and treat hypotension with vasopressors such as ephedrine or metaraminol ± further IV fluid loading.

Taylor's Approach to SAB[44]

1   After obtaining adequate IV access, place the patient in the lateral or sitting position.

2   The point of entry is 1 cm medial and 1 cm caudal to the lower-most prominence of the posterior superior iliac spine. The aim is to pass the spinal needle through the L5–S1 interspace via a lateral oblique approach. Sterilise and drape the skin around the entry site.

3   Anaesthetise the skin at the entry point.

4   Direct the spinal needle medially in a cephalad direction, aiming to enter the subarachnoid space laterally between L5 and S1. If bone is encountered, walk the needle off the sacrum into the subarachnoid space.

Local Anaesthetic Solutions for SAB

Bupivacaine: Either bupivacaine plain 0.5% solution, or bupivacaine 0.5% heavy solution (containing glucose 80 mg/mL), can be used. Heavy bupivacaine, which is hyperbaric in CSF, demonstrates less cephalad spread than plain. These solutions provide subarachnoid blockade for 2–2.5 h. The dose for transurethral resection of prostate (TURP) surgery of either solution is ≈ 3 mL. The dose of heavy or plain bupivacaine 0.5% for LSCS is ≈ 2.5 mL.[45]

Ropivacaine is about 25% less potent than bupivacaine. For hip arthroplasty 3.5 mL of 0.5% solution is effective.

Cinchocaine (Nupercaine, Dibucaine) heavy 0.5% solution contains 60 mg/mL glucose. Effects last ≈ 2 h. A suitable dose for TURP surgery is 1.8–2 mL. About 1.5 mL would be suitable for LSCS.[45]

Tetracaine (Pontocaine): Duration of action longer than bupivacaine. A suitable dose for LSCS is 7–10 mg of hyperbaric solution.

Subarachnoid Opioids

1 Although prolonged effective analgesia is provided, there are significant side effects with intrathecal opioids. The most important of these is delayed respiratory depression.

2 *Morphine*: Give 0.1–0.5 mg depending on the patient's size and physical condition. Onset of analgesia takes ≈ 15–45 min and the effects last about 12–24 h. Pruritis is common, especially in patients undergoing Caesarean delivery (70–85%).[46]

3 *Diamorphine* (heroin): Give 0.3–0.8 mg, depending on the patient's size and physical condition. Effects last up to 22 h.[47]

4 *Fentanyl*: Small doses are useful for enhancing the intra-operative effect of LA solutions, e.g. fentanyl 25 µg + 2.5 mL bupivacaine 0.5% heavy solution is a suitable dose for LSCS. Analgesic effects of intrathecal fentanyl have a rapid onset but there is little evidence for significant postoperative analgesia at a dose of 20–25 µg.[48]

5 *Pethidine*: This is the only opioid with significant LA properties in doses suitable for analgesia. Pethidine can be used as a sole agent for spinal anaesthesia. 1 mg/kg pethidine has been used as a sole agent for LSCS.[49] Subarachnoid pethidine is associated with a high incidence of nausea and vomiting in labouring women.

6 Sufentanil: 2.5–5 µg in adults.

▶ *Adverse Effects of Subarachnoid Opioids*

These include:

1 pruritis
2 nausea and vomiting
3 delayed respiratory depression.

▶ *SAB Needles*

1 *Quincke*: Conventional sharp cutting edge needle. 25 and 26 G needles are available, but even with the 26 G needle the incidence of postdural puncture headache (PDPH) is about 20–25% in the obstetric population.[50] It is recommended to orientate the needle bevel parallel to the longitudinal direction of the dural fibres.

2 *Whitacre*: Pencil-point needle without a cutting edge, intended to reduce the incidence of PDPH. The rounded opening is on the side 2 mm from the tip. The incidence of PDPH with a 22 G Whitacre is ≈ 3.5%[51] and ≈ 1.2% with a 25 G needle.[52]

3 *Sprotte*: A pencil-point variant with, compared to the Whitacre, a gentler conical point angle and a larger hole at the distal end of the shaft. The incidence of PDPH ≈ 3–10% with 24 G Sprotte in the obstetric poulation.[50]

'Saddle' Block

This is a type of SAB aimed at anaesthetising the sacral nerves only. SAB is performed in the sitting position with 1.5 mL of heavy bupivacaine 0.5% and the patient remains sitting for at least 5 min.

Combined Spinal Epidural Anaesthesia

These techniques can be undertaken in several different ways:

1 siting an epidural catheter, then performing a subarachnoid block at a more caudad vertebral interspace.

2 using a 'kit' (e.g. Portex, Mallinckrodt) containing a Tuohy needle with a Huber tip ± a spinal needle 'back-eye' aperture for a 26 or 27 G pencil-point spinal needle and a blind-ended

catheter with three lateral eyes. In another variation the epidural needle may have a separate barrel fused to it for the spinal needle.

3   siting a spinal needle, then, while leaving the obturator in place, siting an epidural catheter at the same interspace.[53]

▶ Use of a Combined Spinal Epidural Kit 'Needle-Through-Needle' Technique

1   It is recommended that the patient be positioned in the lateral decubitus position. This is to avoid/diminish the hypotensive effects of spinal anaesthesia while positioning and securing the epidural catheter.

2   Use the Tuohy needle to identify the epidural space in the usual way.

3   The spinal needle is then passed through the Tuohy needle into the subarachnoid space. A 'popping' sensation may be felt and CSF may or may not be seen returning through the spinal needle. Active aspiration may produce CSF.[54]

4   Inject an appropriate LA dose into subarachnoid space (depending on procedure). See above for dosages.

5   Remove the spinal needle and insert the epidural catheter through the Tuohy needle, then remove the Tuohy needle. Tape the epidural catheter securely.

6   Use epidurally administered LA to supplement subarachnoid block or for postoperative analgesia.

▶ Problems with Combined Spinal Epidural 'Needle-Through-Needle' Technique

1   The spinal needle, when passed through the epidural needle, may be too short to reach the dura, or may be angled by the Huber point of the Tuohy needle to miss the dura completely.

2   The epidural catheter may enter the subarachnoid space although the risk of this is low.[53]

S

3   An epidural 'test-dose' is difficult to interpret in the presence of subarachnoid anaesthesia. The 'best' time to 'test' whether the catheter is in the epidural space is after regression of the spinal block.

4   After subarachnoid anaesthesia has been initiated it may not be possible to pass the epidural catheter or the catheter may pass into a blood vessel, resulting in the unplanned abandonment of the epidural component. Attempts to resite the epidural may result in unplanned 'saddle' block or unilateral block.[53]

5   There is a risk of metallic fragments being created due to friction between the two metal needles.[55]

6   The anaesthetist may be distracted from the undesirable physiological effects of SAB by the process of siting and securing the epidural catheter.

7   One way to negate some of these problems is to use a technique where the subarachnoid space is identified but the stylette is replaced. The epidural catheter is then sited before SAB is attempted either by using a Tuohy needle with a separate spinal needle channel or by separate punctures.[56]

▶ CSE and Labour

CSE is being used increasingly to relieve labour pain. A suggested dose is bupivacaine 2.5 mg plus fentanyl 25 µg. This is effective for about 90 min. This can be followed by an epidural infusion or top-ups as required. See EPIDURAL ANAESTHESIA.

Advantages

1   Rapid onset of analgesia.

2   Little or no motor block.[57]

3   Epidural catheter placement may be more reliable when a CSE technique is used compared with the traditional epidural-only technique.[58]

Disadvantages

1 An 18% incidence of foetal bradycardia has been noted when this technique is used. No increase in the emergency CS rate was seen.[58]

2 The risk of meningitis may be increased due to the proximity of the catheter to the breech in the dura.[56]

3 The risk of damage to the spinal cord and in particular the conus may be increased compared with traditional epidural anaesthesia.[59]

▶ *CSE and CS*

CSE enables prolongation of anaesthesia due to unforeseen circumstances such as the need for post-CS hysterectomy.[56]

However, there is no evidence that CSE is superior to a 'single shot' spinal for CS.[56]

Anticoagulant Therapy and SAB

See *EPIDURAL ANAESTHESIA, Anticoagulant Therapy and Epidurals.*

Continuous Spinal Anaesthesia/Analgesia

Continuous spinal anaesthesia/analgesia is very effective for anaesthesia and managing postoperative pain and cancer pain. This technique is not popular due to the high incidence of post-dural puncture headaches and technical difficulties. For example, fine needles and catheters designed to reduce the incidence of PDPH have a tendency to kink and break. This treatment modality has also been associated with significant neurological injury such as cauda-equina syndrome. To minimise the risks of neurological injury the following are recommended:[60]

1 Insert catheters no more than 3 cm into the subarachnoid space.

2 Avoid caudal placement.

3 Use small doses of plain isobaric LA solutions. Abandon the technique if up to 3 mL of LA is ineffective.[60]

▶ *Advantages*

1   Excellent analgesia.

2   Good cardiovascular stability when small doses of plain solution are used. Hence this technique has been used in patients with severe aortic stenosis.

3   Continuous infusions of opioids can be very effective in treating labour pain in obstetric patients with severe cardiac lesions, e.g. intrathecal sufentanil 10 μg followed by an infusion of 5 μg/h. See *SUFENTANIL*.

▶ *Disadvantages*

1   Risk of cauda-equina syndrome.

2   Risk of PDPH.

3   Increased risk of infection/meningitis.

4   Risk of catheter breakage.

5   Possible increased risk of intrathecal bleeding.

Complications of SAB

1   Hypotension is the most common side effect. Ensure the patient is adequately hydrated, and treat hypotension promptly. Hypotension, severe bradycardia and/or asystole may occur even in young, healthy patients. Prompt treatment with atropine, ephedrine and/or adrenaline is usually effective.[61]

2   Headache. See *SAB needles* above.

3   Nerve injury. Transient radicular radiation may occur with mild to severe back pain radiating to the buttock, usually lasting < 2 days. The incidence of this complication wth bupivacaine is 0–3%.

4   Spinal cord injury and especially injury to the conus medullaris may also occur.[62] Do not inject the solution through a spinal needle that has caused pain on entering the subarachnoid space.[62] If pain occurs when injecting anaesthetic solution, cease injecting and resite the spinal needle. A space no higher than L3/4 should be selected.[59]

S

5   Spinal cord compression due to haemorrhage or infection. The risk of a spinal or epidural haematoma in association with a SAB is about 1:250 000.[63]

6   Transitory deafness can occur in up to 16% of patients having SAB.[64] This may be due to middle ear changes as a result of CSF loss and this complication may be more common in younger patients.[64]

Subarachnoid Haemorrhage

See *CEREBRAL ANEURYSM SURGERY*.

Subclavian Vein Central Line

Technique for Insertion

1   Position patient supine with a rolled towel or bag of fluid between the shoulder blades. Tilt the trolley ≈ 10–15° head down.

2   Sterilise the skin above and below the clavicle, then palpate the inferior edge of the clavicle and identify the border of the subclavius muscle (which runs from the first rib to the inferior surface of the clavicle). This border lies just lateral to the curvature at the midpoint of the clavicle.

3   Anaesthetise the skin and deeper tissues with a 32 mm 23 G needle, aiming towards the sternal notch and keeping the shaft of the needle parallel to the floor.

4   Insert the Seldinger needle with the shaft parallel to the floor, aiming to pass the needle just under the clavicle and aiming towards the sternal notch.

5   If the subclavian artery is entered the needle needs to pass more anteriorly (the artery lies posterior to the vein). See Figure B2, 'Anatomical relations of the superior surface of the first rib', on page 72.

6   Aspirate while advancing the needle. If air is obtained, the needle has passed through the pleura.

S

7   Once the subclavian vein is punctured, remove the syringe and pass the guide wire into the vein and remove the Seldinger needle.

8   Incise the skin with a scalpel to enable the dilator to be passed over the wire, then insert the dilator into the vein, thus allowing easy passage of the catheter. Remove the dilator, then pass the catheter over the wire and into the vein. Remove the wire. Insert the catheter 12 cm for the average adult. Suture the catheter to the skin and cover with a sterile dressing.

9   Organise and review chest X-ray. The tip should lie in the SVC above the cephalic limit of the pericardial reflection.

Never lose visual contact with the wire. Never leave a catheter lumen open to air.

Succinylcholine

See *SUXAMETHONIUM*.

Sufentanil

A synthetic opioid drug that is a derivative of fentanyl. Used for the induction and maintenance of anaesthesia and for postoperative analgesia. Sufentanil is about 5–10 × more potent than fentanyl and has a slightly shorter elimination half-life.

Dose

IV: The appropriate dose required depends on the complexity of surgery, e.g. appendicectomy 1–2 µg/kg, bowel resection 2–8 µg/kg.[65] For cardiac surgery 8–50 µg/kg (with postoperative ventilation).

Epidural dose: 30–50 µg for adults.

Intrathecal dose: In adults 2.5–5 µg. An intrathecal infusion of sufentanil can be considered for labour in obstetric patients with severe cardiovascular disease. A patient with severe pulmonary valve disease received intrathecal sufentanil 10 µg LD, then an infusion of 5 µg/h with good effect.[66]

Superior Laryngeal Nerve (SLN) Block

Anatomy

A branch of the vagus nerve, the *superior laryngeal nerve,* divides into an *external* and *internal* branch. The *external* branch supplies the cricothyroid muscle and the *internal* branch supplies sensation to the interior of the larynx as far down as the vocal cords. The *internal* branch passes around the inferior border of the greater cornu of the hyoid bone and through the *thyrohyoid membrane.*

Technique

1 Palpate the hyoid bone. Sterilise the skin and then use a 32 mm 23 G needle to 'walk' caudad off the hyoid bone's greater cornu near its posterior tip and just through the thyrohyoid membrane.
2 Inject 2–3 mL of LA, e.g. lignocaine 2%.

Superior Vena Cava Syndrome

Description

In this condition the superior vena cava (SVC) is obstructed, usually by malignant masses on the right side such as bronchogenic carcinoma or lymphoma. The effects of obstruction include:

1 oedema of the head, neck and upper extremities
2 cerebral venous congestion with headaches, visual disturbances, raised ICP and altered mentation
3 proptosis
4 dyspnoea, orthopnoea and cough
5 laryngeal oedema.

The condition is exacerbated if the obstruction is below the azygous vein, preventing collaterals forming.

Anaesthetic Implications

1 Management in a head-up position may be helpful.
2 Keep the patient well volume loaded to maintain preload but avoid overhydration.
3 Avoid venodilating drugs.
4 Give drugs and fluids into veins draining into the inferior vena cava. If central venous access is required use the femoral vein.
5 Laryngeal oedema due to venous engorgement may make intubation difficult.
6 The effects of the mediastinal mass causing the obstruction may also be deleterious. See *MEDIASTINAL MASS AND ANAESTHESIA*.

Supine Hypotensive Syndrome

See *PREGNANT SURGICAL PATIENT—ANAESTHETIC IMPLICATIONS*.

Supra-orbital and Supratrochlear Nerve Blocks

See *FOREHEAD BLOCK*.

Supraventricular Tachycardias (SVT)

These tachycardias are usually narrow complex tachycardias and they originate either in the atrium (atrial tachycardias) or the bundle of HIS (junctional tachycardias). However, some SVTs may demonstrate broad QRS complexes (see *BROAD COMPLEX TACHYCARDIA*). Junctional SVTs tend to respond to vagal manoeuvres (such as carotid sinus massage) and adenosine with slowing or termination (breaking) of the tachycardia. Atrial tachycardias tend to respond to vagal manoeuvres and adenosine with a slowing of the ventricular rate (less effective conduction of atrial impulses). This may make diagnosis easier by revealing the nature of the atrial electrical activity.

S

Attempt to diagnose the type of SVT from the patient's history and 12 lead ECG. Possibilities are:

1 *atrial fibrillation*—the tachycardia is irregular
2 *atrial flutter*—flutter waves on the ECG
3 *unifocal atrial tachycardia*—a regular tachycardia with monomorphic abnormal P waves. The rate is usually 130–160.
4 *multifocal atrial tachycardia* (MAT). MAT is uncommon and may be confused with atrial fibrillation due to its irregularity. It can be distinguished from atrial fibrillation by the presence in MAT of P waves of three or more different morphologies. In contrast, atrial fibrillation does not have identifiable P waves.[67]
5 *atrio-ventricular* (AV) node re-entry tachycardia. Re-entry is confined to the AV node. The tachycardia is regular and typically has an abrupt onset and offset. It is a junctional tachycardia so there are no P waves.
6 *AV re-entry tachycardia*—there is an accessory pathway that allows re-entry in addition to the AV node. An example is Wolff-Parkinson-White syndrome. A pre-tachycardia ECG may show typical features of WPW, enabling the diagnosis to be made. See *WOLFF-PARKINSON-WHITE SYNDROME*.

In non-decompensated patients there is often time to obtain a cardiology consultation and a 12 lead ECG. Atrial fibrillation, flutter and WPW are dealt with elsewhere under the relevant headings.

Treatment of Narrow Complex Regular SVT (Presumed to be Junctional) Excluding WPW

▶ *Patients Without Significant Cardiovascular Compromise*

1 If possible, ask the patient or obtain from another source the usual effective treatment for the patient's SVT, e.g. verapamil.
2 In the absence of such information, attempt vagal manoeuvres such as carotid sinus massage, Valsalva manoeuvre, or ice water on the face. This causes slowing of AV conduction which may:

    (a) have no effect, suggesting an atrial tachycardia

    (b) slow the tachycardia or abruptly terminate it, suggesting a junctional tachycardia

    (c) cause a sudden bradycardia, which can trigger ventricular fibrillation, especially in patients with digoxin toxicity or ischaemic myocardium.[68]

3 If vagal manoeuvres are ineffective give adenosine. See *ADENO-SINE*. This drug also slows AV conduction and may produce similar effects as described for carotid sinus massage, i.e. it may be effective in junctional SVT and have little or no effect on atrial SVT. In patients with WPW, adenosine may cause a dangerously rapid ventricular response.[68]

4 If adenosine is ineffective consider an anti-arrythmic drug such as verapamil or a β blocker such as esmolol. Do not use verapamil and a β blocker together in the same patient.

5 If the above treatment is ineffective consider amiodarone, rapid atrial pacing[69] and cardioversion—see below.

▶ Patients with Significant Cardiovascular Compromise

This can be defined as SBP < 90 mmHg, chest pain, heart failure or heart rate > 200 bpm.[70]

    Use DC cardioversion under sedation or anaesthesia. For monophasic defibrillators use energy settings of 50–100 J, 200 J, then 360 J.[67] For biphasic defibrillators about half this energy can be used.[68] If this is unsuccessful give amiodarone, then repeat cardioversion shocks.

Treatment of Narrow Complex Irregular SVT or Unifocal Atrial Tachycardia (Excluding Atrial Fibrillation/flutter)

For patients with atrial fibrillation or atrial flutter see the relevant entries. For patients with MAT or unifocal atrial tachycardia:

1 Carotid sinus massage, adenosine and cardioversion are usually ineffective.

2 There is usually an underlying cause such as chronic airways limitation or electrolyte abnormality. Treatment of the cause may reverse the SVT.

3 Magnesium is the drug of choice for acute control of MAT.[70]

4 Consider verapamil or β blockers to improve rate control by slowing AV conduction. These drugs may also revert the SVT. Do not use verapamil and a β blocker in the same patient.

5 Consider amiodarone or use amiodarone first if the patient has known underlying cardiac dysfunction (i.e. ejection fraction less than 40%).[67]

6 If significant cardiovascular compromise, use DC cardioversion as above. Cardioversion may be ineffective in MAT.[69]

Treatment of Pulseless SVT

Treat as for *CARDIAC ARREST*. Give synchronised DC cardioversion shocks. For monophasic defibrillators use energy settings of 100 J, 200 J, then 360 J. If unsuccessful give amiodarone, then repeat cardioversion shocks.[68] For biphasic defibrillators about half this energy can be used.

Sux Apnoea

In this condition, paralysis due to suxamethonium is prolonged up to several hours. It is due to abnormal or deficient pseudo-cholinesterase (plasma cholinesterase). See *SUXAMETHONIUM*.

Incidence of Abnormal Pseudocholinesterase

In about 0.7% of the population suxamethonium-induced paralysis will be slightly prolonged.[71] In about 1 in 2000 patients the effects of suxamethonium may last several hours.[71]

Investigation of Sux Apnoea: Dibucaine Numbers

The dibucaine number is a measure of the percentage inhibition by dibucaine (cinchocaine) of the activity of normal cholinesterase. The test is done by adding benzocholine to plasma, which

S

pseudocholinesterase breaks down. The addition of dibucaine inhibits the breakdown of benzocholine to varying degrees, depending on the type of pseudocholinesterase present. Normal pseudocholinesterase is inhibited the most. Fluoride or chloride can be used instead of dibucaine.

Dibucaine number	Patient phenotype	Clinical significance
Table S4 Clinical significance of dibucaine number		
80	Normal	Nil
40	Heterozygous	Paralysis prolonged (minutes)
20	Homozygous	Paralysis prolonged (hours)

Management

1 Maintain light anaesthesia and mechanical ventilation until paralysis spontaneously reverses as evidenced by a nerve stimulator.
2 Investigate the patient and near relatives for an inherited pseudocholinesterase abnormality.

Causes of Pseudocholinesterase Deficiency

1 Plasmapheresis, dialysis, cardiac bypass.
2 Drugs such as ecothiopate drops, cytotoxic drugs, chlorpromazine.
3 Exposure to organophosphate compounds.

Suxamethonium

Depolarising neuromuscular blocking drug. It is a dicholine ester of succinic acid.

Dose

Adult: 1.5 mg/kg IV, 2.5 mg/kg IM. For electroconvulsive therapy give ≈ 30 mg.

Child: 2 mg/kg IV, 4 mg/kg IM.

Advantages

1 Produces rapid, profound, reliable paralysis in 30–60 s.
2 Short-acting with a duration of action of 3–5 min. Metabolised by pseudocholinesterase.

Disadvantages

1 Suxamethonium causes a rise in the serum potassium. This rise is exaggerated in certain conditions associated with muscle denervation. Subsequent hyperkalaemia can precipitate cardiac arrest. Suxamethonium is contraindicated in these conditions, which include serious burns, denervation illnesses such as Guillain-Barré, hemiplegia and paraplegia, tetanus and Duchenne's muscular dystrophy.
2 Suxamethonium is also contraindicated in the presence of hyperkalaemia from any cause, e.g. renal failure.
3 This drug can accentuate myotonia in myotonic dystrophy.
4 It is a potent trigger of malignant hyperpyrexia.
5 Suxamethonium can cause prolonged paralysis in patients with deficient/abnormal pseudocholinesterase (plasma cholinesterase). See *SUX APNOEA*.
6 Muscle pains may occur, especially in young women.
7 Suxamethonium can cause severe bradycardia, especially in children. This is most likely to occur when a second dose of suxamethonium is given.
8 Suxamethonium causes a small rise in intra-ocular pressure (IOP), which could, theoretically, place the eye with a penetrating injury at risk. Loss of intra-ocular contents due to suxamethonium has not been reported but loss of contents due

S

to coughing is well-recognised. See *EYE INJURY, PENETRATING*. Narrow angle glaucoma is another condition in which elevation of IOP is undesirable.

9   This drug also causes a rise in intracranial pressure but this is opposed by thiopentone.

10 If suxamethonium is given after the administration of neo-stigmine, muscle paralysis may last up to 50–90 min due to inhibition of plasma cholinesterase.[72]

11 Suxamethonium effects can be prolonged in the presence of some drugs such as ecothiopate iodide.

12 Suxamethonium use has resulted in cardiac arrest and death in a number of children with occult myopathy.[73]

Syntocinon

See *OXYTOCIN*.

Syntometrine

See *ERGOMETRINE MALEATE*.

Tt

Tachycardias

Attempt to make a specific diagnosis. If the QRS complexes are narrow see *SUPRAVENTRICULAR TACHYCARDIAS (SVT)*. If the QRS complexes are broad see *BROAD COMPLEX TACHYCARDIA, VENTRICULAR TACHYCARDIA (VT)*.

Tension Pneumothorax

See *CHEST DRAIN*.

Thiopentone

Thiobarbiturate intravenous general anaesthetic agent and anticonvulsant. Also used for cerebral protection during periods of brain ischaemia, e.g. carotid artery surgery, and for barbiturate coma in severe head injuries.

Dose for IV anaesthesia

Adult: 3–5 mg/kg IV. The drug acts within 1 arm–brain circulation time and its effects last 5–15 min.
Child: 5 mg/kg.

Advantages

1 No pain on injection.
2 Inexpensive.
3 Potent anticonvulsant.
4 Cerebrovascular resistance increases with reduced cerebral blood flow, reduced intracranial pressure and reduced cerebral metabolic O_2 demand.

T

Disadvantages

1 Repeated doses or infusion of thiopentone result in prolongation of recovery time. Recovery becomes dependent on drug metabolism (rather than redistribution as with lower doses), which is slow (elimination $t^1/_2$ 3.4–22 h).

2 Thiopentone has negative inotropic effects; it decreases cardiac output by 20% and mean arterial pressure decreases.[1]

3 Thiopentone may have some bronchoconstrictive effects.[1] Use thiopentone with caution or avoid in asthmatics. See *ASTHMA*.

4 Thiopentone can precipitate neurotoxicity in some types of porphyria (see *PORPHYRIA*).

5 Extravasation of thiopentone may cause tissue necrosis.

6 Intra-arterial thiopentone can cause severe arterial constriction and distal limb gangrene (see *INTRA-ARTERIAL INJECTION*).

7 Thiopentone is associated with a higher incidence of postoperative nausea and vomiting compared with propofol.[2]

8 Severe anaphylactoid reactions can occur with an incidence of about 1 per 20 000.[1]

Thoracic Epidural

See *EPIDURAL ANAESTHESIA*.

Thoracoabdominal and Thoracic Aortic Aneurysm Repair

(More than a brief overview of this highly complex subject is beyond the scope of this manual.)

The Crawford Classification of Thoracoabdominal Aneurysms

• *Type 1*—extends from the proximal descending thoracic aorta (DTA) to the upper abdominal aorta but terminates proximally to the renal arteries.

- *Type 2*—as above but the aneurysm extends beyond the renal arteries.
- *Type 3*—begins in the distal half of the DTA and extends for a variable length into the abdomen.
- *Type 4*—involves most of the abdominal aorta.

Pre-operative Assessment and Preparation

The overall mortality for thoracoabdominal aortic aneurysm repair is about 10%. During thoracic aorta cross-clamping, the kidneys and spinal cord are subject to severe ischaemia. The incidence of paraplegia is about 3–15% and the incidence of renal failure is 18–27%.[3] The pre-operative assessment and preparation is similar to abdominal aortic aneurysm repair (see *ENDOLUMINAL ABDOMINAL AORTIC ANEURYSM REPAIR*) with the following qualifications:

1 Place arterial line and rapid infusion cannula in the right arm. This is because the left arm will be bent up and placed over the shoulders.
2 A double lumen tube will be required.

Physiological Effects of Thoracic Aorta Cross-clamping

1 Thoracic aorta cross-clamping produces severe cardiovascular changes with 50% increase in mean arterial pressure and 40% reduction in ejection fraction, and produces left ventricular wall motion abnormalities in 92% of patients.[3] Myocardial ischaemia may be precipitated.
2 Preload consistently increases with clamping above the coeliac artery.
3 Renal blood flow is severely ($\approx$ 90%) decreased.[3]
4 Blood flow to the spinal cord is greatly diminished. CSF pressure increases.

T

Physiological Effects of Thoracic Aorta Unclamping

1 Systemic vascular resistance and arterial pressure decrease by 70–80%.[3]
2 Cardiac output may increase, decrease or be unchanged.[3]

Strategies to Protect Spinal Cord and Renal Function

1 Femoral vein–femoral artery bypass.
2 Left atrial to left femoral artery bypass.
3 Upper or lower pulmonary vein to distal thoracic or proximal abdominal aorta bypass.[4]
4 External shunt from the left ventricular apex or ascending aorta to the distal aorta beyond the clamp or the femoral artery.
5 Moderate hypothermia to 32°C.
6 Intrathecal papaverine.
7 Drainage of cerebrospinal fluid.
8 Regional spinal cord cooling.
9 Intercostal and lumbar artery re-implantation.[5]
10 Profound hypothermia with cardiopulmonary bypass and circulatory arrest.[6]
11 Minimise cross-clamp time. Spinal cord injury increases dramatically after 30 min of cross-clamp time.
12 Prevent hyperglycaemia.
13 Cold perfusion of the renal arteries.
14 Mannitol and frusemide.

CSF Drainage

CSF is drained via an intrathecal lumbar drain to lower CSF pressure. This reduces intraspinal pressure and therefore increases spinal cord perfusion pressure. Aim to keep CSF pressure at or below 10 mmHg.[4] Continue CSF pressure control for 3 days postoperatively. If delayed paraplegia occurs CSF drainage may produce improvement.

Thromboelastography (TEG)

This technique is a test of coagulation, documenting the interaction of platelets, clotting factors and clot quality (throughout the process of clot formation, strengthening, contraction and lysis). It has been used mainly in liver transplant and cardiac surgery but may find wider applications. The device and the technique involve the following steps:

1 0.35 mL of freshly drawn blood is placed in a cup heated to 37°C.
2 A pin suspended on a torsion wire has its tip in the blood sample.
3 The cup oscillates and while the blood is liquid the pin is not affected.
4 As clot starts to form the pin is twisted and this signal is amplified and recorded on heat-sensitive paper.

TEG Measurements[7]

The following variables can be identified:

1 reaction time (r)—time from sample placement to TEG amplitude reaching 2 mm (NR 6–8 min). This correlates to the time of initial fibrin formation.
2 clot formation time (K)—the time from r to TEG amplitude reaching 20 mm (NR 3–6 min). This is the time for a fixed degree of clot viscoelasticity to be reached.
3 alpha angle (α°)—the angle formed by the slope of the TEG tracing between r and K (NR 50–60°). This is an indication of the speed at which a solid clot forms.
4 maximum amplitude (MA)—the widest point of the TEG (NR 50–60 mm). This reflects the absolute strength of the fibrin clot.
5 A_{60} is the amplitude of the tracing 60 min after MA is achieved (NR MA—5 mm). This is a measure of clot lysis or retraction.
6 clot lysis index (CLI)—the A_{60} divided by (MA × 100) and expressed as a percentage. This value measures amplitude as a function of time and reflects lysis destruction of clot integrity.

T

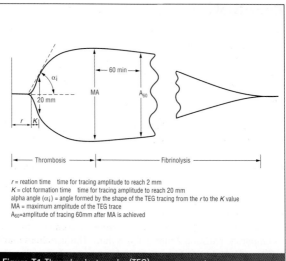

r = reaction time   time for tracing amplitude to reach 2 mm
K = clot formation time   time for tracing amplitude to reach 20 mm
alpha angle (α_i) = angle formed by the shape of the TEG tracing from the r to the K value
MA = maximum amplitude of the TEG trace
A_{60} = amplitude of tracing 60mm after MA is achieved

Figure T1 Thromboelastgraphy (TEG) measurements

Interpretation of Results

1   Reaction time (r) prolongation may be due to coagulation factor deficiencies, anticoagulants or hypofibrinoginaemia. A short reaction time suggests a hypercoagulable state.

2   Coagulation time (K) reflects intrinsic clotting factors, fibrinogen and platelet function.

3   A decreased value of the alpha angle ($\alpha°$) suggests hypo-fibrinoginaemia or thrombocytopenia.

4   Maximum amplitude (MA) is significantly reduced by platelet abnormalities or deficiency.

Thrombophilia

See *DEEP VENOUS THROMBOSIS (DVT) PROPHYLAXIS.*

Thyroid Storm/Thyrotoxic Crisis

Thyroid storm is a hypermetabolic clinical syndrome resulting from excessive thyroid hormone and causing life-threatening multiorgan dysfunction. These effects typically include:

1 tachycardia and other tachydsrhythmias, hypertension, pulmonary oedema and congestive cardiac failure
2 tachypnoea and hypercapnia
3 delirium, stupor and coma—seizures may occur
4 respiratory and metabolic acidosis
5 electrolyte derangements such as hypokalaemia, hyper-calcaemia, hypomagnasaemia and hyponatraemia
6 hyperthermia
7 nausea, vomiting, diarrhoea and abdominal pain.

Thyroid storm can be triggered by thyroid surgery, withdrawal of antithyroid drugs and intercurrent illness such as infection. It is more likely to occur postoperatively than intra-operatively.

Prevention of Thyroid Storm in Hyperthyroid Patients for Elective Thyroidectomy

1 Patients should be rendered euthyroid with a 6–8 week course of antithyroid drug.
2 Give potassium iodide for 1–2 weeks before surgery.
3 Add a β blocker drug for tachycardia if present.

Prevention of Thyroid Storm During Emergency Surgery[8]

In patients undergoing emergency surgery, the risk of thyroid storm can be reduced by:

1 β adrenergic blocker drugs such as propranolol or esmolol

T

2 antithyroid drugs such as propylthiouracil (PTU) 200–400 mg PO 6 h

3 hydrocortisone 40 mg IV 6 h. Glucocorticoids decrease peripheral conversion of T_4 to T_3.

4 potassium iodide 5 drops PO 6 h or Lugol's solution 30 drops 6 h. These inhibit release of T_4 and T_3.

Do not give aspirin, which displaces thyroid hormones from binding proteins.

Treatment of Thyroid Storm

Treatment can be divided into supportive measures and drug therapy.

1 Ensure adequate airway, breathing and circulation. Intubation and ventilation may be required.

2 IV fluid therapy, including glucose solution. Significant dehydration may occur.

3 Normalise glucose and electrolytes.

4 Treat hyperthermia with cooling blankets, icepacks and cold lavage of body cavities. Paracetamol can be given, but not aspirin.

5 Give an antithyroid drug such as propylthiouracil (PTU). Give 1 g PO, then 200 mg PO 6 h. Alternatively, use carbimazole 60–120 mg PO. These can be given by a nasogastric tube. Effects usually begin in 1 h.

6 Potassium iodide or Lugol's solution. This can be given 1 hour after the antithyroid drug. Give potassium iodide 500 mg PO 8 h or 200 mg in 500 mL N/S over 2 h every 12 h. Iodine can increase thyroid hormone release if it is not given *after* PTU. If a patient is allergic to iodine, use lithium carbonate 300 mg PO 6 h.

7 Propranolol or other β adrenergic blocker drug. Give propranolol 40 mg PO 8 h or 1 mg IV as required. Aim for a heart rate of 90 bpm.

T

TIME FREQUENCY BALANCED SPECTRAL ENTROPY

8 Glucocorticoid drug such as hydrocortisone 100 mg IV 6 h. This will treat adrenal insufficiency and decrease T_4 release and conversion to T_3.

9 Guanethidine or reserpine therapy should be considered in propranolol-resistant thyroid storm or in patients unable to tolerate β blockers. The doses are reserpine 2.5–5 mg/kg 4–6 h or guanethidine 1–2 mg/kg/day in divided doses.

10 Consider plasmapheresis, plasma exchange, dialysis or charcoal haemoperfusion in refractory cases to remove thyroid hormone.

11 Consider dantrolene if the above measures are unsuccessful.

Thyromental Distance

See *DIFFICULT AIRWAY MANAGEMENT*.

Tibial Nerve Sheath Catheter

A technique for postoperative analgesia in which the surgeon inserts a catheter into the tibial nerve sheath during surgery for a below-knee amputation. The nerve block is established with 20 mL of bupivacaine 0.25% or ropivacaine 10 mg/mL. This is followed by an infusion of bupivacaine 0.25% run at 10 mL/h.

Ticlopidine

Potent antiplatelet drug with significant anaesthetic and surgical implications. See *PLATELET ADENOSINE DIPHOSPHATE (ADP) RECEPTOR ANTAGONISTS*.

Time Frequency Balanced Spectral Entropy

Entropy is a measure of disorder in a system. A signal with maximum irregularity has an entropy value of 1 and a completely regular predictable signal (e.g. a sine wave) has an entropy value of 0.

Westmead Pocket Anaesthetic Manual   551

In the awake patient EEG signals are highly irregular and therefore have high entropy. In the anaesthetised subject the EEG becomes more regular and the entropy value falls. The Datex-Ohmeda S/5 Entropy module (M-ENTROPY) measures the level of 'disorder' (signal unpredictability) in the EEG and the frontalis muscle electromyelogram, and uses this information to calculate the level of consciousness. This information is used to provide a measure of hypnosis during anaesthesia and to detect possible awareness.

Some Terms Explained

The theory behind entropy algorithms is extremely complex and beyond the scope of this manual. However, a brief explanation of some key terms is offered.

▶ *Time Frequency*

This term refers to the system using 'time windows' or epochs to look at different signal frequencies. Low-frequency signals require more time to analyse than high frequency signals. A single time window of fixed length is not optimal for examining the extremely wide EEG/EMG frequency range ($\approx$ 0.5–50 Hz). Multiple time windows of different lengths are therefore used by the monitoring system to examine the wide frequency range of the EEG and EMG more speedily.

▶ *State Entropy (SE)*

State entropy is computed over the frequency range of 0.8–32 Hz. As it includes the EEG-dominant part of the spectrum, it primarily reflects the cortical state of the patient (level of hypnosis).[9] State entropy provides a stable indicator of the effects of anaesthetic/hypnotic drugs on the cortex similar to BIS monitoring. (See *BISPECTRAL INDEX (BIS) EEG MONITOR.*)

▶ *Response Entropy (RE)*

Response entropy is computed over a frequency range of 0.8–47 Hz
and includes the EEG- and EMG-dominant part of the spectrum.
Response entropy measurement is designed to respond to fast
changes. For example, when patients during anaesthesia become
aroused RE rises first with muscle activation and SE changes a few
seconds later. On average, RE indicates emergence from anaesthesia
7 s faster than SE.[10]

▶ *RE and SE*

The system normalises RE and SE in such a way that RE becomes
equal to SE when the EMG power (sum of spectral power between
32 and 47 Hz) is equal to zero. The RE–SE difference then serves as
an indication of EMG activation.[9] EMG data are used in addition
to EEG information because the sudden appearance of EMG signals
appears to provide an early warning of nociception and light
anaesthesia.

Practical Aspects of Entropy Monitoring

The measurement range of the device is 0–100 (to avoid decimal
numbers with a 0–1 range). Response entropy ranges from 0–100
while state entropy varies from 0–91.

Application of the Electrodes

1 The skin on the forehead and temple is carefully wiped with an
   alcohol wipe and allowed to dry.
2 A disposable Entropy Sensor is placed with three electrodes
   applied to the forehead and temple.

Interpretation of Measurements

1 Two numbers are displayed: the SE and RE.
2 RE between 45 and 70 indicates a surgical depth of hypnosis.
   RE and SE numbers can be interpreted in a similar way to the
   equivalent BIS monitoring numbers. See *BISPECTRAL INDEX
   (BIS) EEG MONITOR*.

T

Sources of Error[9]

1   *NDNMBDs*: Electrical activity in the facial muscles is very resistant to neuromuscular blocking drugs.
2   *Electrocautery*: In most cases, the hardware of the entropy module is able to ignore electrocautery signals. The device can also detect that electrocautery interference is occurring and reject the data.
3   *Cardiac pacemakers*: No effect.
4   *Blinking and eye movement*: The monitor is able to detect and reject these signals.

Tonsillectomy, Bleeding after Surgery

The main anaesthetic issues are:

1   hypovolaemia and anaemia due to haemorrhage, requiring resuscitation ± blood transfusion
2   'full stomach' due to swallowing of blood
3   potential difficulty to intubate the patient due to blood, oedema and distortion of airway anatomy
4   potential underlying bleeding disorder.

Pre-anaesthetic Phase

1   Adequately resuscitate the patient's intravascular volume. Transfuse blood if required.
2   Obtain skilled assistance and notify the surgeon who must be present in the operating theatre.
3   Ensure at least two separate suction units are working and accessible.

Anaesthetic Phase

The main anaesthetic options are:

1   gaseous induction with the patient in the left lateral position with intubation when the patient is 'deep' and still lateral

2 rapid sequence induction with thiopentone, suxamethonium and cricoid pressure. See *RAPID SEQUENCE INDUCTION (RSI)*.

Perform nasogastric drainage of blood from the stomach before extubation.

Torsade De Pointes

This is a polymorphic ventricular tachycardia. The QRS complexes appear to twist around the baseline on the ECG. When the patient is in sinus rhythm this condition is associated with a long Q-T interval and U waves. A ventricular beat during the Q-T interval initiates the ventricular tachycardia.

These abnormalities can be congenital or acquired due to electrolyte abnormalities or drugs. Patients with sick sinus syndrome, AV block, and those who have had a right radical neck dissection tend to have an increased incidence of prolongation of the Q-T interval.[11]

Patient Medications Associated with a Long Q–Tc[12]

1 Anti-arrhythmic drugs such as quinidine, procainamide, disopyramide, amiodarone and sotalol.
2 Phenothiazines.
3 Tricyclic antidepressants, haloperidol.
4 Lithium.
5 Cisapride.
6 Terfenadine.
7 Erythromycin.

Electrolyte Abnormalities Associated with a Long Q–Tc[12]

1 Hypokalaemia.
2 Hypomagnasaemia.
3 Hypocalcaemia.

See *ELECTROCARDIOGRAPHY*.

Prevention of Torsade de Pointes in Patients with a Prolonged Q–Tc Interval

Avoid drugs which prolong the Q–T interval, such as isoflurane, sevoflurane and droperidol.[13] Halothane shortens the Q–Tc interval. Propofol shortens the Q–T interval but not the Q–Tc.

Treatment

1 Cease aggravating factors such as sevoflurane (see *SEVOFLU-RANE*). Use a propofol infusion to maintain anaesthesia if surgery cannot be terminated.

2 Torsade frequently resolves spontaneously but ventricular fibrillation can occur.

3 Overdrive transvenous pacing is probably the treatment of choice in the non-compromised patient but is difficult to organise rapidly.[14] While this is being organised consider increasing the heart rate with a bolus of isoprenaline 20 µg, then an infusion. See *ISOPRENALINE*.

4 The drug treatment of choice is magnesium sulphate.[14] Give 2 g IV (4 mL of the 50% solution) over 10–15 min. Follow this dose with an infusion of 0.5–0.75 g/h for 12–24 h.

5 Increasing the heart rate with atropine is suggested if there is an underlying bradycardia.[14] However, this may be counter-productive as atropine (and glycopyrronium) may increase the Q–T interval.[15]

6 Lignocaine may be useful.[14] Give 75–100 mg over 1–2 min, then an infusion. See *LIGNOCAINE*.

7 If cardiovascular collapse occurs treat as for ventricular fibrillation. See *CARDIAC ARREST*.

8 Correct the underlying disturbance if possible, e.g. hypokalaemia.

Total Intravenous Anaesthesia (TIVA)

See *PROPOFOL*.

Total 'Spinal'

See *EPIDURAL ANAESTHESIA*.

Tracheal Intubation, Attenuating Hypertensive Response to

See *HYPERTENSIVE RESPONSE TO INTUBATION (ATTENUATION OF)*.

Tracheostomy, Elective

Anaesthetic Management of the Intubated Patient

1   Position the patient with a 1 L bag of fluid between the scapulae. Have the neck extended and the head resting on a head ring. Ensure that the patient is adequately paralysed.

2   Deflate the endotracheal tube cuff when the surgeon is just about to incise the trachea. If the surgeon ruptures the endotracheal tube cuff during the dissection, change to a bag ventilation technique, which is easier to control than the ventilator. If the leak is too large, ask the surgeon to 'plug' the tracheal stoma to improve the seal.

3   Increase the FiO_2 to 100% 5 min before the tracheal tube is inserted and ensure that the patient is adequately paralysed. There is an increased risk of tracheal fire when 100% O_2 is used. O_2 and N_2O also support combustion. However, the risk of airway fire must be weighed against the risk of desaturation if complications occur with tracheal tube insertion. Precautions against airway fire in this situation include:[16]

   (a) filling the cuff of the endotracheal tube with saline
   (b) ensuring there is no cuff leak
   (c) pushing the cuff of the endotracheal tube to just above the carina.

   If a fire occurs:
   (a) Disconnect the endotracheal tube from the O_2 supply.

T

(b) Extinguish the fire, e.g. cut a large hole in a litre bag of N/S and pour an adequate amount over the fire to extinguish it.

(c) When the fire is extinguished and the charred tube fragments are removed, reintubate the patient.

(d) Evaluate the extent of fire injury by bronchoscopy and laryngoscopy.

(e) Manage the patient postoperatively in the intensive care unit.

4   When the surgeon is ready to insert the tracheal tube, pull the endotracheal tube back slowly under your direct vision until the tube is just cephalad to the tracheal stoma. This way, if there is a problem with tracheal tube insertion the endotracheal tube can be easily reinserted into the trachea.

Tramadol Hydrochloride

Tramadol is an atypical opiod analgesic drug that is also useful for treating postoperative shivering. See *SHIVERING POSTOPERATIVELY*. A synthetic 4-phenyl-piperidine analogue of codeine, tramadol has a mu opioid receptor agonist action and also blocks the neuronal reuptake of monoamine oxidase, noradrenaline and serotonin.[17] Tramadol has 10–15% of the potency of morphine parenterally.[17] Tramadol is inferior to morphine for treating severe pain.[18]

Dose

Adult PO, IM, PR dose: 50–100 mg 4–6 h. The maximum recommended daily dose is 600 mg. Oral dose requires ≈ 20 min–1 h to have an effect and the effect peaks after ≈ 2 h.

Adult IV/IM bolus dose: 50–100 mg IV over 2–3 min or IM 4–6 h. For severe pain follow a 100 mg bolus with 50 mg boluses every 10–20 min to a maximum total dose of 250 mg.

Adult IV infusion dose: Give an initial bolus dose of 100 mg over 2–3 min. Load 200 mg of tramadol in 500 mL of N/S. Run an infusion of 15 mg/h (= 38 mL/h). Reduce the rate after 6 h.

Adult patient-controlled analgesia: Give an initial bolus dose of 100 mg over 2–3 min. Load 300 mg of tramadol in 60 mL N/S. Begin with a bolus dose of 20 mg with a 5 minute lockout.

Adult epidural dose: 100 mg in 10 mL N/S epidurally can provide effective postoperative analgesia. This dose can be repeated as required to a maximum of 400 mg/day.[19]

Paediatric dose: 1–2 mg/kg PO, IM or total IV dose 4–6 h.

Advantages

1   Tramadol has a relative lack of serious side effects compared with opioids and non-steroidal anti-inflammatory drugs. There is a low potential for respiratory depression and dependence.[20]

2   The drug is well-absorbed orally.

3   Tramadol does not cause spasm of the sphincter of Oddi.[18] Urinary retention and constipation is less likely than with other opioids.

4   Tramadol does not cause morphine effects or a withdrawal effect in patients on methadone.[21]

5   Tramadol is thought to be safe to use in labour, and is unlikely to cause birth defects during pregnancy.[21]

Disadvantages

1   Tramadol is mainly metabolised by the liver with 30% excreted in the urine as unchanged drug.[18]

2   60% of tramadol's metabolites are excreted in the urine. Therefore use the drug cautiously in the presence of renal/liver impairment.

3   There is a risk of seizures if the patient is receiving drugs that lower the seizure threshold, such as tricyclic antidepressants and monoamine oxidase inhibitors, or if the patient has a history of seizures.[18]

4   There is a risk of serotonin syndrome if tramadol is given with a drug that increases serotonin levels in the CNS, e.g. selective

T

serotonin reuptake inhibitors such as sertraline, tricyclic anti-depressants, meclobemide, venlafaxine and St John's wort.[22]

5   Tramadol can cause dizziness, nausea, confusion, drowsiness and headache. Nausea caused by tramadol is not antagonised by ondansetron.[21]

6   Rapid IV injection of tramadol may cause hypotension due to peripheral vasodilation.[23]

Tranexamic Acid

This is an antifibrinolytic drug that decreases bleeding and trans-fusion requirements during cardiac surgery.[24] The drug acts by attaching to the lysine binding site on the plasmin molecule, displacing plasminogen from fibrin.[25] A suggested dosage is 10 mg/kg loading dose, then an infusion of 1 mg/kg/h.[26]

Transcutaneous Cardiac Pacing

See *PACEMAKERS AND ANAESTHESIA*.

Transtracheal Jet Ventilation

Facilitated by a device such as a Sanders injector. This device consists of a length of high pressure tubing connected directly to the 'wall' O_2 outlet and the distal end to the injector. The injector is hand-held with a button that, when depressed, releases high pressure O_2. A second length of pressure tubing is attached to the injector and has a luer lock at its distal end. This can be used to attach the tubing to a cannula placed in the trachea. Half-second 'bursts' of O_2 are usually sufficient to ventilate an adult. Look for chest inflation to help judge jet ventilation time. One person must concentrate solely on maintaining the cannula in place. Insufflation of the tissues is a constant risk.

Transurethral Resection of Prostate (TURP)

The main challenges associate with TURP surgery are blood loss and TURP syndrome due to excessive absorption of glycine. The transfusion rate is about 6%.[27]

Anaesthesic Technique

A regional or general anaesthetic technique is equally satisfactory.[28] It is important that the patient does not cough as this makes surgery more difficult. If regional anaesthesia is used, anaesthesia to T9 is required.[29] An appropriate dose of heavy bupivacaine 0.5% is 3 mL for most patients. It is very important to minimise the absorption of bladder irrigation fluid and prevent hyponatraemia.

Methods of achieving these aims and other important aspects of anaesthetic care include the following:

1 Limit the height of the irrigation bag to 60 cm above the prostate.[30] The bag should *not* be pressurised and frequent bladder emptying should occur. Ensure that only 1.5% glycine is used for bladder irrigation, *not water*.

2 Limit resection time to ≤ 1 h.[30]

3 Give prophylactic gentamicin 120–240 mg, especially if the patient is chronically catheterised.

4 Only use N/S for IV fluid replacement.

5 Treat hypotension associated with spinal anaesthesia with vasopressors rather than large volumes of IV crystalloid solution.[31]

6 Erection can interfere with surgery. If persistent spray the base of the penis with ethyl chloride. If erection persists, consider an injection of metaraminol 0.5 mg in 10 mL of N/S injected into the corpus cavernosum, with a tourniquet around the base of the penis.[32]

T

TURP Syndrome

This is due to excessive absorption of glycine and consists of:

1 *hyponatraemia*, leading to a decreased level of consciousness and/or seizures. Severe reactions are usually associated with serum Na$^+$ < 120 mmol/L. For a description of ECG changes associated with hyponatraemia see *ELECTROCARDIOGRAPHY*.
2 *hypervolaemia*, resulting in problems such as pulmonary oedema
3 *ventricular tachycardia or fibrillation*, if serum Na$^+$ falls to 100 mmol/L or less
4 *visual disturbances, haemolysis and coagulopathy*.

Treatment of TURP Syndrome

1 Ensure adequate airway, ventilation and satisfactory pulse rate and mean arterial pressure.
2 Cease glycine infusion as soon as possible.
3 Measure serum Na$^+$. If this is > 120 mmol/L and the patient is asymptomatic, treat with fluid restriction and N/S as sole IV replacement fluid.
4 If serum Na$^+$ < 120 mmol/L and the patient is symptomatic, give 50–100 mL boluses of hypertonic saline over 1 h. Recheck serum Na$^+$ after each bolus. Rapid correction of hyponatraemia may cause central pontine myelinolysis. Correct serum Na$^+$ to 120 mmol/L only, and do not increase serum Na$^+$ by more than 12 mmol/L per day. If hypertonic saline is not available consider boluses of *sodium bicarbonate*.[31]
5 Treat pulmonary oedema in the usual way; give O$_2$ therapy, sit the patient up and give *frusemide* 40 mg IV. See *PULMONARY OEDEMA*.

Laser Prostatectomy

Using a Neodymium:Yag laser, laser prostatectomy is associated with minimal blood loss and minimal irrigation fluid absorption.[33]

Tricuspid Regurgitation and Ebstein's Anomaly

Tricuspid Regurgitation

▶ Aetiology

Causes of tricuspid regurgitation include:

1 functional, being secondary to dilation of the right ventricle as occurs in pulmonary hypertension and right ventricular volume overload due to aortic stenosis
2 rheumatic fever. There is usually tricuspid stenosis as well.

Infective endocarditis is often associated with IV drug use.

▶ Pathophysiology

Tricuspid regurgitation causes right atrial volume overload, which is usually well-tolerated. Associated conditions such as pulmonary hypertension are more important to consider. See *PULMONARY HYPERTENSION*.

▶ Anaesthetic Considerations[34]

Tailor the anaesthetic as for the underlying condition, e.g. aortic stenosis or pulmonary hypertension. In general:

1 Provide antibiotic prophylaxis (see *BACTERIAL ENDOCARDITIS PROPHYLAXIS*).
2 Maintain intravascular volume and CVP in the high normal range to maintain RV stroke volume.
3 Avoid high intrathoracic pressure.
4 Avoid factors that increase pulmonary vascular resistance (see *PULMONARY HYPERTENSION*).

Ebstein's Anomaly

▶ Description

This is a congenital condition characterised by the following:[34]

1 Malformed tricuspid valve leaflets which may be displaced downwards into the right ventricle may be present.
2 The part of the right ventricle adjacent to the valve is atrialised and the remaining functional RV is thus small.
3 The tricuspid valve is usually regurgitant but may be stenotic.
4 There is usually an inter-atrial communication (80%) such as an ASD or patent foramen ovale through which there may occur right to left shunting of blood.

▶ Clinical Features

The condition may cause a wide spectrum of effects from congestive cardiac failure in neonates to asymptomatic adults.

Clinical effects include:
1 heart murmur, usually systolic
2 supraventricular and ventricular dysrhythmias. Wolff-Parkinson-White syndrome may occur in up to 20% of patients.[35]
3 cyanosis
4 paradoxical embolism through the inter-atrial communication
5 congestive cardiac failure
6 ECG usually showing tall wide P waves and first degree AV block
7 possible massive enlargement of the right atrium. A cardio-thoracic ratio on CXR of > 0.65 is a predictor of sudden death.[36]

▶ Anaesthetic Management

Due to the rarity of this condition it is difficult to provide clear anaesthetic guidelines from the literature.

1 Provide antibiotic prophylaxis (see *BACTERIAL ENDOCARDITIS PROPHYLAXIS*).
2 Use appropriate monitoring (e.g. arterial line, CVP), depending on the severity of the patient's condition and the nature of the surgery. PA catheter insertion may provoke life-threatening dysrhythmias.[37] When inserting a central line ensure that the

Seldinger wire and the tip of the CVP line stay within the SVC. CVP lines may increase the risk of bacterial endocarditis.[36]

3 Induction times may be prolonged due to pooling of induction drugs in the enlarged right atrium.[36]

4 Provide cardiovascular stability by maintaining preload, afterload and sinus rhythm. Tachycardia is poorly tolerated due to reduced filling of the small RV.

5 Factors which increase right-to-left shunt (if present) must be avoided. These include hypotension, raised intrathoracic pressure and pulmonary vasoconstriction. See *PULMONARY HYPERTENSION* and *EISENMENGER'S SYNDROME*.

6 IPPV may cause increased right to left shunting due to increased intrathoracic pressure.

7 An opioid-based 'cardiac' anaesthetic may help provide optimal CVS stability more effectively than volatile agents.

8 Avoid introducing any intravascular air due to the risk of paradoxical emboli.

▶ *Obstetric Implications*

1 There should be close consultation between anaesthetist, cardiologist and obstetrician.

2 The extra cardiovascular stress of pregnancy can precipitate symptoms or cause life-threatening deterioration in patients with Ebstein's anomaly. This deterioration may include RV failure, worsening right-to-left shunting and worsening dysrhythmias.

3 In the absence of cyanosis and dysrhythmias, pregnancy tends to be well-tolerated.[37]

4 Epidural anaesthesia has been used successfully in these patients for labour and delivery.[37,38] Establishment of the block should be done slowly and carefully with appropriate monitoring, e.g. arterial line, central line, ECG monitoring.

5 Use epidural opioids to help minimise epidural LA requirements. Consider intrathecal opioids.

6   Do not use adrenaline-containing LA solutions.
7   It is very important to minimise the risk of intravascular air due to the risk of paradoxical embolism. For example, do not use a loss-of-resistance-to-air technique when siting the epidural.
8   Aorto-caval compression must be avoided.
9   SAB anaesthesia for CS is contraindicated in patients significantly affected by Ebstein's anomaly.[35]
10 Syntocinon should be used cautiously due to its vasodilating effects and prostaglandin $F_{2\alpha}$ is suggested as a possible alternative.[35] Ergometrine should be avoided due to its vasoconstrictive effects on the pulmonary vasculature.[35]

Trimetaphan

This is a monoquaternary sulfonium derivative and acts as a ganglion blocker at sympathetic and parasympathetic ganglia. It does this by competing with acetylcholine at cholinergic receptor sites. It also has some direct vasodilating properties and causes histamine release.[39] Used for its hypotensive effects.

Dose

Adults: Mix 500 mg in 250 mL of 5% glucose. Give trimetaphan by infusion, starting at a rate of 25 µg/kg/min and titrate to response. In a 70 kg patient = 50 mL/h. Can also give boluses of 1–4 mg (0.5–2 mL of above solution). Acts rapidly and effects wear off ≈ 30 min after cessation of infusion.
Note: Do not use in asthma (releases histamine).[39]

Tropisetron

5-HT$_3$ receptor antagonist antiemetic drug.
Adult dose: 2 mg IV over at least 30 s once daily.

Uu

Umbilical Vein Catheterisation

See *NEONATAL RESUSCITATION*.

Uterine Atonia, Postpartum

See *POSTPARTUM HAEMORRHAGE*

Uterine Inversion

This is an obstetric emergency associated with:

1 severe haemorrhage/exsanguination
2 cardiovascular instability due to haemorrhage and vasovagal reflexes secondary to traction on the peritoneum.[1] There may also be traction on sympathetic nerves producing neurogenic shock.
3 severe pain.

Treatment

1 An attempt should be made by the obstetrician to *immediately* push the uterus back to its normal position. However, the constricted cervix may prevent this. Urgently transfer the patient to the operating theatre.
2 Resuscitate the patient with IV fluid volume replacement via large bore IV cannulas, using crystalloid/colloid/blood as appropriate.
3 Provide analgesia for the patient's often severe pain.
4 Induce GA with a rapid sequence induction (see entry).
5 Provide uterine relaxation with increased inhaled concentration of volatile anaesthetic agent. If insufficient relaxation effect give

U

glyceryl trinitrate IV or sublingually as described for *UTERINE RELAXATION FOR RETAINED PLACENTA* below.

6   Rarely, laparotomy may be required to replace the uterus.

Uterine Relaxation for Retained Placenta

Uterine relaxation may be required for a retained placenta, external version of the second twin and uterine inversion. Uterine relaxation can be obtained by giving an increased concentration of volatile inhalational anaesthetic agent during general anaesthesia. Rapid uterine relaxation can also be obtained by giving IV glyceryl trinitrate (GTN) 50 μg boluses[2] or sublingual metered dose spray (e.g. 800 μg).[1]

Preparation of IV Glyceryl Trinitrate for Uterine Relaxation

Remove 1 mL from an ampoule containing 50 mg of glyceryl trinitrate in 10 mL (5 mg) and dilute to 10 mL with N/S. Take 1 mL (500 μg) from this solution and dilute to 10 mL, resulting in a final concentration of 50 μg/mL. Give 1 mL boluses as required. The dose required is variable but 100–200 μg is usually effective.[3]

Uterine Rupture

Description

The incidence of uterine rupture is about 0.05% of all deliveries with a maternal mortality of about 10% and a foetal mortality of about 20%.[4] Risk factors include uterine scar, use of oxytocics to augment labour, prolonged labour, and breech extraction.

Symptoms and Signs

1   Abdominal pain which is often atypical.
2   Acute foetal bradycardia or sudden profound foetal distress may be seen.

3   PV blood loss.
4   Hypovolaemic shock.
5   Change in abdominal shape.
6   Haematuria.

Anaesthetic Management

1   Ensure adequate patient airway and breathing.
2   Resuscitate the patient's intravascular volume with appropriate IV fluids (crystalloid, colloid, blood).
3   Immediate laparotomy is usually required.
4   General anaesthesia is usually required but, if the mother and foetus are stable, regional anaesthesia can be considered.[5]

U

Vv

Valdecoxib

Long-acting oral COX2 selective NSAID. Also available as a parenteral prodrug, Parecoxib.

Vasa Previa

In this condition the umbilical vessels run through the membranes between the foetal presenting part and the cervix. Normal vaginal delivery is impossible and foetal death from haemorrhage is very likely once the membranes rupture. Management is elective CS in cases diagnosed prelabour and emergency CS in cases diagnosed during labour.

Vasopressin

Acts by causing vasoconstriction through activation of V1 receptors. Also causes antidiuresis through its actions on V2 receptors in the distal tubule of the kidney. This drug is useful:

1   for the treatment of vasodilatory shock associated with severe sepsis unresponsive to a noradrenaline infusion
2   for the treatment of vasodilatory shock related to post-cardiopulmonary bypass unresponsive to a noradrenaline infusion
3   for the treatment of uncontrolled bleeding oesophageal varices
4   as an alternative vasopressor to adrenaline in the management of shock-resistant VF.

Dose

For vasodilatory shock, administer as an IV infusion, preferably through a central line. Mix 20 units (u) of vasopressin with 40 mL of 5% glucose run at 0.08–0.1 units/min = 10–12 mL/h. For VF cardiac arrest give 40 u as a single dose. See *CARDIAC ARREST*.

Vecuronium

NDNM blocking bis-quaternary aminosteroid analogue of pancuronium.

Dose

0.1 mg/kg IV with recovery occurring in about 30 min. Can also be given by infusion at a rate of 50–80 µg/kg/h.

Advantages

1 Vecuronium is very cardiovascularly stable, lacking the tachycardic effects of pancuronium.
2 Low potential for histamine release.
3 May be lower risk of allergic reaction than rocuronium. See *ROCURONIUM*.

Disadvantages

1 Effects of vecuronium may be prolonged in renal and liver failure. About 25% of the vecuronium dose is excreted unchanged by the kidney; the rest is metabolised by the liver.
2 Must be reconstituted from powder form at the time of injection.
3 Slower onset than rocuronium.

Veins of the Upper Limb

See Figure V1 overleaf.

V

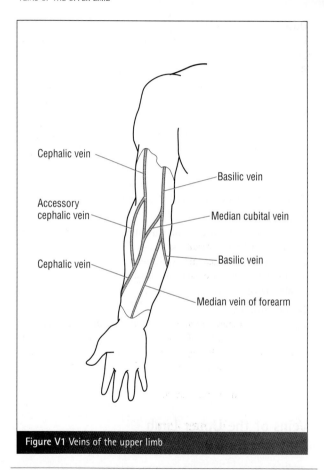

Figure V1 Veins of the upper limb

Venous Gas Embolism

See *GAS EMBOLISM, VENOUS*.

Ventricular Ectopic Beats (VEBs)

VEBs are not life-threatening if there is no underlying heart disease. VEBs after a myocardial infarction may precede ventricular fibrillation but treatment of VEBs is probably *not* beneficial (IV lignocaine is *no longer* recommended).[1] Ensure electrolytes are normal and treat any other possible underlying cause such as myocardial ischaemia. β blockers may be tried in patients who are symptomatic from VEBs, e.g. *atenolol* 25–50 mg PO 12–24 h.

Ventricular Ejection Fraction

See *CARDIAC INVESTIGATIONS*.

Ventricular Fibrillation

See *CARDIAC ARREST*.

Ventricular Tachycardia (VT)

Defined as > two consecutive ventricular ectopic beats. Termed sustained ventricular tachycardia if the duration of the tachycardia is more than 30 seconds.[2] Subdivided into monomorphic and polymorphic VT.[2]

Monomorphic VT

(QRS complexes have the same morphology.) It is the most common cause of broad complex tachycardia, but supraventricular tachycardia (SVT) with aberrant conduction can look similar. See *BROAD COMPLEX TACHYCARDIA*. Always seek early expert cardiology assistance.

V

Treatment of Monomorphic VT in the Cardiovascularly Compromised Patient

1 *If pulseless VT, give immediate non-synchronised DC shocks 200 J, 300 J, 360 J (see CARDIAC ARREST).*

2 If the patient has adverse signs defined as SBP < 90 mmHg, chest pain, heart failure, or a heart rate > 150 bpm, cardiovert the patient under sedation or anaesthesia.[3] Use synchronised monophasic shocks of 100 J, 200 J, 360 J. If using biphasic cardioversion, about half the energy of monophasic defibrillation is required.

3 If the initial cardioversion is unsuccessful give an anti-arrhythmic drug such as sotalol (possibly the drug of choice)[4] or amiodarone and repeat cardioversion.

4 Identify and treat the cause of the VT if possible, e.g. give IV potassium and magnesium if hypokalaemia is present.

5 Overdrive RV pacing may be effective.[5]

Treatment of Monomorphic VT in the Cardiovascularly Stable Patient

1 If the patient is cardiovascularly stable give sotalol 1–1.5 mg/kg IV over 5 min. Give a repeat dose of 0.5–0.75 mg/kg if needed. Alternatively, use amiodarone 5 mg/kg IV over 30 min, then IV infusion of 10–15 mg/kg over 24 h.

2 Procainamide can be considered.

3 If pharmacotherapy unsuccessful perform R wave synchronised DC monophasic cardioversion 100 J under sedation or anaesthesia. If using biphasic cardioversion, about half the energy of monophasic defibrillation is required.

4 Overdrive RV pacing may be effective.[4]

Polymorphic VT Treatment

1 *If pulseless VT, give immediate non-synchronised DC shocks 200 J, 300 J, 360 J (see CARDIAC ARREST).*

2 If the patient has adverse signs as described above first decide if the Q-T interval is prolonged. If yes, the patient may be suffering from torsade de pointes. See *TORSADE DE POINTES*. Look at the rhythm tracing for the distinctive pattern of torsades—a widening and narrowing pattern.

3 If the Q-T interval is not prolonged treat as for monomorphic VT.

Verapamil

Calcium channel blocking drug useful for the treatment of:

1 hypertension
2 angina
3 dysrhythmias such as supraventricular tachycardia (SVT), atrial fibrillation and atrial flutter.

Dose

Adult: For the treatment of dysrhythmias give 1 mg IV increments to a maximum of 10 mg.

Problems with Verapamil—Contraindications and Interactions

1 Adenosine rather than verapamil is now the drug of choice for treating SVT. Several fatalities have occurred from giving verapamil to patients with broad complex tachycardia in the mistaken belief that an SVT rather than VT was occurring. *Verapamil must never be given in the presence of an undiagnosed broad complex tachycardia.*[6]

2 Patients given verapamil while receiving β receptor blocking drugs or inhalational agents may suffer severe bradycardias.[7]

3 Verapamil and dantrolene, in combination, may cause severe hyperkalaemia and resultant ventricular fibrillation.[8]

4 Verapamil is contraindicated in AF associated with Wolff-Parkinson-White syndrome, sick sinus syndrome and second or third degree heart block. It is also contraindicated in heart failure, cardiogenic shock and porphyria.[9]

V

Ww

Warfarin

Synthetic coumarin derivative used as an anticoagulant for the treatment and prevention of venous and arterial thromboembolism. Acts by preventing the synthesis of vitamin K dependent clotting factors II, VII, IX and X.

Dose

Adult: Give 10 mg PO on day 1 of therapy, then daily at the estimated daily maintenance dose, usually 5 mg/day. After day 3, adjust the dose depending on the measured prothrombin time, INR and the therapeutic target. If giving heparin or low molecular weight (LMW) heparin, overlap heparin with warfarin for at least 5 days and do not cease heparin or LMW heparin until the INR is in the target range. See Table W1.

Table W1 Target INR for various disease states	
Diagnosis	**Desirable INR range**
Prosthetic heart valve	2.5–3.5
Recurrent severe DVT/PE, arterial thrombo-embolic disease	2.5–3.5
DVT, PE, valve lesions, prevention of thrombo-embolus after MI, AF, TIAs	2.0–3.0
Tissue heart valves for 3 months after insertion	2.0–3.0
DVT prophylaxis	2.0–2.5

W

Warfarin and Surgery

An INR < 1.5 is 'safe' for surgery to proceed. If INR > 1.5 warfarin effects can be reversed with fresh frozen plasma and vitamin K. See *FRESH FROZEN PLASMA (FFP)*. Vitamin K 1 mg IV slowly will antagonise the effects of warfarin but 8–12 h is required. Although IV vitamin K has been associated with anaphylactic reactions a new product with a mixed micelle formation called Konakion MM is thought to be much safer.[1]

Weights of Children

Table W2 Estimated weights and ages of children	
Average age	Estimated weight (kg)
Neonate	3
4 months	6
1–8 years	(2 × age) + 9
9–13 years	3.3 × age

Whole Blood

Defined as blood collected with an anticoagulant and without further processing. Platelets and white cells in whole blood become non-viable after a few days. There are few indications for whole blood, such as neonatal exchange transfusions.

Leukocyte-depleted whole blood has been filtered to remove most of the white cells. It is indicated:

1 for patients who have febrile non-haemolytic transfusion reactions

W

2   to reduce the risk of HLA alloimmunisation in patients who are likely to have repeated transfusions
3   to reduce the risk of transmission of white cell carried infections such as cytomegalovirus.

Wolff–Parkinson–White Syndrome

This is a pre-excitation syndrome producing tachyarrhythmias. An accessory atrio-ventricular connection pathway enables atrial depolarisation to be conducted to the ventricles much faster than through the atrio-ventricular (AV) node. Characteristic ECG findings are:

1   PR interval < 0.12 s (3 mm)
2   slurred upstroke on QRS complex (delta wave), QRS is prolonged
3   secondary ST segment and T wave changes.

These patients are prone to the following dysrhythmias:

1   supraventricular tachycardia (80%). In 85% the QRS complexes are narrow and in 15% they are widened.
2   atrial fibrillation/atrial flutter (20%). These can be life-threatening because ventricular rate can be very fast. QRS complexes are irregular and wide.

Treatment of WPW Syndrome Dysrhythmias

▶ *Regular Narrow Complex SVT*

1   Seek expert cardiology advice early. Contact the patient's cardiologist if possible. Find out what treatments have been used successfully in the past.
2   If the patient is cardiovascularly stable, aim to decrease the rate of AV node conduction. Try vagal manoeuvres such as carotid sinus massage.
3   If unsuccessful give adenosine (see *ADENOSINE*). Verapamil or a β blocker drug may be helpful. Procainamide may work in resistant episodes.[2]

W

4 Use synchronised DC cardioversion with sedation or anaesthesia if the patient becomes unstable or the above treatment is not successful.

▶ *Atrial Fibrillation or Irregular Wide Complex Tachycardia Thought to be Atrial Fibrillation*

There is usually marked variation in the width of the QRS complex and variability in the tachycardia. This dysrhythmia should not be treated by drugs decreasing AV node conduction. *Do not use digoxin or verapamil.*[3] This can lead to very fast ventricular rates due to rapid conduction down the accessory pathway. This can in turn lead to degeneration into ventricular fibrillation. Treatment includes the following:

1 Procainamide is the drug of choice.[2]
2 Adenosine may temporarily break the re-entrant cycle but is usually not effective in converting the atrial fibrillation.[4]
3 Use synchronised DC cardioversion with sedation or anaesthesia if the patient becomes unstable or the above treatment is not successful.
4 Prior electrophysiological studies may have indicated which drugs are effective in individual patients. If possible discuss drug therapy with the patient's cardiologist.

▶ *Long-term Treatment*

1 Chronic oral therapy with amiodarone or sotalol may reduce recurrence rates.
2 Radio-frequency catheter ablation of the accessory pathway or surgical ablation may provide a cure.

Wrist Blocks

The median, ulnar and radial nerves can all be blocked at the wrist. For the distribution of these nerves in the hand see *ELBOW BLOCKS*.

Distal arm blocks are not recommended when a tourniquet is used, except for short procedures.[5]

Technique

▶ *Median Nerve*

Lies between the tendon of palmaris longus (roughly in the middle of the wrist) and flexor carpi radialis (just lateral to palmaris longus).

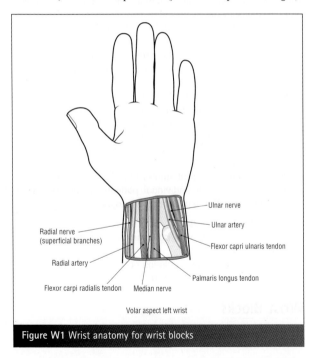

Ulnar nerve

Ulnar artery

Flexor capri ulnaris tendon

Radial nerve
(superficial branches)

Radial artery

Palmaris longus tendon

Flexor carpi radialis tendon   Median nerve

Volar aspect left wrist

Figure W1 Wrist anatomy for wrist blocks

W

Mark the point 2 cm proximal from the most distal wrist crease, between these tendons. Insert 25 G needle through to the deep fascia at this point and paraesthesia should be obtained at a depth of < 1 cm.[6] Inject 5 mL of LA as the needle is withdrawn.

▶ *Ulnar Nerve*
Insert the needle on the ulnar side of the ulnar artery (between the ulnar artery and flexor carpi ulnaris) to the ulnar styloid. Inject 5 mL of LA as the needle is withdrawn.

▶ *Radial Nerve*
Insert the needle just lateral to the radial artery 2.5 cm proximal to the wrist joint. Inject 3 mL of LA, then inject a superficial ring of LA solution dorsally over the border of the wrist into the 'anatomical snuff box' area (between the extensor tendons of thumb).

Xx

Xenon

'Inert' noble gas with potent anaesthetic properties at atmospheric pressure that may provide a practical alternative to N_2O.

Physical Properties and MAC

Blood:gas solubility coefficient	0.14
Oil:gas solubility coefficient	1.9
Boiling point	–107.1°C
MAC	71

Advantages

1   Xenon probably does not undergo biotransformation.
2   Rapid induction and emergence from anaesthesia.
3   Not thought to be teratogenic.[1]
4   Does not trigger malignant hyperthermia.[2]
5   Xenon has minimal effects on the cardiovascular system.[2]

Disadvantages

1   Xenon is very expensive ($60/L)[3] as it must be prepared from air. Xenon's concentration in air is only 0.0000087%.[4]
2   Cerebral blood flow is increased by xenon concentration > 60%.[2]

Zz

Ziconotide

Omega conotoxin calcium channel blocking drug isolated from a type of Philippino sea snail. Useful for postoperative analgesia and does not produce tolerance.

Zolpidem

Imidazopyridine hypnotic drug useful for sedation. Acts by binding selectively to the $omega_1$ benzodiazepine receptor subtype.

Dose
Adults: 10 mg PO.

Appendix 1: Drug Infusion Regimes Summary

Adrenaline

Mix 6 mg adrenaline with 100 mL N/S; start infusion at 5 mL/h. Titrate to effect.

Dobutamine

Mix 250 mg dobutamine with 100 mL N/S.

Dose range 0.5–40 µg/kg/min. For a 70 kg patient = 1–60 mL/h (usual range required 5–20 mL/h).

Dopamine

Mix 200 mg dopamine with 100 mL N/S.

Dose range 1–20 µg/kg/min. For a 70 kg patient = 2–40 mL/h.

Esmolol

Presented as a solution containing 10 mg/mL.

Give LD 0.5 mg/kg over 1 min, then infusion 50–150 µg/kg/min. For a 70 kg patient = 21–63 mL/h.

Isoprenaline

Mix 2 mg in 50 mL 5% glucose. Start infusion at 1.5 mL/h; dose range for adults is 1–10 µg/min (1.5–15 mL/h).

Glyceryl Trinitrate

Mix 250 mg GTN with 500 mL 5% glucose.

In adults run at 10–400 µg/min = 1–40 mL/h.

Noradrenaline

Mix 6 mg noradrenaline with 100 mL 5% glucose.

In adults start infusion at 5 mL/h and titrate to effect.

Phenytoin

Mix 15–18 mg/kg phenytoin with 100 mL N/S (not glucose). Infuse no faster than 50 mg/min.

Sodium Nitroprusside

Mix 50 mg SNP with 100 mL 5% glucose.
Dose range 0.3–6 µg/kg/min. For a 70 kg patient run at 2.5–50 mL/h (up to 80 mL/h in an emergency).

Appendix 2: Some Important Biochemical and Haematological Reference Ranges

Sodium	136–146 mmol/L
Potassium	3.2–5.5 mmol/L
Chloride	94–107 mmol/L
Carbon dioxide	24–31 mmol/L
Anion gap	12–20 mmol/L
Urea	2.5–6.5 mmol/L
Creatinine	60–125 µmol/L
Total bilirubin	2–21 µmol/L
Total protein	63–84 g/L
Albumin	35–53 g/L
Alkaline phosphatase	30–115 U/L
Gamma-glutamyl transpeptidase	8–43 U/L
Alanine aminotransferase	10–47 U/L
Prothrombin time	11–18 s
Activated partial thromboplastin time	25–36 s
White cell count	4–11×10^9/L
Haemoglobin	130–180 g/L
Platelets	150–400×10^9/L
Troponin levels	0–0.05 µg/L no myocardial damage 0.05–0.1 µg/L minor cardiac damage > 0.1 µg/L significant cardiac damage

References

A

1   Katz DJ, Stanley JC, Zelenock GB. Operative mortality rates for intact and ruptured abdominal aortic aneurysms in Michigan: an eleven-year statewide experience. *J Vasc Surg* 1994;19:804–15.

2   Halfpenny M, Rushe C, Breen P, Cunningham AJ, Boucher-Hayes D, Shorten GD. The effects of fenoldopam on renal function in patients undergoing elective aortic surgery. *Eur J Anaesthesiol* 2002;19:32–9.

3   Gelman S. The pathophysiology of aortic cross-clamping and unclamping. *Anesthesiology* 1995;82:1026–60.

4   Wallace A, Layug B, Tateo I et al. Prophylactic atenolol reduces post-operative myocardial ischaemia. *Anesthesiology* 1998;88:7–17.

5   Davies MJ, Silbert BS, Mooney PJ, Dysart RH, Meads AC. Combined epidural and general anaesthesia versus general anaesthesia for abdominal aortic surgery: a prospective randomized trial. *Anesth Intensive Care* 1993;21:790–4.

6   Walker GV, Beattie C. Abdominal Aortic Aneurysm Repair. In: Roizen MF, Fleisher LA (eds.). *Essence of Anesthesia Practice*. WB Saunders, Philadelphia, 1997, p. 337.

7   Cunningham AJ. Anaesthesia for abdominal aortic surgery—a review (part 1). *Can J Anaesth* 1989;36:426–44.

8   McCroy C, Cunningham AJ. Low dose dopamine: will there ever be a scientific rationale? *Br J Anaesth* 1997;78:350–1.

9   Rubin LA, Rosner HL. Abdominal Aortic Aneurysm Repair Resection and Postoperative Pain Management. In: Yao F-SF. (ed.). *Yao and Artusio's Anesthesiology: Problem Orientated Patient Management*. Lippincott-Raven, Philadelphia, 1998, pp. 296–315.

10   Cunningham AJ. Anaesthesia for abdominal aortic surgery—a review (part 2). *Can J Anaesth* 1989;36:568–77.

11 Baker AB, Lloyd G, Fraser TA, Bookalil MJ, Yezerski SD. Retrospective review of 100 cases of endoluminal aortic stent-graft surgery from an anaesthetic perspective. *Anaesth Intensive Care* 1997;25:378–84.

12 Baxendale BR, Baker DM, Hutchinson A, Chuter TAM, Wenham PW, Hopkinson BR. Haemodynamic and metabolic response to endovascular repair of infra-renal aortic aneurysms. *Br J Anaesth* 1996; 77:581–5.

13 Brimacombe J, Berry A. A review of anaesthesia for ruptured abdominal aortic aneurysm with special emphasis on preclamping fluid resuscitation. *Anaesth Intensive Care* 1993;21:311–23.

14 Ernst CB. Abdominal aortic aneurysm. *New Eng J Med* 1993;328:1167–72.

15 Crawford ES. Ruptured abdominal aortic aneurysm: an editorial. *J Vasc Surg* 1991;13:348–50.

16 Obstetrical Haemorrhage. In: Cunningham FG, MacDonald PC, Gant NF et al. (eds.). *Williams Obstetrics*, 20th edn. Stamford, CT, Appleton and Lange, 1997, p. 746.

17 Ross BK. Critical care issues in obstetric anesthesia. *Audio Digest Anesthesiology* 1999;41.

18 Terui K. Antepartum Haemorrhage. In: Birnbach DJ, Gatt SP, Datta S. *Textbook of Obstetric Anesthesia*. Churchill Livingstone, Philadelphia, 2000, p. 401.

19 Schwarte LA, Hartmann M. Intentional circulatory arrest to facilitate surgical repair of a massively bleeding artery. *Anesth Analg* 2003;97:339–40.

20 *Cardiovascular Drug Guidelines*, 2nd edn, Victorian Medical Post Graduate Foundation Inc. Australia, 1995, p. 119.

21 McDonogh AJ. The use of steroids and nebulized adrenaline in the treatment of viral croup over a seven year period in a district hospital. *Anaesth Intensive Care* 1994;22:175–8.

22 MacDonnell SPJ, Timmins AC, Watson JD. Adrenaline administered via a nebulizer in adult patients with upper air way obstruction. *Anaesthesia* 1995;50:35–6.

23 O'Connell AJ, Keneally J P. Paediatric burns. *Curr Anaesth Crit Care* 1994;5:209–17.

24 Benumof JL. Airway exchange catheters: Simple concept, potentially great danger (Editorial). *Anesthesiology* 1999;91:342–4.

25 Matejtschuk P, Dash CH, Gascoigne EW. Production of human albumin solution: a continually developing colloid. *Br J Anaesth* 2000;85: 887–95.

26 Cochrane Injuries Group Albumin Reviewers. Human albumin administration in critically ill patients: systematic review of randomized controlled trials. *Br Med J* 1998;317:235–40.

27 The SAFE Study Investigators. A comparison of albumin and saline for fluid resuscitation in the intensive care unit. *N Eng J Med* 2004;350(22):2247–56.

28 Levy JH. *Anaphylactic Reactions in Anesthesia and Intensive Care*, 2nd edn. Butterworth-Heinemann, Boston, 1992, p. 133.

29 Kudenchuk PJ, Cobb LA, Copass MK et al. Amiodarone for resuscitation after out of hospital cardiac arrest due to ventricular fibrillation. *N Eng J Med* 1999;341:871–8.

30 Silfast T, Pettila V. Amiodarone versus lidocaine for shock resistant ventricular fibrillation. *N Eng J Med* 2002;347:368–70.

31 Stern R. *Drugs, Diseases and Anaesthesia.* Lippincott-Raven, Philadelphia, 1997, pp. 9–10.

32 Morgan M. Amniotic fluid embolism. *Anaesthesia* 1979;34:30–2.

33 Davies MG, Harrison JC. Amniotic fluid embolism: maternal mortality revisited. *Brit J Hosp Med* 1992;47:775–6.

34 Cattaneo AN. Air and amniotic fluid embolus. In: Birnbach DJ, Gatt SP, Datta S (eds.). *Textbook of Obstetric Anaesthesia.* Churchill Livingstone, Philadelphia, 2000, pp. 435–54.

35 Fisher M. Clinical observations on the pathophysiology and treatment of anaphylactic cardiovascular collapse. *Anaesth Intensive Care* 1986;14:17–21.

36 Laxenaire MC, Mertes PM. Anaphylaxis during anaesthesia. Results of a 2 year survey in France. *Br J Anaesth* 2001;87:549–58.

37 Mertes PM, Laxenaire M-C, Allergic reactions during anaesthesia. *Eur J Anaesthesiol* 2002;19:240–62.

38 Guidelines 2000 for cardiopulmonary resuscitation and emergency cardiovascular care. *Circulation* 2000;102(suppl):I-41–I-243.

39 Fisher MM. Anaphylaxis. In: Bersten AD, Soni N, Oh TE (eds.). *Oh's Intensive Care Manual*, 5th edn. Butterworth-Heinemann, Edinburgh, 2003, pp. 617–20.

40 Fischer M, Baldo BA. The diagnosis of fatal anaphylactic reactions during anaesthesia: employment of immunoassays for mast cell tryptase and drug reactive IgE antibodies. *Anaesth Intens Care* 1993;21:353–7.

41 Mulroy MF. *Regional Anaesthesia; An Illustrated Procedural Guide*, 2nd edn. Little, Brown and Company, Boston, 1996, p. 212.

42 Kearon C, Hirsh J. Management of anticoagulation before and after elective surgery. *N Eng J Med* 1997;336;21:1506–11.

43 Souto JC, Oliver A, Zazu-Jausoro I, Vives A, Fontcuberta J. Oral surgery in anticoagulated patients without reducing the dose of oral anticoagulant. *J Oral Maxillofacial Surg* 1996;54:27–32.

44 Otley CC, Fewkes JL, Frank W, Olbricht SM. Complications of cutaneous surgery in patients who are taking warfarin, aspirin or non-steroidal anti-inflammatory drugs. *Arch Dermatol* 1996;132:161–6.

45 Dujardin KS, Enriquez-Sarano M, Schaff HV et al. Mortality and morbidity of aortic regurgitation in clinical practice. A long term follow-up study. *Circulation* 1999;99:1851–7.

46 ACC/AHA Guideline update for perioperative cardiovascular evaluation for noncardiac surgery—executive summary: A report by the ACC/AHA task force on practice guidelines (Committee to update the 1996 guidelines on perioperative cardiovascular evaluation for noncardiac surgery). *J Am Coll Cardiol* 2002;39:542–53.

47 O'Keefe JH Jr, Shub C, Retkke SR. Risk of noncardiac surgical procedures in patients with aortic stenosis. *Mayo Clin Proc* 1989;64:400–5.

48 Mason R. *Anaesthesia Databook*, 3rd edn. Greenwich Medical Media Limited, London, 2001, p. 46.

49 Brighouse D. Anaesthesia for Caesarean section in patients with aortic stenosis: the case for regional anaesthesia. *Anesthesia* 1998;53:107–9.

50 Whitfield A, Holdcroft A. Anaesthesia for Caesarean section in patients with aortic stenosis: the case for general anaesthesia. *Anesthesia* 1998;53:109–11.

51 Levy JH. Novel pharmacological approaches to reduce bleeding. *Can J Anesth (supplement)* 2003;50:S26–S30.

52 Peters DC, Noble S. Aprotinin: an update of its pharmacology and therapeutic use in open heart surgery and coronary artery bypass surgery. *Drugs* 1999;57:233–60.

53 Janssens M, Joris J, David JL et al. High dose aprotinin reduces blood loss in patients undergoing total hip replacement surgery. *Anesthesiology* 1994;80:23–9.

54 Kirby RR, Taylor RW, Civetta JM. *Pocket Companion of Critical Care: Immediate Concerns.* JB Lippincott Company, Philadelphia, 1990, pp. 35–7.

55 Aitkenhead AR, Smith G (eds.). *Textbook of Anaesthesia,* 2nd edn. Churchill Livingstone, Edinburgh, 1990, pp. 338–9.

56 Teabeault JR. Aspiration of gastric contents: Experimental study. *Am J Pathol* 1952;28:51–67.

57 Tuxon DV. Aspiration syndromes. In: Oh TE (ed.). *Intensive Care Manual,* 3rd edn. Butterworths, Oxford, 1990, p. 216.

58 Yao F-SF. Aspiration Pneumonitis and Acute Respiratory Failure. In: Yao F-SF (ed.). *Yao and Artusio's Anesthesiology: Problem Orientated Patient Management,* 4th edn. Lippincott-Raven, Philadelphia, 1998, pp. 53–85.

59 Bishop MJ. Anaesthesia for patients with asthma. *Anesthesiology* 1996;85:455–6.

60 Mason R. *Anaesthesia Databook,* 3rd edn. Greenwich Medical Media Limited, London, 2001, p. 55.

61 Hirshman C. Perioperative management of the asthmatic patient. *Can J Anaesth* 1991;38:4:26–32.

62 Kablin CS, Yarnold PR, Grammer LC. Low complication rate of corticosteroid treated asthmatics undergoing surgical procedures. *Arch Intern Med* 1995;155:1379–84.

63 Tait AR, Knight PR. Intraoperative respiratory complications in patients with upper respiratory tract infections. *Can J Anaesth* 1987;34:300–3.

64 Goff MJ, Shahbaz RA, Ficke DJ, Uhrich TD, Ebert TJ. Absence of bronchodilation during desflurane anaesthesia. *Anesthesiology* 2000;93:404–8.

65 McAlpine LG, Thomson NC. Lidocaine-induced bronchoconstriction in asthmatic patients. Relation to histamine airway responsiveness and effect of preservatives. *Chest* 1989;96:1012–15.

66 Kim ES, Bishop MI. Endotracheal intubation, but not laryngeal mask airway insertion, produces reversible bronchoconstriction. *Anesthesiology* 1999;90:391–4.

67 Mashford ML, Cosolo W, Day RO et al. *Therapeutic Guidelines: Analgesic,* 3rd edn. Therapeutic Guidelines Limited on behalf of the Victorian Drug Use Advisory Committee, Melbourne, 1997, p. 61.

68 Fodale V, Santamaria LB. Laudanosine, an atracurium and cisatracurium metabolite. *Eur J Anesthesiol* 2002;19:466–73.

69 Nathanson MH, Gajraj NM. Review article: The perioperative management of atrial fibrillation. *Anaesthesia* 1998;53:665–76.

70 Sanyhavi S, Rayner-Klein J. Management of pre arrest arrhythmia. *Br J Anaesth COPD Reviews* 2002;4:104–12.

71 Mittal S, Ayati S, Stein KM et al. Transthoracic cardioversion of atrial fibrillation. Comparison of rectilinear biphasic versus damped sine wave monophasic shocks. *Circulation* 2000;101:1282–7.

72 *Cardiovascular Drug Guidelines,* 2nd edn. Victorian Medical Post Graduate Foundation Inc., Australia, 1995, p. 115.

73 Holt A. Management of Cardiac Arrhythmias. In: Bersten AD, Soni N, Oh TE (eds.). *Oh's Intensive Care Manual,* 5th edn. Butterworth-Heinemann, Edinburgh 2003, pp. 157–205.

74 Cobcroft MD, Forsdick C. Awareness under anaesthesia: the patient's point of view. *Anaesth Care* 1993;21:837–43.

75 Schwender D, Klasing S, Daunderer M, Madler C, Poppel E, Peter K. Awareness during general anesthesia. Definition, incidence, clinical relevance, causes, avoidance and medicolegal aspects. *Anaesthestist* 1995;44:743–54.

76 Ottevaere JA. Awareness During Anaesthesia. In: Duke J (ed.). *Anesthesia Secrets,* 2nd edn. Hanley and Belfus Inc, Philadelphia, 2000, pp. 165–8.

77 Jenkins K, Baker AB. Review article: Consent and anaesthetic risk. *Anaesthesia* 2003;58:962–84.

78 Bailey AR, Jones JG. Patient's memories of events during general anaesthesia. *Anaesthesia* 1997;52:460–76.

B

1 Prevention of bacterial endocarditis. Recommendations by the American Heart Association. *JAMA* 1997;277:1794–801.

2 *Antibiotic Guidelines,* 9th edn. Victorian Medical Post Graduate Foundation Inc., Australia, 1996, pp. 92–5.

3   Prasad A, Fraser AG. Prevention of infective endocarditis: enthusiasm tempered by realism. *Br J Hosp Med* 1995;54:341–6.

4   Mulroy MF. *Regional Anaesthesia; an Illustrated Procedural Guide*, 2nd edn, Little Brown and Company, Boston 1996, p. 186.

5   Roscow CE. Can we measure the depth of anaesthesia? *American Society of Anesthesiologists 50th Annual Refresher Course lectures* 1999;114:1–7.

6   Bloom MJ, Whitehurst S, Mandel M, Policare R. Bispectral index as an EEG measure of the sedative effects of isoflurane (Abstract). *Anesthesiology* 1995;83(3A):A195.

7   Glass P, Gan TJ, Sebel PS, Rosow C, Kearse L, Bloom M, Manberg P. Comparison of the bispectral index (BIS) and measured drug concentrations for the monitoring effects of propofol, midazolam, alfentanil and isoflurane. (Abstract). *Anesthesiology* 1995;83(3A):A374.

8   Kearse L, Rosow C, Connors P, Denman W, Dershwitz M. Propofol sedation/hypnosis and bispectral EEG analysis in volunteers. (Abstract). *Anesthesiology* 1995;83(3A):A506.

9   Gan TJ, Glass PS, Windsor A, Payne F, Roscow C, Sebel P, Manberg P and the BIS Utility Study Group. Bispectral index monitoring allows faster emergence and improved recovery from propofol, alfentanil, and nitrous oxide anaesthesia. *Anesthesiology* 1997;87:808–15.

10 Myles PS, Leslie K, McNeil J, Forbes A, Chan MTV. Bispectral Index monitoring to prevent awareness during anaesthesia: the B-Aware randomized controlled trial. *Lancet* 2004;363:1757–63.

11 Yli-Hankala A, Vakkuri A, Annila P, Korttila K. EEG bispectral index monitoring in sevoflurane or propofol anaesthesia: analysis of direct costs and immediate recovery. *Acta Anesthesiol Scand* 1999;43:545–9.

12 Mathes DD. Bleomycin and hyperoxia exposure in the operating room. *Anesth Analg* 1995;81:624–9.

13 Gorbock MS. Inflation of the endotracheal tube cuff as an aid to blind nasal intubation. (Letter) *Anesth Analg* 1987;66:913.

14 American College of Surgeons, Committee on Trauma. *Advanced Life Support Course Manual*. Chicago, American College of Surgeons, 1989.

15 *Paediatric Trauma Service Manual* for the New Children's Hospital 1996, p. 23.

16   Brimacombe J, Berry A. A review of anaesthesia for ruptured abdominal aortic aneurysm with special emphasis on preclamping fluid resuscitation. *Anaesth Intensive Care* 1993;21:311–23.

17   Bond AC, Davies CK. Ketamine and pancuronium for the shocked patient. *Anaesthesia* 1974;29:59–62.

18   Sessler DI. Symposium article; deliberate mild hypothermia. *J Neurosurg Anesthesiology* 1995;7:38–46.

19   Ramsa JG. Methods of reducing blood loss and non blood substitutes. *Can J Anaesth* 1991;38:592–612.

20   Monk TG. Alternatives to allogenic blood transfusions. *Can J Anesth* 1999;46:R3–6.

21   Goodnough LT, Monk TG, Andriole GL. Erythropoietin therapy. *N Engl J Med* 1997;336:933–8.

22   Report by the ASA task force on blood component therapy. Practice guidelines for blood component therapy. *Anesthesiology* 1996;84:732–47.

23   Crosby ET. Review article: Perioperative haemotherapy part 1, indications for blood component transfusion. *Can J Anaesth* 1992;39:695–707.

24   Goodnough LT, Brecher ME, Kanter MH, Aubuchon JP. Transfusion medicine (first of two parts) Blood transfusion. *N Eng J Med* 1999;340:438–47.

25   Goskowicz R. Massive transfusion: problems and solutions in blood conservation/massive transfusion. *Audio Digest* 1996;38:23.

26   Trauma Committee of the Royal Australian College of Surgeons. *Early Management of Severe Trauma Course Manual.* 1992, p. 61.

27   Lovric VA. Alterations in blood components during storage and their clinical significance. *Anesth Intensive Care* 1984;12:246–51.

28   Benumof JL. Sleep apnoea and the obese patient. *Audio Digest: Anesthesiology* 2000;42.

29   Al-Haddad MF, Coventry DM. Brachial plexus blockade. *Br J Anaesth CEPD Reviews* 2002:33–6.

30   Lavoie J, Martin R et al. Axillary brachial plexus block using a peripheral nerve stimulator: single or multiple injections. *Can J Anaesth* 1992;39:583–6.

31   Wagner PJ, Sharrock NE. Update in regional anaesthesia for shoulder surgery. *Curr Opin Anaesthesiology* 1998;11:503–6.

32   Sukhani R, Barclay J, Aasen M. Prolonged Horner's syndrome after interscalene block: a management dilemma. *Anesth Analg* 1994;79:601–3.

33   Bridenbaugh LD. The upper extremity: somatic blockade. In: Cousins MJ, Bridenbaugh PO (eds.). *Neural Blockade in Clinical Anaesthesia and Management of Pain*, 2nd edn. JB Lippincott Company, Philadelphia, 1988, pp. 387–416.

34   Pham-Dang C, Gunst J-P, Gouin F et al. A novel supraclavicular approach to brachial plexus block. *Anesth Analg* 1997;85:111–16.

35   Wilson JL, Brown DL, Wong GY et al. Infraclavicular brachial plexus block: parasagittal anatomy important to the coracoid technique. *Anesth Analg* 1998;87:870–3.

36   Kilka HG, Geiger P, Mehrkens HH. Infraclavicular vertical brachial plexus blockade. A new method for anaesthesia of the upper extremity. An anatomical and clinical study. *Anaesthestist* 1995;44:339–44.

37   Poon L. The use of naropin (ropivacaine HCL) for interscalene blocks using a catheter for post operative pain relief. *AstraZeneca Block of the Month educational leaflet*, 2003.

38   Carling A, Simmonds M. Complications from regional anaesthesia for carotid endarterectomy. *Br J Anaesth* 2000;84:797–800.

39   Devitt JH. Refresher Course outline: Blunt thoracic trauma: anaesthesia, assessment and managenment. *Can J Anaesth* 1993;40: R29–34.

40   Guidelines 2000 for cardiopulmonary resuscitation and emergency cardiovascular care. *Circulation* 2000;102(suppl):I-237–I-240.

41   Hemmingsen C, Kielson P, Ordorico J. Ketamine in the treatment of bronchospasm during mechanical ventilation. *Am J Emerg Med* 1994;12:417–20.

42   Hirshman CA. Perioperative management of the asthmatic patient. *Can J Anaesth* 1991;38:R26–32.

43   Goff MJ, Shahbaz RA, Ficke DJ, Uhrich TD, Ebert TJ. Absence of bronchodilation during desflurane anaesthesia. *Anesthesiology* 2000;93:404–8.

44 Patel A, Harrison E, Durward A, Murdoch IA. Intrathecal recombinant human deoxyribonuclease in acute life-threatening asthma refractory to conventional treatment. *Br J Anaesth* 2000;84:505–7.

45 Manthous CA, Hall JB, Caputo MA et al. Heliox improves pulsus paradoxus and peak expiratory flow in nonintubated patients with severe asthma. *Am J Respir Crit Care Med* 1995;151:310–14.

46 Covino BG. Recent advances in local anaesthesia. *Can J Anaesth* 1991;38:R26–32.

47 Juels AN. Anesthesia and burns. In: Duke J, Rosenberg SG (eds.). *Anesthesia Secrets*. Hanley & Belfus, Inc, Philadelphia, Mosby, St Louis, 1996, pp. 352–5.

48 Miller RD, Savarese JJ. Pharmacology of muscle relaxants and their antagonists. In: Miller RD (ed.). *Anesthesia*, 3rd edn. Churchill Livingstone, New York, 1990, pp. 414–15.

49 Hilton PJ, Hepp M. The immediate care of the burned patient. *Br J Anaesth CEPD Reviews* 2001;1:113–16.

50 Shaw A, Anderson J et al. The early management of large burns. *Br J Hosp Med* 1995;53:247–50.

51 O'Connell AJ, Keneally JP. Paediatric burns. *Current Anaesth and Crit Care* 1994;5:209–17.

52 Mackie DP. Burns. In: Bernsten AD, Soni N, Oh TE (eds.). *Oh's Intensive Care Manual*, 5th edn. Butterworth-Heinemann, Oxford, 2003, pp. 755–62.

53 Oxer HF. Hyperbaric oxygen—an interest for anaesthetists? *Australasian Anaesthesia* 1992;25–33.

54 Gorman DF, Clayton D, Gilligan JE, Webb RK. A longitudinal study of 100 consecutive admissions for carbon monoxide poisoning to the Royal Adelaide Hospital. *Anaesth Intensive Care* 1992;20:311–16.

55 Brogan TV, Sharar SR. Toxic gas, fume, and smoke inhalation. In: Parrillo JE (ed.). *Current Therapy in Clinical Care Medicine*, 3rd edn. Mosby, St Louis, 1997, pp. 258–63.

56 Atkinson RS, Rushman GB, Davies NJH. *Lee's Synopsis of Anesthesia*, 11th edn. Butterworth-Heinemann, Oxford, 1993, pp. 851–2.

57 Sykes MK, Vickers MD, Hull CJ, Winterburn PJ, Shepstone BJ. *Principles of Measurement and Monitoring in Anaesthesia and Intensive Care*, 3rd edn. Blackwell Scientific Publications, Oxford, 1991, p. 265.

58 Pace N, Strajman E, Walker EL. Acceleration of carbon monoxide elimination in man by high pressure oxygen. *Science* 1950;111:652.

59 Hartmann GS. Burns. In Yao F-SF (ed.). *Anesthesiology: Problem Orientated Patient Management*, 4th edn. Lippincott-Raven, Philadelphia 1998, pp. 898–918.

C

1 Department of Health and Social Security. *Report on Confidential Enquiries into Maternal deaths in the United Kingdom*, 1994–1996. London HSMO, 1999.

2 Hawkins JL, Koonin LM, Palmer SK, Gibbs CP. Anaesthesia related deaths during obstetric delivery in the United States, 1979–1990. *Anesthesiology* 1997;86:277–84.

3 Barnardo PD, Jenkins JG. Failed tracheal intubation in obstetrics: a 6 year review in a UK region. *Anaesthesia* 2000;55:685–94.

4 Preston R. Editorial: The evolving role of the laryngeal mask airway in obsterics. *Can J Anesth* 2001;48:1061–5.

5 Han T-H, Brimacombe J, Lee E-J. The laryngeal mask airway is effective (and probably safe) in selected healthy parturients for elective Caesarean section: a prospective study of 1067 cases. *Can J Anesth* 2001;48:1117–21.

6 Morris S. Management of difficult and failed intubation in obstetrics. *Br J Anaesth CEPD Reviews* 201;4:117–21.

7 Hewett E, Livingstone P. Management of failed endotracheal intubation at caesarean section. *Anaesth Intensive Care* 1990;18:330–5.

8 Setayesh AR, Kholdebarin AR, Moghadam MS, Setayesh HR. The Trendelenberg position increases the spread and accelerates the onset of epidural anaesthesia for Caesarean section. *Can J Anesth* 2001;48:890–3.

9 Policy statement 4.3. 5 July 1997. Australian Resucitation Council.

10 Policy statement 6.3. 3 February 2002. Australian Resucitation Council.

11 Paradis NA, Martin GB, Goetting MG et al. Simultaneous aortic, jugular bulb and right atrial pressure during cardiopulmonary resuscitation in humans: insight into mechanisms. *Circulation* 1989;80:361–8.

12 Policy statement 11.2. 2 July 1999. Australian Resuscitation Council.

13 Gullo A. Cardiac arrest, chain of survival and Utstein style. *Eur J Anaesthesiol* 2002;19:624–33.

14 Revised policy statement 11. 3 July 2002. Australian Resuscitation Council.

15 Vincent R. Drugs in modern resuscitation. *Br J Anaesth* 1997;79:188–97.

16 Kudenchuk PJ, Cobb LA, Copass MK et al. Amiodarone for resuscitation after out-of-hospital cardiac arrest due to ventricular fibrillation. *New Eng J Med* 1999;341:871–8.

17 Cass DP, Schwartz B, Cooper R, Gelaznikas R, Barr A. Amiodarone as compared with lignocaine for shock-resistant ventricular fibrillation. *New Eng J Med* 2002;346:884–90.

18 Rosen KR, Elizabeth H, Casto S, Casto J. Basic and advanced life support, acute resuscitation, and cardiac resuscitation. *Curr Opin Anaesthiology* 2001;14:177–84.

19 Riley DP, Hales PA. Transcutaneous cardiac pacing for asystole during permanent pacemaker lead repositioning. *Anaesth Intensive Care* 1992;20:524–5.

20 Policy statement 5. 4 July 1991. Australian Resuscitation Council.

21 Policy statement 6.2. 3 July 1997 Australian Resuscitation Council.

22 Guidelines 2000 for cardiopulmonary resuscitation and emergency cardiovascular care. *Circulation* 2000;102 (suppl I): I-247–I-249.

23 Younberg JA. Anesthetic considerations for major vascular surgery. Annual refresher course lecture. *American Society of Anesthesiologists* 1997;245:1–7.

24 Fleisher LA, Barash PG. Review article. Preoperative cardiac evaluation for noncardiac surgery: a functional approach. *Anesth Analg* 1992;74:586–958.

25 Older P. *CPX: Testing: Who Needs It.* Anaesthetic Continuing Education Seminar notes printed by the Australian Society of Anaesthetists and the Australian and New Zealand College of Anaesthetists, July 1995.

26 Palacios IF, Miller SW. Coronary arteriography and left ventriculography. In: Eagle KA, Haber E, DeSanctis RW, Austen WG (eds.). *The Practice of Cardiology*, 2nd edn. Little, Brown and Company, 1989, pp. 1644–7.

27 Soni N. *Practical Procedures in Anaesthesia and Intensive Care*. Butterworth-Heinemann, Oxford, 1994, p. 79.

28 ACC/AHA Guideline update for perioperative cardiovascular evaluation for noncardiac surgery—executive summary: A report by the ACC/AHA task force on practice guidelines (Committee to update the 1996 guidelines on perioperative cardiovascular evaluation for noncardiac surgery). *J Am Coll Cardiol* 2002;39:542–53.

29 Chassot P-G, Delabays A, Spahn DR. Preoperative evaluation of patients with, or at risk of, coronary artery disease undergoing noncardiac surgery. *Br J Anaesth* 2002;89:747–59.

30 Mathes DD, Stone DJ, Dent JM. Special article: preoperative cardiac risk stratification: ritual or requirement. *J Cardiothoracic Vascular Anaesthesia* 2001;15:626–30.

31 Kaluza GL, Joseph J, Lee JR, Raizner ME, Raizner AE. Catastrophic outcomes of noncardiac surgery soon after coronary stentng. *J Am Coll Cardiol* 2000;35:1288–94.

32 Poldermans D, Boersma E, Bax JJ et al. Dutch Echocardiographic Cardiac Risk Evaluation Applying Stress Echocardiography Study Group. Bisoprolol reduces cardiac death and myocardial infarction in high risk patients as long as 2 years after successful major vascular surgery. *Eur Heart J* 2001;22:1353–825.

33 Park KW. Review article: Perioperative cardiology consultation. *Anesthesiology* 2003;98:754–62.

34 Olympio MA. The preoperative evaluation of symptomatic carotid endarterectomy: a debated issue. *J Neurosurgical Anesthesiol* 1996;8:310–3.

35 Mazer CD. Con: Combined coronary and vascular surgery is not better than separate procedures. *J Cardiothoracic Vascular Anesth* 1998;12:228–30.

36 Davies MJ, Dysart RH, Silbert BS, Scott DA Cook RJ. Prevention of tachycardia with atenolol pre-treatment for carotid endarterectomy under cervical plexus blockade. *Anaesth Intensive Care* 1992;20:161–4.

37 Lineberger C, Lubarsky DA. Anesthesia for carotid endarterectomy. *Current Opin in Anaesthesiol* 1998;11:479–84.

38 Wilke HJ, Ellis JE, McKinsey JF. Carotid endarterectomy: perioperative and anaesthetic considerations. *J Cardiothoracic Vasc Anesth* 1996;7:928–49.

39 Lien CA, Van Poznak A. Carotid Endarterectomy. In: Yao F-SF (ed.). *Yao and Artusio's Anesthesiology: Problem Orientated Patient Management*, 4th edn. Lippincott-Raven 1998, pp. 455–81.

40 Gottlieb A, Satariano-Hayden P, Schoenwald P, Rykman J, Piedmonte M. The effects of carotid sinus nerve blockade on hemodynamic stability after carotid endarterectomy. *J Cardiothoracic Vasc Anesth* 1997;11:67–71.

41 Wilkes M, Hickey N. Anaesthesia for carotid surgery. *Br J Hosp Med* 1995;53:31–4.

42 Stoneham MD, Knighton JD. Review article: regional anaesthesia for carotid endarterectomy. *Br J Anaesth* 1999;82:910–19.

43 Lewis MP, Thomas P, Wilson LF, Mulholland RC. The 'whoosh' test. A clinical test to confirm correct needle placement in caudal epidural injections. *Anaesthesia* 1992;47:1002–3.

44 Prentiss JE. Cardiac arrest following caudal anaesthesia. *Anesthesiology* 1979;50:51.

45 Sinclair JC, Fox HA, Lentz JF, Fuld GL et al. Intoxication of the foetus by a local anaesthetic. A newly recognised complication of maternal caudal anaesthesia. *N Eng J Med* 1965;273:1173.

46 Murphy PM. *Essays and MCQs in Anaesthesia and Intensive Care*. Edward Arnold, London 1995, p. 88.

47 Gravlee GP. Blood conservation strategies. *Audio Digest* 1996;38:23.

48 National heart, lung and blood institute autologous transfusion symposium working group. Autologous transfusion: current trends and research issues. *Transf* 1995;35:525–30.

49 Brown V. Clinical strategies to avoid blood transfusion. *Anaesthesia and Intensive Care Medicine* 2004;5:68–70.

50 Cull RE, Will RG. Diseases of the Nervous System. In Edwards CRW, Bouchier IAD, Haslett C, Chilvers ER (eds.). *Davidson's Principles and Practice of Medicine*, 17th edn. Churchill Livingstone, Edinburgh, 1995, pp. 1022–115.

51 Hunt WE, Hess RM. Surgical risk as related to time of intervention in the repair of intracranial aneurysms. *J Neurosurg* 1968;28:14–20.

52 Sutcliffe AJ. Subarachnoid haemorrhage due to cerebral aneurysm. *Br J Anaesth CEPD Reviews* 2002;2:45–8.

53 Guy J, McGrath BJ, Borel Co et al. Perioperative management of aneurysmal subarachnoid haemorrhage: Part 1. Operative management. *Anesth Analg* 1995;81:1060–72.

54 Rayner K, Choi P. Concurrent subarachnoid haemorrhage and myocardial injury. *Can J Anaesth* 1997;44:515–19.

55 Archer DP, Leblanc RL. Haemodynamic considerations in the management of patients with subarachnoid haemorrhage. *Can J Anaesth* 1991;38:454–70.

56 Young WL. Cerebral aneurysms: current anaesthetic management and future horizons. *Can J Anaesth* 1998;45:R17–24.

57 Bedfort NM, Hardman JG, Nathanson MH. Cerebral hemodynamic response to the introduction of desflurane: a comparison with sevoflurane. *Anesth Analg* 2000;91:152–5.

58 Mack PF. Cerebral Aneurysm. In Yao F-SF (ed.). *Anesthesiology: Problem Orientated Patient Management*, 4th edn. Lippincott-Raven, Philadelphia, 1998, pp. 504–24.

59 Traill R. Neurosurgical anaesthesia. *Bailliere's Clinical Anaesth* 1993;7:2:399–422.

60 Emery G, Handley G, Davies MJ, Mooney PH. Incidence of phrenic nerve block and hypercapnia in patients undergoing carotid endarterectomy under cervical plexus block. *Anesth Intensive Care* 1998;26:377–81.

61 Kam AC, O'Brien M, Kam PCA. Pleural drainage systems. *Anaesthesia,* 1993;48:154–61.

62 Savarese JJ, Deriaz H et al. The pharmacodynamics of cisatracurium in healthy adults. *Curr Opin Anaesthesiology* 1996;9:(suppl 1): s16–22.

63 Fodale V, Santmaria LB. Review: Laudanosine, an atracurium and cisatracurium metabolite. *Eur J Anaesthesiol* 2002;19:466–73.

64 Pollard BJ. Rocuronium and cisatracurium. *Br J Hosp Med* 1997;57:346–8.

65 Eisenach J, De Kock M, Klimscha W. Alpha 2 adrenergic agonists for regional anaesthesia; a clinical review of clonidine (1984–1995). *Anesthesiology* 1996;85:655–74.

66 Aantaa R, Scheinin M. Alpha 2 adrenergic agents in anaesthesia. *Acta Anaesthesiol Scand* 1993;37:433–48.

67 Goldsack C, Scuplak S, Smith M. A double-blind comparison of codeine and morphine for postoperative analgesia following intracranial surgery. *Anaesthesia* 1996;51:1029–32.

68 Hirsch N. Advances in neuroanaesthesia. *Anaesthesia* 2003;58:1162–203.

69 Williams DG, Hatch DJ, Howard RF. Review article: Codeine phosphate in paediatric medicine. *Br J Anaesth* 2001;86:413–21.

70 Eichinger S, Schreiber W, Heinz T et al. Airway management in a case of neck impalement: use of the oesophageal tracheal combitube airway. *Br J Anaesth* 1992;68:534–5.

71 *Cardiovascular Drug Guidelines*, 2nd edn. Victorian Medical Postgraduate Foundation Therapeutics Committee, Melbourne, 1995, p. 133.

72 Dobb CJ. Cardiogenic shock. In: Oh TE (ed.). *Intensive Care Manual*, 4th edn. Butterworth-Heinemann, Oxford, 1997, pp. 146–52.

73 Johnson MR. Congestive heart failure. In: Parrillo JE (ed.). *Current Therapy in Clinical Care Medicine*, 3rd edn. Mosby, St Louis, 1997, pp. 109–15.

74 Francis GS. Congestive heart failure: Inotropic agents. In: Parrillo JE (ed.). *Current Therapy in Clinical Care Medicine*, 3rd edn. Mosby, St Louis, 1997, pp. 116–21.

75 Runciman WB, Webb RK, Klepper ID et al. Crisis management— validation of an algorithm by an analysis of 2000 incident reports. *Anaesth Intensive Care* 1993;21:579–92.

76 Bowyer M. Blood products and coagulation. In: Parsons PE, Wiener-Kronish JP (eds.). *Critical Care Secrets*. Hanley & Belfus, Inc, Philadelphia, Mosby-Year Book, Inc, St Louis, 1992, p. 263.

77 Forbes AM. Colloids and blood products. In: Oh TE (ed.). *Intensive Care Manual*, 4th edn. Butterworth-Heinemann, Oxford, 1997, p. 756.

78 Bowyer MW. Blood products and coagulation. In: Parsons PE, Weiner-Kronish JP (eds.). *Critical Care Secrets*. Hanley & Belfus, Philidelphia Mosby-Year Book, St Louis, 1992, pp. 267–70.

D

1   Yentis SM, Hirsch NP, Smith GB. *Anaesthesia and Intensive Care A–Z*, 2nd edn. Butterworth-Heineman, Oxford, 2000, p. 216.

2   The National Working Party on the Management and Prevention of Venous Thromboembolism. (Booklet) *Prevention of Venous Thromboembolism Best Practice Guidelines for Australian and New Zealand,* 2nd edn. HEMI, 2001.

3   Bullingham A, Strunin L. Prevention of postoperative venous thromboembolism. *Br J Anaesth* 1995;75:622–30.

4   Hertzberg M, Koutts J, Guy D et al. *Guidelines for Anticoagulation.* Prepared by the Drug Committee, Westmead Hospital and Community Health Services, 1999.

5   Mittal S, Ayati S, Stein KM et al. Comparison of a novel rectilinear biphasic waveform with a damped sine wave monophasic waveform for transthoracic ventricular defibrillation. *J Am Coll Cardiol* 1999;34:1595–601.

6   Bardy GH, Marchlinski FE, Sharma AD et al. Multicenter comparisons of truncated biphasic shocks and standard damped sine wave monophasic shocks for transthoracic ventricular defibrillation. *Circulation* 1996;94:2507–14.

7   Valenzuela TD, Roe DJ Nichol G et al. Outcomes of rapid defibrillation by security officers after cardiac arrest in casinos. *N Eng J Med* 2000;343:1206–9.

8   Guidelines 2000 for cardiopulmonary resuscitation and emergency cardiovascular care. *Circulation* 2000;102 (suppl I):I-40.

9   Guidelines 2000 for cardiopulmonary resuscitation and emergency cardiovascular care. *Circulation* 2000;102 (suppl I):I-320.

10 Apfelbaum JL. The new inhaled agents. *Audio Digest Anesthesiology* 1996;21.

11 Goff MJ, Shahbaz RA, Ficke DJ, Uhrich TD, Ebert TJ. Absence of bronchodilation during desflurane anaesthesia. *Anesthesiology* 2000;93:404–8.

12 Bedfort NM, Hardman JG, Nathanson MH. Cerebral hemodynamic response to the introduction of desflurane: a comparison with sevoflurane. *Anesth Analg* 2000;91:152–5.

13 Frink EJ. Toxicologic potential of desflurane and sevoflurane. *Acta Anaesthesiol Scand* 1995;120–1.

14 Ramsey JG. Methods of reducing blood loss and non blood substitutes. *Can J Anaesth* 1991;3:595–612.

15 Levy JH. Novel pharmacologic approaches to reduce bleeding. *Can J Anaesth (Suppl)* 2003;50:S26–S30.

16 Coloma M, Duffy LL, White P, Tongier WK, Huber PJ. Dexamethasone facilitates discharge after outpatient anorectal surgery. *Anesth Analg* 2001;92:85–8.

17 Wang JJ, Ho ST, Liu HS, Ho CM. Prophylactic antiemetic effect of dexamethasone in women undergoing ambulatory laparoscopic surgery. *Br J Anaesth* 2000;84:459–62.

18 Aouad MT, Siddik SS, Rizk LB et al. The effect of dexamethasone on postoperative vomiting after tonsillectomy. *Anesth Analg* 2001;34:684–8.

19 Tramér MR. A rational approach to the control of postoperative nausea and vomiting: evidence from systemic reviews. Part 1. Efficacy and harm of antiemetic interventions, and methodological issues. *Acta Anaesthesiol Scand* 2001;45:4–13.

20 Hall JE, Uhrich TD, Barney JA et al. Sedative, amnestic, and analgesic properties of small dose dexmedetomidine infusions. *Anesth Analg* 2000;90:699–705.

21 Van Heerden PV. Sedation, Analgesia and Muscle Relaxation in the Intensive Care Unit. In: Bersten AD, Soni N, Oh TE (eds.). *Oh's Intensive Care Manual*, 5th edn. Butterworth-Heinemann, Edinburgh, 2003, pp. 833–40.

22 Aantaa R, Scheinin M. Alpha2-adrenergic agents in anaesthesia. *Acta Anaesthesiol Scand* 1993;37:433–48.

23 Aantaa R, Kanto J, Scheinin M. Intramuscular dexmedetomidine, a novel alpha2-adreno receptor agonist, as premedication for minor gynaecological surgery. *Acta Anaesthesiol Scand* 1991;35:283–8.

24 Sasada MP, Smith SP. *Drugs in Anaesthesia and Intensive Care*, 2nd edn. Oxford University Press, Oxford, 1998, pp. 96–7.

25 Pleuvry BJ. Plasma expanders. *Anaesthesia and Intensive Care Medicine* 2002;3:228–31.

26 Miller RD. Transfusion therapy. In Miller RD (ed.). *Anesthesia.* Vol. 2, 3rd edn, Churchill Livingstone, New York, 1990, p. 1495.

27 Gold BS. Anaesthetic care of patients with diabetes mellitus for ambulatory surgery. *ASA Refresher Courses in Anesthesiology* 1999;27:73–81.

28 Roizen MF. Perioperative management of the diabetic patient. ASA refresher course lecture notes, Atlanta, 1995;412:1–6.

29 Milaskiewicz RM, Hall GM. Diabetics and anaesthesia: The past decade. *Br J Anaesth* 1992;69:198–206.

30 Van de Velde M. What is the best way to provide analgesia after Caesarean section? *Curr Opin Anesthesiology* 2000;13:267–70.

31 Wood M. Opioid agonists and antagonists. In: Wood M, Wood A, (eds.). *Drugs and Anesthesia, Pharmacology for Anesthesiologists,* 2nd edn. Williams and Wilkins, Baltimore, 1990, pp. 145–6.

32 *British National Formulary.* British Medical Association and the Pharmaceutical Press;22;1991;73.

33 Tarkkila P, Rosenberg PH. Perioperative analgesia with non-steroidal analgesics. *Curr Opin Anesthesiology* 1998;11:407–10.

34 Crosby ET, Cooper RM, Douglas MJ et al. The unanticipated difficult airway with recommendations for management. *Can J Anaesth* 1998;45:757–76.

35 Murphy GS, Vender JS. ASA scientific papers emphasise patient safety. *APSF Newsletter* Winter 2001–2;16(4):49–64.

36 Samsoon GLT, Young JRB. Difficult tracheal intubation: a retrospective study. *Anaesthesia* 1987;42:487–90.

37 Cobley M, Vaughan RS. Recognition and management of difficult airway problems. *Br J Anaesth* 1992;68:90–7.

38 Mathew M, Hanna LS, Aldrete JA. Pre-operative indices to anticipate difficult tracheal intubation. *Anesth Analg* 1989;68:S187.

39 Bond A, Nussey A. Clinical prediction of a difficult intubation. *Anaesth Intensive Care* 1993;21:358–60.

40 Wilson ME, Spiegelhalter D, Robertson JA, Lesser P. Predicting difficult intubation. *Br J Anaesth* 1988;61:211–16.

41 Nath G, Sekar M. Predicting difficult intubation—a comprehensive scoring system. *Anaesth Intensive Care* 1997;25:482–6.

42 Knill RL. Difficult laryngoscopy made easy with a 'BURP'. *Can J Anaesth* 1993;40:798–9.

43 Tamura M, Ishikawa T, Kato R, Isono S, Nishino T. Mandibular advancement improves the laryngeal view during direct laryngoscopy performed by inexperienced physicians. *Anesthesiology* 2004;100:598–601.

44 Benumof JL. Laryngeal mask airway and the ASA difficult airway algorithm. *Anesthesiology* 1996;84:686–99.

45 Brimacombe J, Keller C, Judd DV. Gum elastic bougie-guided insertion of the ProSeal laryngeal mask airway is superior to the digital and introducer tool techniques. *Anesthesiology* 2004;100:25–9.

46 Heath ML, Allagain J. Intubation through the laryngeal mask—a technique for unexpected difficult intubation. *Anaesthesia* 1991;46:545–8.

47 Lim SL, Tay DHB, Thomas E. A comparison of three types of tracheal tube for use in the laryngeal mask assisted blind orotracheal intubation. *Anaesthesia* 1994;49:255–7.

48 White M. Disseminated Intravascular Coagulation. In Parsons PE, Wiener-Kronish JP (eds.). *Critical Care Secrets*. Hanley & Belfus Inc, Philadelphia, 1992, pp. 267–70.

49 Horne MK. Hemorrhagic and Thrombotic Disorders. In Parrillo JE (ed.). *Current Therapy in Clinical Care Medicine*, 3rd edn. Mosby, St Louis, 1997, pp. 357–8.

50 Feinstein DI. Treatment of disseminated intravascular coagulation. *Semin Thromb Hemost* 1988;14:351–62.

51 Bouwmeester FW, Jonkhoff AR, Verheijen RH, van Geijn HP. Successful treatment of life-threatening postpartum haemorrhage with recombinant activated factor VII. *Obstet Gynecol* 2003;101:1174–6.

52 Moscardo F, Perez F, de la Rubia J et al. Successful treatment of severe intra-abdominal bleeding associated with disseminated intravascular coagulation using recombinant activated factor VII. *Br J Haematol* 2001;14:174–6.

53 Chuansumrit A, Chantarojanasiri T, Isarangkura P, Teeraratkul S, Hongeng S, Hathirat P. Recombinant activated factor VII in children with acute bleeding resulting from liver failure and disseminated intravascular coagulation. *Blood Coagul Fibrinolysis* 2000;11 (Suppl 1):S101–5.

54 *Cardiovascular Drug Guidelines*, 2nd edn. Victorian Medical Post Graduate Foundation Inc. Melbourne, 1995, p. 111.

55 Cuthbertson BH, Hunter J, Webster NR. Inotropic agents in the critically ill. *Br J Hosp Med* 1996;56:386–98.

56 McCrory C, Cunningham AJ. Low-dose dopamine: will there ever be a scientific rationale? (Editorial). *Br J Anaesth* 1997;78:350–1.

57 Bonde J, Lauritsen K, Stenberg M, Kamp-Jensen M, Olsen NV. Low-dose dopamine in surgical and intensive care unit patients. *Acta Anaesthesiol Scand* 1996;40:326–30.

58 Hill RP, Lubarsky DA, Phillips-Bute et al. Cost-effectiveness of prophylactic antiemetic therapy with ondansetron, droperidol or placebo. *Anesthesiology* 2000;92:958–67.

59 Shaw A, Matthews EE. Postoperative neuroleptic malignant syndrome. *Anaesthesia* 1995;50:246–7.

60 Tramér MR. A rational approach to the control of postoperative nausea and vomiting: evidence from systemic reviews. Part II. Recommendations for prevention and treatment, and research agenda. *Acta Anaesthesiol Scand* 2001;45:14–19.

E

1 Foster JMG, Jones RM. The anaesthetic management of Eisenmenger syndrome. *Annals of the Royal College of Surgeons of England* 1984;66:353–5.

2 Temelcos C, Kuhn R, Stribley C. Sterilization of women with Eisenmenger syndrome: report of 4 cases. *Aust NZ Obstet Gynaecol* 1997;37:121–3.

3 Pollack KL, Chestnut DH, Wenstrom KD. Anesthetic management of a parturient with Eisenmenger's syndrome. *Anesth Analg* 1990;70:212–5.

4   Morray JP, Lynn AM, Stamm SJ, Herndon PS, Kawabori I, Stevenson
     JG. Hemodynamic effects of ketamine in children with congenital
     heart disease. *Anesth Analg* 1984;62:895–9.

5   Jones P, Patel A. Anaesthetic dilemma: Eisenmenger's syndrome and
     problems with anaesthesia. *Brit J Hosp Med* 1995;54:214.

6   Sammut MS, Paes ML. Anaesthesia for laparoscopic cholecystectomy
     in a patient with Eisenmenger's syndrome. *Br J Anaesth*
     1997;79:810–12.

7   Hytens L, Alexander JP. Maternal and neonatal death associated
     with Eisenmenger's syndrome. *Acta Anaesthesiologica Belgica*
     1986;37:45–51.

8   Smedstad KG. Morison DH. Pulmonary hypertension and pregnan-
     cy a series of eight cases. *Can J Anaesth* 1994;41:6:502–12.

9   Yentis SM, Steer PJ, Plaat F. Eisenmenger's syndrome in pregnancy:
     maternal and fetal mortality in the 1990s. *Br J Obstet Gynaecol*
     1998;105:921–2.

10   Spinnato JA, Kraynack BJ, Cooper MW. Eisenmenger's syndrome in
     pregnancy: epidural anaesthesia for elective Caesarean section. *N
     Eng J Med* 1981;20:1215–17.

11   Stoelting RK, Dierdorf SF. *Anesthesia and Co-existing Disease*, 4th edn.
     Churchill-Livingstone, Philadelphia, 2002, p. 58.

12   Mason R. *Anaesthesia Data Book—A Perioperative and Peripartum
     Manual*, 3rd edn. Greenwich Medical Media Limited, London, 2001,
     p. 166.

13   Bridenbaugh LD. The upper extremity: somatic blockade. In:
     Cousins MJ, Bridenbaugh PO (eds.). *Neural Blockade in Clinical
     Anaesthesia and Management of Pain*, 2nd edn, Lippincott,
     Philadelphia, 1988, pp. 408–11.

14   Messick JM, MacKenzie RA, Nugent M. Anesthesia in remote loca-
     tions. In: Miller RD (ed.). *Anesthesia,* 3rd edn. Churchill Livingstone,
     New York, 1990, p. 2084.

15   Skoyles JR, Sherry KM. Pharmacology, mechanisms of action and
     uses of selective phosphodiesterase inhibitors. *Br J Anaesth*
     1992;68:293–302.

16   Loisance D, Benvenuti C, Dubois Rande JL et al. Enoximine improves
     selection of candidates for urgent cardiac transplantation.
     International J Cardiol 1990;28:S23–S27.

17 Sasada MP, Smith SP. *Drugs in Anaesthesia and Intensive Care*, 2nd edn. Oxford University Press, Oxford, 1998, pp. 138–9.

18 Hines RL. New cardiovascular drugs. *ASA Refresher Courses in Anesthesiology* 1999;27:92.

19 Scott DB, Hibbard BM. Serious non-fatal complications associated with extradural block in obstetric practice. *Br J Anaesth* 1990;64:537–41.

20 Hlavin ML, Kaminski HJ, Ross JS et al. Spinal epidural abscess: a 10 year perspective. *Neurosurgery* 1990;27:177–84.

21 Yuste M, Canet J, Garcia M, Gil MA, Vidal F. Case Report: An epidural abscess due to resistant *Staphylococcus aureus* following epidural catheterisation. *Anaesthesia* 1997;52:150–68.

22 Brookman CA, Rutledge MLC. Epidural abscess: case report and literature review. *Regional Anaesth and Pain Med* 2000;25:428–31.

23 Del Curling O, Gower DJ, McWhorter JM. Changing concepts in spinal epidural abscess: a report of 29 cases. *Neurosurgery* 1990;27:185–92.

24 Danner RL, Hartman BJ. Update of spinal epidural abscesses: 35 cases and review of the literature. *Reviews of Infectious Diseases* 1987;9:477–94.

25 Heusner AP. Nontuberculous spinal epidural infections. *N Eng J Med* 1948;239:845–54.

26 Brown DL, Wedel DJ. Spinal, epidural and caudal anaesthesia. In: Miller RD (ed.). *Anaesthesia,* 3rd edn, Churchill Livingstone, New York, 1990, p. 1397.

27 Blomberg RG, Lofstrom JB. The test dose in regional anaesthesia. *Acta Anaesthesiol Scand* 1991;35:465–8.

28 Goodman EJ, Dehorta E, Taguiam JM. Safety of spinal and epidural anaesthesia in parturients with chorioamnionitis. *Reg Anesth* 1996;21:436–41.

29 De Lem-Casasola OA, Lema MJ. Postoperative epidural opioid analgesia:What are the choices? *Anesth Analg* 1996;83:867–75.

30 El-Behesy JD, Koh KF, Hirsch N, Yentis SM. Distinguishing cerebrospinal fluid from saline used to identify the extradural space. *Br J Anaesth* 1996;77:784–5.

31 Collier CB. Complications of regional anaesthesia. In: Birnbach DJ, Gatt S (eds.). *Textbook Of Obstetric Anesthesia*. Churchill Livingstone, New York, 2000, pp. 504–23.

32 Kuczkowski KM, Benumof JL. Decrease in the incidence of post-dural puncture headache: maintaining CSF volume. *Acta Anaesthesiol Scand* 2003;47:98–100.

33 Gielen MJM. Post dural puncture headache: a review. *Regional Anaesthesia* 1989;14:101–6.

34 Carp H, Sing PJ, Vadhera R, Jayaram A. Effects of serotonin-receptor agonist sumatriptin on postdural headache: report of 6 cases. *Anesth Analg* 1994;79:180–2.

35 Morgan P. Review article: Spinal anaesthesia in obstetrics. *Can J Anaesth* 1995;42:1145–63.

36 Rivindran RS. Epidural autologous blood patch on an outpatient basis. *Anesth Analg* 1984;63:962.

37 Beards SC, Jackson A, Griffiths AG, Horsman EL. Magnetic resonance imaging of extradural blood patches: appearances from 30 min to 18 h. *Br J Anaesth* 1993;71:182–8.

38 Hardman JG, Gajraj NM. Epidural blood patch. *Br J Hosp Med* 1996;56:268–9.

39 Southorn P, Vasdev GM, Chantigin RC, Lawson GM. Reducing the potential morbidity of an unintentional spinal anaesthesia by aspirating cerebrospinal fluid. *Br J Anaesth* 1996;76:467–9.

40 Tsui BCH, Malherbe S, Koller J, Aronyk K. Reversal of an unintentional spinal anaesthetic by cerebrospinal lavage. *Anesth Analg* 2004;98:434–6.

41 Wildsmith JAW, McClure JH. Editorial. *Anaesthesia* 1991;46:613–4.

42 Haljamoe H. Thromboprophylaxis, coagulation disorders and regional anaesthesia. *Acta Anaesthesiol Scand* 1996;40:1024–40.

43 Horlocker TT. Low molecular weight heparin and neuraxial blockade. *Thrombosis Research* 2001;101:V141–54.

44 Sage DJ. Epidurals, spinals and bleeding disorders in pregnancy: A review. *Anaesth Intensive Care* 1990;18:319–26.

45 Horlocker TT et al. Perioperative antiplatelet therapy does not increase the risk of spinal haematoma associated with regional anaesthesia. *Anesth Analg* 1995;80:303–9.

46 Scott DB, Hibbard BM. Serious non-fatal complications associated with extradural block in obstetric practice. *Br J Anaesth* 1990;64:537–41.

47 Macarthur AJ, Macarthur C, Weeks SK. Is epidural anaesthesia in labor associated with chronic low back pain? A prospective cohort study. *Anesth Analg* 1997;85:1066–70.

48 Vandermeulen EP, Van Aken H, Vermylen J. Anticoagulants and spinal-epidural anaesthesia. *Anesth S Analg* 1994;79:1165–77.

49 Wulf H. Epidural anaesthesia and spinal haematoma. *Can J Anaesth* 1996;43:1260–71.

50 Schmidt A, Nolte H. Subdural and epidural haematomas following epidural anaesthesia. A literature review. *Anaesthestist* 1992;41:276–84.

51 Kelly BJ. Status Epilepticus. In Parsons PE, Weiner-Kronish JP (eds.). *Critical Care Secrets*, Hanley & Belfus, Philadelphia, 1992, pp. 284–7.

52 Lowenstein DH, Alldredge BK. Status epilepticus at an urban public hospital in the 1980s. *Neurology* 1993;43:483–8.

53 Thomas G, Hirsch N. Generalised convulsive status epilepticus. *Anaesth Intensive Care* 2003;4:120–2.

54 Opdam H. Status Epilepticus. In Bersten AD, Soni N, Oh TE (eds.). *Oh's Intensive Care Manual*, 5th edn. Butterworth-Heinemann, Edinburgh, 2003, pp. 485–93.

55 Hall RI. Editorial. Esmolol—just another beta blocker? *Can J Anaesth* 1992;39:757–64.

56 Malinow AM. Anaesthetic considerations for pre-eclamptic patient. *Audio Digest, Anesthesiology* 1995;37:21.

57 Glass PS, Leiman BC, Reves JG. Etomidate: what is its present role in anesthesia. *Seminars in Anaesthesia* 1988;7:143–51.

58 Anathanam JJK, Francis RI. How to do a peri-bulbar block: the transconjunctival approach modified for the anxious patient. *Br J Hosp Med* 1994;52:295–8.

59 Wong DHW. Regional anaesthesia for intraocular surgery. *Can J Anaesth* 1993;40:635–57.

60 Berry CB, Murphy PM. Regional anaesthesia for cataract surgery. *Br J Hosp Med* 1993;49:10;689–701.

61 Corke PJ, Baker J, Cammack R. Comparison of 1% ropivacaine and a mixture of 2% lignocaine and 0.5% bupivacaine peribulbar anaesthesia in cataract surgery. *Anesth Intensive Care* 1999;27:248–52.

62 Guise PA. Single quadrant sub-tenon's block. Evaluation of a new local anaesthetic technique for eye surgery. *Anaesth Intensive Care* 1996;24:241–4.

63 Ferrari LR. The injured eye. *Anesthesiology Clinics of North America* 1996;14:1:125–49.

64 Libonati MM, Leaky JJ, Ellison N. The use of succinylcholine in open eye surgery. *Anesthesiology* 1985;62:637–40.

F

1 Stoelting RK. 'NPO' and aspiration: new perspectives. American Society of Anesthesiologists refresher course lectures 1997;111:1–7.

2 Stoelting RK. NPO: Fact and fiction. *Audio-Digest* 1995;37:15.

3 Phillips S, Daborn AK, Hatch DJ. Preoperative fasting and paediatric anaesthesia. *Br J Anaesth* 1994;73:529–36.

4 Fourme TC, Vieillard-Baron A, Loubieres Y et al. Early fat embolism after liposuction. *Anesthesiology* 1988;89:782–4.

5 Lafont ND, Kalonjii MK, Barre J, Guillaume C, Boogaerts JG. Clinical features and echocardiography of embolism during cemented hip arthroplasty. *Can J Anaesth* 1997;44:112–17.

6 Colonna DM, Kilgus D, Brown W, Challa V, Stump DA, Moody DM. Acute brain fat embolization occurring after total hip arthroplasty in the absence of a patent foramen ovale. *Anesthesiol* 2002;96:1027–9.

7 Mason R. *Anaesthesia Data Book—A Perioperative and Peripartum Manual*, 3rd edn. Greenwich Medical Media Limited, London, 2001, p. 194.

8 Byrick RJ. Editorial: Cement implantation syndrome: a time limited embolic phenomenon. *Can J Anaesth* 1997;44:107–11.

9 Corke PJ. Anaesthesia for Caesarean section on a patient with acute fatty liver of pregnancy. *Anaesth Intensive Care* 1995;23:215–18.

10 Long CJ. Hepatic Disease. In Birnbach DJ, Gatt SP, Datta S (eds.). *Textbook of Obstetric Anesthesia*. Churchill Livingstone, Philadelphia, 2000, pp. 607–16.

11 Lim W, Kennedy N. Hemiarthroplasty of the hip under triple nerve block. *Anaesth Intensive Care* 1994;22:722–3.

12 Halfpenny M, Rushe C, Breen P, Cunningham AJ, Boucher-Hayes D, Shorten GD. The effects of fenoldopam on renal function in patients undergoing elective aortic surgery. *Eur J Anaesthesiol* 2002;19:32–9.

13 Bovill JG. Which new potent opioid? Important criteria for selection. *Hospital Therapeutics* 1987;June:5–20.

14 Palmer CM, Cork RC, Hays R, Van Maren G, Alves D. The dose-response relation of intrathecal fentanyl for labor analgesia. *Anesthesiology* 1998;88:355–61.

15 Striebel HW, Krämer J, Lubmann I, Rohierse-Hohler I, Rieger A. Pharmacokinectics of intranasal fentanyl (German) *Der Schmerz* 1993;7:122–5.

16 Yentis SM, Hirsch NP, Smith GB. *Anaesthesia and Intensive Care A–Z*, 2nd edn. Butterworth-Heinemann, Oxford, 2000, p. 216.

17 Mazzei WJ. Cardiovascular monitoring. *Audio Digest. Anesthesiology* 1996;38:5.

18 Australian Red Cross Blood Service, *Circular of Information—an Extension of Blood Component Labels*, The Australian Red Cross Blood Service, Melbourne, 2003, pp. 26–7.

19 Downes KA, Yomtovian R, Sarode R. Serial measurements of clotting factors in thawed plasma stored for 5 days. *Transfusion* 2001;41:570.

20 Hardy J, Belisle S, Robitaille D. Blood Products: when to use them and how to avoid them. *Can J Anaesth* 1994;41:5:R52–61.

G

1 Webber S, Andrzejowski J, Francis G. Gas embolism in anaesthesia. *Br J Anaesth CEPD Reviews* 2002;2:53–7.

2 Gabba DM, Fish JF, Howard SK. *Crisis Management in Anesthesiology.* Churchill Livingstone, New York, 1994, pp. 116–19.

3 Chui PT, Gin T, Oh TE. Anaesthesia for laparoscopic general surgery. *Anaesth Intensive Care* 1993;21:163–71.

4 Powell CG, Unsworth DJ, McVey FK. Severe hypotension associated with angiotensin-converting enzyme inhibition in anaesthesia. *Anaesth Intensive Care* 1998;26:107–9.

5   Teasdale G, Jennett B. Assessment of coma and impaired consciousness: A practical scale. *Lancet* 1974;2:81–3.

6   Mason RA. *Anaesthesia Databook: A Clinical Practice Compendium.* Churchill Livingstone, New York, 1990, pp. 112–14.

7   Stoelting RK, Dierdorf SF. *Anaesthesia and Co-existing Disease*, 3rd edn. Churchill Livingstone, New York, 1993, pp. 399–40.

8   Klein L. Cardiogenic shock. In: Parrillo JE (ed.). *Current Therapy in Critical Care Medicine*, 3rd edn. Mosby, St Louis, 1997, pp. 72–8.

9   Axemo P, Fu X, Lindberg B, Ulmsten U, Wessen A. Intravenous nitroglycerine for rapid uterine relaxation. *Acta Obstet Gynecol Scand* 1998;77:50–3.

10   Dawson NJ, Gabbott DA. Use of sublingual glyceryl trinitrate as a supplement to volatile inhalational anaesthesia in a case of uterine inversion. *International Journal of Obstetric Anaesthesia* 1997;6:135–7.

11   Cass N, Cass L. *Pharmacology for Anaesthetists.* Churchill Livingstone, Edinburgh, 1994, p. 53.

H

1   Pleuvry BJ. Plasma expanders. *Anaesthesia and Intensive Care Med* 2002;3:228–31.

2   Forbes AM. Colloids and blood products. In Oh TE (ed.). *Intensive Care Manual*, 4th edn. Butterworth-Heinemann, Oxford, 1997, pp. 754–9.

3   Harrison BA, Vasdev G. Anesthesia for Bronchoscopy. In Faust RJ, Cucchiara RF, Rose SH et al. (eds.). *Anesthesiology Review*, 3rd edn. Churchill Livingstone, Philadelphia, 2002, p. 513.

4   Hirsch IB, McGill JB, Cryer PE, White PF. Perioperative management of surgical patients with diabetes mellitus. *Anesthesiology* 1991;74:346–59.

5   *Cardiovascular Drug Guidelines*, 2nd edn, Victorian Medical Post Graduate Foundation Inc., Australia, 1995, p. 127.

6   Broomhead C. Management of patients with a cardiac transplant. *Br J Hosp Med* 1995;54:571–3.

7   Cheng DCH, Ong DD. Anaesthesia for non-cardiac surgery in heart-transplanted patients. *Can J Anaesth* 1993;40:981–6.

8   Shaw IH, Kirk AJB, Conacher ID. Anaesthesia for patients with transplanted hearts and lungs undergoing non-cardiac surgery. *Br J Anaesth* 1991;67:772–8.

9   Morgan-Hughes NJ, Hood G. Anaesthesia for a patient with a cardiac transplant. *Br J Anaesth CEPD Reviews* 2002;2:74–8.

10 Bullingham A, Strunin L. Prevention of postoperative venous thromboembolism. *Br J Anaesth* 1995;75:622–30.

11 Yentis S, Hirsch N, Smith GB. *Anaesthesia and Intensive Care*, 2nd edn. Butterworth-Heinemann, Oxford, 2000, p. 257.

12 Grant IS. Intercurrent disease and anaesthesia. In Aitkenhead AR, Smith G (eds.). *Textbook of Anaesthesia*, 2nd edn. Churchill Livingstone, New York, 1990, pp. 645–76.

13 Mason RA. Anaesthesia Databook. *A Clinical Practice Compendium.* Churchill Livingstone, New York, 1990, p. 136.

14 Hodges PJ, Kam PCA. Review article: the peri-operative implications of herbal medicines. *Anaesthesia* 2002;57:889–99.

15 Gunning K. Echinacea in the treatment and prevention of upper respiratory tract infections. *Western Journal of Medicine* 1999;171:198–200.

16 Rose KD, Croissant PD, Parliament CF. Spontaneous spinal epidural haematoma with associated platelet dysfunction from excessive garlic ingestion: a case report. *Neurosurgery* 1990;26:880–2.

17 Burnham BE. Garlic as a possible risk for postoperative bleeding. *Plastic and Reconstructive Surgery* 1995;95:213.

18 Miller LG. Herbal medicines. Selected clinical considerations focusing on known or potential drug-herb interactions. *Arch Internal Med* 1999;159:1857–8.

19 *Australian Prescriber* 2002;25:19.

20 Shann F. *Drug Doses*, 11th edn. Collective Pty Ltd 2001, p. 34.

21 Sarhill N, Walsh D, Nelson KA. Hydromorphone: pharmacology and clinical applications in cancer patients. *Support Care Cancer* 2001;9:84–96.

22 Latta KS, Ginsberg B, Barkin RL. Meperidine: a clinical review. *American J Therapeutics* 2002;9:53–68.

23 Goodarzi M. Comparison of epidural morphine, hydromorphone and fentanyl for postoperative pain control in children undergoing orthopaedic surgery. *Paediatr Anaesth* 1999;419–22.

24 Coda BA, O'Sullivan B, Donaldson G, Bohl S, Chapman CR, Shen D. Comparative efficacy of patient-controlled administration of morphine, hydromorphone, or sufentanil for the treatment of oral mucositis pain following bone marrow transplantation. *Pain* 1997;72:333–46.

25 Pleuvry BJ. Plasma expanders. *Anaesthesia and Intensive Care Med* 2002;3:228–31.

26 Thornberry EA. Perioperative fluids. *Anaesthesia and Intensive Care Medicine* 2002:3;414–17.

27 Mack PF. Cerebral Aneurysm. In Yao F-SF (ed.). *Anesthesiology Problem Orientated Patient Management*, 4th edn, Lippincott-Raven, Philadelphia 1998, pp. 504–24.

28 Barclay K, Kluger MT. Effect of bolus dose of remifentanil on haemodynamic response to tracheal intubation. *Anaesth Intensive Care* 2000;28:403–7.

29 Elliott P, O'Hare R, Bill KM, Phillips AS, Gibson FM, Mirakhur RK. Severe cardiovascular depression with remifentanil. *Anesth Analg* 2000;91:58–61.

30 Hall RI. Editorial. Esmolol—just another beta blocker? *Can J Anaesth* 1992;39:757–64.

31 Yao F-S, Yao F. Hypertension. In Yao F-S (ed.). *Anesthesiology: Problem Orientated Patient Management*, 4th edn. Lippincott-Raven, Philadelphia, 1998, pp. 316–33.

32 Sia-Kho E. Pregnancy-induced Hypertension. In Yao F-S (ed.). *Anesthesiology: Problem Orientated Patient Management*, 4th edn. Lippincott-Raven, Philadelphia, 1998, pp. 681–703.

33 Elliott PM, McKenna WJ. Management of hypertrophic cardiomyopathy. *Br J Hosp Med* 1996;55:419–23.

34 Loubser P, Suh K, Cohen S. Adverse effects of spinal anesthesia in a patient with idiopathic hypertrophic subaortic stenosis. *Anesthesiology* 1984;60:228–30.

35 Wynn J, Braunwald E. The Cardiomyopathies and Myocarditides. In: Isselbacher KJ, Braunwald E, Wilson JD, Martin JB, Fauci AS, Kasper D (eds.). *Harrison's Principles of Internal Medicine*, 13th edn. McGraw-Hill Inc, New York,1994, pp. 1088–93.

36 Mason R. *Anaesthesia Data Book—A Perioperative and Peripartum Manual*, 3rd edn. Greenwich Medical Media Limited, London, 2001, p. 82.

37 Shah DM, Sunderji SG. Hypertrophic cardiomyopathy and pregnancy: report of a maternal mortality and review of the literature. *Obstetrical and Gynecological Survey* 1985;40:444–8.

38 Stoelting RK, Dierdorf S. *Anaesthesia and Co-existing Disease*, 4th edn. Churchill Livingstone, Philadelphia, 2002, pp. 120–5.

39 Baraka A, Jabbour S, Itani I. Severe bradycardia following epidural anaesthesia in a patient with idiopathic hypertrophic subaortic stenosis. *Anesth Analg* 1987;66:1337–8.

40 Paix B, Cyna A, Belperio P, Simmons S. Epidural analgesia for labour and delivery in a parturient with congenital hypertrophic obstructive cardiomyopathy. (Case report) *Anaesth Intensive Care* 1999;27:59–62.

41 Edmends S, Ghosh S. Hypertrophic obstructive cardiomyopathy complicating surgery for cerebral aneurysm clipping. *Anaesthesia* 1994;49:608–9.

42 Tessler MJ, Hudson R, Naugler-Colville MA et al. Pulmonary oedema in two patients with hypertrophic obstructive cardiomyopathy (HOCM). *Can J Anaesth* 1990;37:469–73.

43 Minnich ME, Quirk JG, Clark RB. Epidural anaesthesia for vaginal delivery in a patient with idiopathic hypertrophic subaortic stenosis. *Anesthesiology* 1987;67:590–2.

44 Boccio RV, Chung JH, Harrison DM. Anesthetic management of Caesarean section in a patient with idiopathic hypertrophic subaortic stenosis. *Anesthesiology* 1986;65:663–5.

45 Oakley GDG, McGarry K, Limb DG et al. Management of pregnancy in patients with hypertrophic cardiomyopathy. *Brit Med J* 1979;1:1749–59.

46 Autore C, Brauneis S, Apponi F et al. Epidural anaesthesia for Caesarean section in patients with hypertrophic cardiomyopathy: a report of three cases. *Anesthesiology* 1999;90:1205–7.

I

1   Sparkes CJ, Rudkin GE, Agiomea K, Fa'arondo JR. Inguinal field block for adult inguinal hernia repair using a short bevelled needle. *Anaesth Intensive Care* 1995;23:143–8.

2   Murphy DE. Intrapleural analgesia. *Br J Anaesth* 1993;3:426–34.

3   Schuster M. Nave H, Piepenbrock S, Pabst R, Panning B. The carina as a landmark in central venous catheter placement. *Br J Anaesthesia* 2000;85;192–4.

4   Waldmann C, Barnes R. Cannulation of central veins. *Anaesthesia and Intensive Care Medicine.* 2004;5:6–9.

5   Collier PE, Blocker SH, Graff DM, Doyle P. Cardiac tamponade from central venous catheters. *Am J Surg* 1998;176:212–4.

6   Harte FA, Chalmers PC, Walsh RF, Danker PR, Shiekh FM. Intraosseous infusions: a parenteral alternative in pediatric resuscitation. *Anesth Analg* 1987;66:687–9.

7   Gouny P, Gaitz JP, Vayssairat M. Acute hand ischaemia secondary to intraarterial buprenorphine injection: treatment with iloprost and dextran-40. *Angiology* 1999;50:605–6.

8   Glass PS, Leiman BC, Reves JG. Etomidate: what is its present role in anesthesia? *Seminars in Anaesthesia* 1988;7:143–51.

9   McGrath P. Accidental intra-arterial flucloxacillin: management using guanethidine. *Anaesth Intensive Care* 1992;20:518–19.

10   Iatrou C, Robinson S, Rosewarne F. Inadvertent intra-arterial midazolam. (letter) *Anaesth Intensive Care* 1997;25:431.

11   Sivalingam P. Inadvertent cannulation of an aberrant radial artery and intra-arterial injection of midazolam. (letter) *Anaesth Intensive Care* 1999;27:424–5.

12   Brimacombe J, Gandin D, Bashford L. Transient decrease in arm blood flow following accidental intra-arterial injection of propofol into the left brachial artery. *Anaesth Intensive Care* 1994;22:291–2.

13   Evans JM, Latto IP, Ng WS. Accidental intra-arterial injection of drugs: A hazard of arterial cannulation. *Br J Anaesth* 1974;460–3.

14   Trail R. Acute head injuries: anaesthetic considerations. In: Keneally J (ed.). *Australasian Anaesthesia.* ANZCA, Melbourne, 1996, pp. 145–50.

15   Craen RA, Gelb AW. The anaesthetic management of neurosurgical emergencies. *Can J Anaesth* 1992;39:5:R29–R34.

16   Frenette L, Bourdreault D, Guay J. Interpleural analgesia improves pulmonary function after cholecystectomy. *Can J Anaesth* 1991;38:171–4.

17   Engdahl O, Boe J, Sandstedt S. Intrapleural bupivacaine for analgesia during chest drainage treatment of pneumothorax. *Acta Anaesthesiol Scand* 1993;37:149–53.

18   Weiner C. The obstetric patient and disseminated intravascular coagulation. *Clin Perinatol* 1986;13:705.

19   Kleinsasser A, Kuenszberg E, Loekinger A et al. Sevoflurane, but not propofol, significantly prolongs the QT interval. *Anesth Analg* 2000;90: 25–7.

J

1   *Jehovah's Witnesses Guidelines for Their Non-blood Medical Management.* Provided by the Jehovah's Witnesses Hospital Liaison Services, Sydney 2000. (Used with permission.)

2   Cox M, Lumley J. Editorial. No blood or blood products. *Anaesthesia* 1995;50:583–5.

3   McIlveney F, Pace NA. Jehovah's Witnesses. A*naesthesia and Intensive Care Medicine* 2004;5:57–9.

K

1   Gurnani A, Sharma PK, Rautela RS, Bhattacharya A. Analgesia for acute musculo-skeletal trauma: low dose subcutaneous infusion of ketamine. *Anesth Intensive Care* 1996;22:34–6.

2   White PF, Way WL, Trevor AJ. Ketamine—its pharmacology and therapeutic uses. *Anesthesiology* 1982;56:119–36.

3   Rainey L, Van Der Walt JH. The anaesthetic management of autistic children. *Anaesth Intensive Care* 1998;26:682–6.

4   Gutstein HB, Johnson KL, Heard MB, Gregory GA. Oral ketamine preanaesthetic medication in children. *Anesthesiology* 1992;76: 28–33.

5   Filatov SM, Baer GA, Rorarius MG, Oikkonen M. Efficacy and safety of premedication with oral ketamine for day-case adenoidectomy compared with rectal diazepam/diclofenac and EMLA. *Acta Anaesthesiol Scand* 2000;44:118–24.

6   Smith K, Halliwell RMT, Lawrence S, Klineberg PL, O'Connell P. Acute renal failure associated with intramuscular ketorolac. *Anaesth Intensive Care* 1993;21:700–3.

L

1   Brimacombe J, Berry A. A review of anaesthesia for ruptured abdominal aortic aneurysm with special emphasis on preclamping fluid resuscitation. *Anaesth Intensive Care* 1993;21:311–23.

2   Dubois F, Berthelot G, Levard H. Cholecystectomie par coelioscopie. *Presse Med* 1989;18:980–2.

3   Duffy BL. Regurgitation during pelvic laparoscopy. *Br J Anaesth* 1979;51:1089–90.

4   Biswas TK, Pembroke A. Asystolic cardiac arrest during laparoscopic cholecystectomy. *Anaesth Intensive Care* 1994;22:289–92.

5   Inada T, Uesugi F, Kawachi S, Takubo K. Changes in tracheal tube position during laparoscopic cholecystectomy. *Anaesthesia* 1996;51:823–6.

6   Chui PT, Gin T, Oh TE. Anaesthesia for laparoscopic general surgery. *Anaesth Intensive Care* 1993;21:163–71.

7   Salonen M, Mäkinen J, Saraste M, Parkkola R. Is laparoscopic hysterectomy bad for the brain? *Gynaecol Endoscopy* 1999;8:161–4.

8   Hagen P, Scholz D, Edwards W. Incidence and size of patent foramen ovale during the first 10 decades of life. *Mayo Clin Proc* 1984;59:17–20.

9   Tuppurainen T, Mäkinen J, Salonen M. Reducing the risk of systemic embolization during gynecologic laparoscopy—effect of volume preload. *Acta Anaesthesiol Scand* 2002;46:37–42.

10   Koivusalo AM, Lindgren L. Effects of carbon dioxide pneumoperitoneum for laparoscopic cholecystectomy. *Acta Anaesthesiol Scand* 2000;44:834–41.

11 Han T-H, Brimacombe J, Lee E-J. The laryngeal mask airway is effective (and probably safe) in selected healthy parturients for elective Caesarean section: a prospective study of 1067 cases. *Can J Anesth* 2001;48:1117–21.

12 Devitt JH, Wenstone R, Noel AG, O'Donnell MP. The laryngeal mask airway and positive pressure ventilation. *Anesthesiology* 1994;80: 550–5.

13 Keller C, Brimacombe J, Raedler C, Puehringer F. Do laryngeal mask airway devices attenuate liquid flow between the oesophagus and the pharynx? A randomized, controlled cadaver study. *Anesth Analg* 1999;88:904–7.

14 *LMA-ProSeal Instruction Manual.* The Laryngeal Mask Company Limited, 2000 (with permission).

15 Brimacombe J, Keller C, Judd DV. Gum elastic bougie-guided insertion of the ProSeal laryngeal mask airway is superior to the digital and introducer tool techniques. *Anesthesiology* 2004;1:25–9.

16 Maltby JR, Beriault MT, Watson NC, Liepert D, Fick GH. The LMA-ProSeal is an effective alternative to tracheal intubation for laparoscopic cholecystectomy. *Can J Anaesth* 2002;49:857–62.

17 Brain AIJ, Verghese C, Addy EV, Kapila A. The intubating laryngeal mask. I: development of a new device for intubation of the trachea. *Br J Anaesth* 1997;79:699–703.

18 Brain AIJ, Verghese C, Addy EV, Kapila A, Brimacombe J. The intubating laryngeal mask. II: a preliminary clinical report of a new means of intubating the trachea. *Br J Anaesth* 1997;79:704–9.

19 van Vlymen JM, Coloma M, Tongier WK. Use of the intubating laryngeal mask airway: are muscle relaxants necessary? *Anesthesiology* 2000;93:340–5.

20 Asai T, Wagle AU, Stacey M. Placement of the intubating laryngeal mask is easier than the laryngeal mask during manual in-line neck stabilization. *Br J Anaesth* 1999;82:712–14.

21 Kihara S, Watanabe S, Brimacombe J, Taguchi N, Yaguchi Y, Yamasaki Y. Segmental cervical spine movement with the intubating laryngeal mask during manual in-line stabilization in patients with cervical pathology undergoing cerevical spine surgery. *Anesth Analg* 2000;91:195–200.

22 Ocker H. Wenzel V, Schmucker P, Steinfath M, Dörges V. A comparison of the laryngeal tube with the laryngeal mask airway during routine surgical procedures. *Anesth Analg* 2002;95:1094–7.

23 Gabbott DA. Recent advances in airway technology. *Br J Anaesth CEPD Reviews* 2001;1:76–80.

24 Cormack RS, Lehane J. Difficult tracheal intubation in obstetrics. *Anaesthesia* 1984;39:1105–11.

25 Rampil IJ. Anesthetic considerations for laser surgery. *Anesth Analg* 1992;74:424–35.

26 Mertes PM, Laxenaire M-C, Allergic reactions during anaesthesia. *Eur J Anaesthesiol* 2002;19:240–62.

27 Protocol for the management of latex allergy, Flinders Medical Centre, Adelaide. In: Keneally J, Jones M (eds.). *Australasian Anaesthesia 1996*. Australian and New Zealand College of Anaesthetists, 1996, pp. 130–4.

28 Fisher MM. Latex allergy during anaesthesia: cautionary tales. *Anaesth Intensive Care* 1997;25:302–3.

29 Holzman RS. Latex allergy: an emerging operating room problem. *Anesth Analg* 1993;76:635–41.

30 McAleer P, Barker D. Latex Allergy: a review. In: Keneally J, Jones M (eds.). *Australasian Anaesthesia 1996*. Australian and New Zealand College of Anaesthetists, 1996, pp. 123–34.

31 Schwartz HA, Zurowski D. Anaphylaxis to latex in intravenous fluids. *J Allergy Clin Immunol* 1993;92:358–9.

32 McLeod GA, Burke D. Review article: Levobupivacaine. *Anaesthesia* 2001;56:331–41.

33 Hung RO, Stewart RD. Lightwand intubation: 1—a new lightwand device. *Can J Anaesth* 1995;42:820–5.

34 Djordjevic D. Trachlight—learning tips (letter). *Can J Anesth* 1999;46:615–17.

35 Albrecht A, Hogg M, Robinson S. Transient radicular irritation as a complication of spinal anaesthesia with hyperbaric 5% lignocaine. *Anaesth Intensive Care* 1996;24:508–10.

36 Neff SP, Merry AF, Anderson B. Airway management in Ludwig's angina. *Anaesth Intensive Care* 1999;27:659–61.

37 Gray H, Pead M. Ludwig's angina. *Anaesthesia and Intensive Care Medicine* 2002;3:250–2.

38 Mulroy MF. *Regional Anesthesia; an Illustrated Procedural Guide*, 2nd edn. Little, Brown and Company, Boston, 1996, pp. 199–200.

M

1 Gomez MN. Magnesium and cardiovascular disease. *Anesthesiology* 1988;89:222–40.

2 Donovan KD, Hockings BEF. Antiarrhythmic Drugs. In: Oh TE (ed.). *Intensive Care Manual*, 4th edn. Butterworth-Heinemann, Oxford, 1997, p. 102.

3 Fagan C, Phelan D. Severe convulsant hypomagnesaemia and short bowel syndrome. *Anaesth Intensive Care* 2001;29:281–3.

4 Breen TW, Yang T. The changing role of magnesium sulphate therapy. *Current Opinion in Anaesthesiology* 1999;12:283–7.

5 Patteson SK, Chesney JT. Anesthetic management for magnetic resonance imaging: problems and solutions. *Anesth Analg* 1992;74:121–8.

6 McBrien ME, Winder J, Smyth L. Anaesthesia for magnetic resonance imaging: a survey of current practice in the UK and Ireland. *Anaesthesia* 2000;55:737–43.

7 Rosewarne F. *Anaesthetic equipment*, 2nd edn. Self-published 1999, pp. 259–65.

8 Langton JA, Wilson I, Fell D. Use of the laryngeal mask airway during magnetic resonance imaging. *Anaesthesia* 1992;47:532–3.

9 Gronert GA. Malignant hyperthermia. *Anesthesiology* 1980;53:396.

10 Ellis FR, Halsall PJ. Malignant hyperthermia. *Anaesthesia and Intensive Care Medicine* 2002;3:222–5.

11 Pollock NA, Langton EE. Management of malignant hyperthermia susceptible parturients. *Anaesth Intensive Care* 1997;25:398–440.

12 Strazis KP, Fox AW. Malignant hyperthermia: A review of published cases. *Anesth Analg* 1993;77:297–304.

13 *Guidelines from the Malignant Hyperpyrexia Association of the United States*—revised 1993.

14 Kaplan RF. *Malignant Hyperpyrexia*. ASA annual meeting refresher course lectures. 1993, p. 522.

15 Australian and New Zealand College of Anaesthetists Policy Document, *Monitoring during Anaesthesia*. Review P18, 1995.

16 Sims C. Masseter spasm after suxamethonium in children. *Br J Hosp Med* 1992;47:2:139–43.

17 Mackie AM et al. Anaesthesia and mediastinal masses. *Anaesthesia* 1984;39:899–903.

18 Pullerits J, Holzman R. Anaesthesia for patients with mediastinal masses. *Can J Anaesth* 1989;36:681–8.

19 Neumann GG, Weingarten AE, Abramowitz RM, Kushins LG, Ladner W. The anesthetic management of the patient with an anterior mediastinal mass. *Anesthesiology* 1984;60:144–7.

20 Lewer BMF, Torrance JM. Anaesthesia for a patient with a mediastinal mass presenting with acute stridor. *Anaesth Intensive Care* 1996;24:605–8.

21 Azizkhan RG, Dudgeon DL, Buck JR et al. Life threatening airway obstruction as a complication to the management of mediastinal masses in children. *J Pediatr Surg* 1985;20:816–22.

22 Hirshman C. Perioperative management of the asthmatic patient. *Can J Anaesth* 1991;38:4:26–32.

23 Cass N, Cass L. *Pharmacology for Anaesthetists*. Churchill Livingstone, Edinburgh, 1994, p. 89.

24 Henzi I, Walder B, Tramér MR. Metoclopramide in the prevention of postoperative nausea and vomiting—a quantitative systemic review of randomized placebo-controlled studies. *Br J Anaesth* 1999;83:761–71.

25 Kim MH, Lee YM. Intrathecal midazolam increases the analgesic effects of spinal blockade with bupivacaine in patients undergoing haemorrhoidectomy. *Br J Anaesth* 2001;86:77–9.

26 Tucker AP, Lai C, Nadeson R, Goodchild CS. Intrathecal midazolam I: A cohort study investigating safety. *Anesth Analg* 2004;98:1512–20.

27 Bozkurt P, Tunali Y, Kaya G, Okar I. Histological changes following epidural injection of midazolam in the neonatal rabbit. *Paediatr Anaesth* 1997;7:385–9.

28 Erdine S, Yucel A, Ozyalci S et al. Neurotoxicity of midazolam in the rabbit. *Pain* 1999;80:419–23.

29 Johansen MJ, Gradert TL, Satterfield WC et al. Safety of continuous intrathecal midazolam infusion in the sheep model. *Anesth Analg* 2004;98:1528–35.

30 Bharti N, Madan R, Mohanty PR, Kaul HL. Intrathecal midazolam added to bupivacaine improves the duration and quality of spinal anaesthesia. *Acta Anaesthesiol Scand* 2003;47:1101–5.

31 Yaksh TL, Allen JW. The use of intrathecal midazolam in humans: a case study in progress. *Anesth Analg* 2004;98:1536–45.

32 Kim MH, Lee YM. Intrathecal midazolam increases the analgesic effects of spinal blockade with bupivacaine in patients undergoing haemorrhoidectomy. *Brit J Anaesth* 2001;86:77–9.

33 Borg PA, Krijinen HJ. Long term intrathecal administration of midazolam and clonidine. *Clin J Pain* 1996;12:63–8.

34 Donnell CG, Harte S, O'Driscoll J, O'Loughlin, Van Pelt FD, Shorten GD. Forum: The effects of concurrent atorvastatin therapy on the pharmacokinetics of intravenous midazolam. *Anaesthesia* 2003;58:874–910.

35 Skoyles JR, Sherry KM. Pharmacology, mechanisms of action and uses of selective phosphodiesterase inhibitors. *Br J Anaesth* 1992;68:293–302.

36 Jaski BE, Fifer MA, Wright RF et al. Positive inotropic and vasodilator actions of milrinone in patients with severe congestive heart failure. Dose-response relationships and comparison to nitroprusside. *J Clin Invest* 1985;75:643–9.

37 Stoelting RK, Dierdorf SF. *Anesthesia and Co-existing disease,* 4th edn. Churchill Livingstone, New York, 2002, pp. 32–5.

38 Mason R. *Anaesthesia Databook; A Perioperative and Peripartum Manual,* 3rd edn. Greenwich Medical Media Limited, London, 2001, pp. 322–8.

39 Mangano DT. Anesthesia for the Pregnant Cardiac Patient. In: Hughes SC, Levinson G, Rosen MA (eds.). *Schnider and Levison's Anaesthesia for Obstetrics.* Lippincott Williams & Wilkins, Philadelphia, 2002, pp. 455–86.

40 Ngan Kee WD, Shen J, Chui ATO et al. Combined spinal epidural anaesthesia in the management of labouring parturients with mitral stenosis. *Anaesth Intensive Care* 1999;27:523–6.

41 Schroeder JS, Harrison DC. Repeated cardioversion during pregnancy: Treatment of refractory paroxysmal atrial tachycardia during three successive pregnancies. *Am J Cardiol* 1971;27:445–6.

42 Feldman S. Drug focus—mivacurium. *Br J Hosp Med* 1997;57:199–200.

43 Bevan DR. The new relaxants: are they worth it? (Refresher course outline). *Can J Anesth* 1999;46:R88–R94.

44 Goudsouzian NG, d'Hollander AA, Viby-Morgensen J. Prolonged neuromuscular block from mivacurium in two patients with cholinesterase deficiency. *Anesth Analg* 1993;77:183–5.

45 Cade L, Kakulas P. Mivacurium in daycase surgical patients. *Anaesth Intensive Care* 1997;25:133–7.

46 Morris JGL. Selective monoamine oxidase inhibitors—clinical applications in neurology. *Australian Prescriber* 1993;16:3:57–8.

47 Malhotra V. Brachial Plexus Block. In: Yao FSF, Artusio JF (eds.). *Anesthesiology: Problem Orientated Patient Management,* 4th edn. JB Lippincott-Raven, Philadelphia, 1998, p. 535.

48 Lippman S, Nash K. Monoamine oxidase inhibitor uptake—potential adverse food and drug reactions. *Current Therapeutics* 1991, February:76–82.

49 Mcfarlane HJ. Anaesthesia and the new generation of monoamine oxidase inhibitors. *Anaesthesia* 1994;49:597–9.

50 Cousins MJ, Mather LE. Intrathecal and epidural opioids. *Anesthesiology* 1984;61:276–310.

51 Stoelting RK. Intrathecal morphine—an underused combination for postoperative pain management (Editorial). *Anesth Analg* 1989;68:707–9.

52 Murphy PM, Stack D, Kinirons B, Laffey JG. Optimising the dose of intrathecal morphine in older patients undergoing hip arthroplasty. *Anesth Analg* 2003;97:1709–15.

53 Chaney MA. Review article: Side effects of intrathecal and epidural opioids. *Can J Anaesth* 1995;42:891–903.

54 Glynn CJ. Intrathecal and epidural administration of opioids. *Bailliere's Clinical Anaesthesiology* 1987;1:4:915–30.

55 Borgeat A, Wilder-Smith OHG, Suter PM. The non-hypnotic therapeutic applications of propofol. *Anesthesiology* 1994;80:642–56.

56   Borgeat A, Stirnemann HR. Ondansetron is effective to treat spinal or epidural morphine-induced pruritus. *Anesthesiology* 1999;90:432–6.

57   Yeh H-M, Chen L-K, Lin C-J et al. Prophylactic intravenous ondansetron reduces the incidence of intrathecal morphine-induced pruritis in patients undergoing cesarean delivery. *Anesth Analg* 2000;91:172–5.

58   Tramér MR. A rational approach to the control of postoperative nausea and vomiting: evidence from systemic reviews. Part II. Recommendations for prevention and treatment, and research agenda. *Acta Anaesthesiol Scand* 2001;45:14–19.

59   Lien CA, Poznak AV. Myasthenia Gravis. In: Yao FSF, Artusio JF (eds.). *Anesthesiology: Problem Orientated Patient Management*, 4th edn. JB Lippincott-Raven, Philadelphia, 1998, p. 535.

60   Ossermann KE, Genkins G. Studies in myasthenia gravis. Review of a twenty-year experience in over 1200 patients. *Mt Sinai J Med* 1971;38:497–538.

61   Alley C, Dierdorf SF. Myasthenia gravis and muscular dystrophies. *Curr Opin Anaesthesiol* 1997;10:248–53.

62   Baraka A. Anesthesia and myasthenia gravis. *Can J Anaesth* 1992;39:476–86.

63   Mongano DT. Perioperative cardiac morbidity. *Anesthesiology* 1990;72:153–84.

64   Yao F-S F. Ischaemic Heart Disease and Noncardiac Surgery. In: Yao FSF, Artusio JF (eds.). *Anesthesiology: Problem Orientated Patient Management*, 4th edn. JB Lippincott-Raven, Philadelphia, 1998, pp. 385–404.

65   ACC/AHA Guideline update for perioperative cardiovascular evaluation for noncardiac surgery—executive summary. A report by the ACC/AHA task force on practice guidelines (Committee to update the 1996 guidelines on perioperative cardiovascular evaluation for noncardiac surgery.) *J Am Coll Cardiol* 2002;39:542–53.

66   Steen P, Tinker JH, Tarhan S. Myocardial reinfarction after anaesthesia and surgery. *JAMA* 1972;220:451.

67   Rao TLK, Jacobs KH, El-Etr AA. Reinfarction following anesthesia in patients with myocardial infarction. *Anesthesiology* 1983;59:499–505.

68 DeGeare VS, Dangas G, Stone GW, Grines CL. Interventional procedures in acute myocardial infarction. *Am Heart J* 2001;131: 15–24.

69 Stone JG, Foex P, Sear JW et al. Myocardial ischaemia in untreated hypertensive patients: effects of a single small oral dose of a beta-adrenergic blocking agent. *Anesthesiology* 1988;68:495–500.

70 Wallace A, Layug B, Tateo I et al. Prophylactic atenolol reduces post operative myocardial ischaemia. *Anesthesiology* 1998;88:7–17.

71 Mangano DT, Layug EL, Wallace A, Tateo IM. Effects of atenolol on mortality and cardiovascular morbidity after noncardiac surgery. The multicenter study of Perioperative Ischaemia Research Group. *N Engl J Med* 1996;335:1713–20.

72 Dodds TM, Stone JG, Coromilas J et al. Prophylactic nitroglycerin infusion during noncardiac surgery does not reduce perioperative ischaemia. *Anesth Analg* 1993;76:705–13.

N

1 Tramér MR. A rational approach to the control of postoperative nausea and vomiting: evidence from systemic reviews. Part 1. Efficacy and harm of antiemetic interventions, and methodological issues. *Acta Anaesthesiol Scand* 2001;45:4–13.

2 Divatia J, Vaidya JS, Badwe RA, Hawaldar RW. Omission of nitrous oxide during anaesthesia reduces the incidence of postoperative nausea and vomiting. A meta-analysis. *Anesthesiology* 1996;85:1055–62.

3 Sneyd JR, Carr A, Byron WD, Bilski AJT. A meta-analysis of nausea and vomiting following maintenance of anaesthesia with propofol or inhalational agents. *Eur J Anaesthesiol* 1998;15:433-445.

4 Harmon D, Bajwa S. Supplemental oxygen for the prevention of nausea and vomiting. *Anesthesiology* 2000;93:584–5.

5 Wilkes M, Hickey N. Anaesthesia for carotid surgery. *Br J Hosp Med* 1995;53:31–4.

6 Marcus R. Surveillance of health care workers exposed to blood from patients infected with human immunodeficiency virus. *New Eng J Med* 1988;89:1362–72.

7   Diprose P, Deakin CD, Smedley J. Ignorance of post-exposure pro-
    phylaxis guidelines following HIV needlestick injury may increase
    the risk of seroconversion. *Br J Anaesth* 2000;84(6):767–70.

8   Katz MH, Gerberding JL. Post exposure treatment of people exposed
    to the human immunodeficiency virus through sexual contact or
    injection drug use. *New Engl J Med* 1997;336:1097–9.

9   Shoret LJ, Bell DM. Risk of occupational infection with blood-borne
    pathogens in operating and delivery room settings. *Am J Infect
    Control* 1993;21:343–50.

10 Liddle C. Hepatitis C. *Anesth Intens Care* 1996;24:180–3.

11 Duke J. Airway Management. In: Duke J (ed.). *Anesthesia Secrets,* 2nd
    edn. Hanley and Belfus, Philadelphia, 2000, pp. 33–42.

12 Roy RN, Betheras R. The Melbourne chart—a logical guide to neona-
    tal resuscitation. *Anaesth Intensive Care* 1990;18:348–57.

13 Elliott RD. Neonatal resuscitation: the NRP guidelines. *Can J Anaesth*
    1994;41:742–53.

14 Wyllie J. Resuscitation of the newborn. *Anaesth Intensive Care Med*
    2002;3:3:88–91.

15 Van de Velde M. What is the best way to provide analgesia after
    Caesarean section? *Curr Opin Anesthesiol* 2000;13:267–70.

16 Craen RA, Gelb AW. The anaesthetic management of neurosur-
    gical emergencies. *Can J Anaesth* 1992;39:5:R29–34.

17 Artu AA. Nitrous oxide plays a direct role in the development
    of tension pneumocephalus intraoperatively. *Anesthesiology*
    1982;57:59–61.

18 Domino KB, Hemstad JR, Lam AM et al. Effect of nitrous oxide on
    intracranial pressure after cranial-dural closure in patients undergo-
    ing craniotomy. *Anesthesiology* 1992;77:421–5.

19 Isert P. Control of carbon dioxide levels during neuroanaesthesia:
    current practice and an appraisal of our reliance on capnography.
    Anaesth Intensive Care 1994;22:435–41.

20 Giebler R, Kollenberg B, Pohlen G, Peters J. Effect of positive end-expi-
    ratory pressure on the incidence of venous air embolism and on the
    cardiovascular response to the sitting position during neurosurgery.
    Br J Anaesth 1998;80:30–5.

21 Young WL. Cerebral aneurysms: management and future horizons. *Can J Anaesth* 1998;45:R17–R24.

22 Traill R. Neurosurgical anaesthesia. *Bailliere's Clinical Anaesth* 1993;7:2:399–422.

23 Abe K. Vasodilators during cerebral aneurysm surgery. *Can J Anaesth* 1993;40:775–90.

24 Gaitini L, Fradis M, Vaida S, Krimerman S, Beny A. Plasmapheresis in neuroleptic malignant syndrome. (Case report.) *Anaesthesia* 1997;52:165–8.

25 Tomson CRV. Neurolept malignant syndrome associated with inappropriate antidiuresis and psychogenic polydypsia. *Brit Med J* 1986;292;171.

26 Shaw MB. Postoperative neuroleptic malignant syndrome. *Anaesthesia* 1995;50:246–7.

27 Nishiyama T. Matsukawa T, Hanaoka K, Conway CM. Interactions between nicardipine and enflurane, isoflurane, and sevoflurane. *Can J Anaesth* 1997;44:10:1071–6.

28 *Cardiovascular Drug Guidelines*, 2nd edn. Published by the VMPF Therapeutics Committee on Behalf of the Victorian Drug Usage Advisory Committee, 1995, p. 68.

29 Sutcliffe AJ. Subarachnoid haemorrhage due to cerebral aneurysm. *Br J Anaesth CEPD Review* 2002;2:45–9.

30 Stenqvist O, Husum B, Dale O. Nitrous oxide: an ageing gentleman. *Acta Anaesthsiol Scand* 2001;45:135–7.

31 Dale O, Husum B. Nitrous oxide: from frolics to global concern in 150 years. *Acta Anaesthesiol Scand* 1994;38:749–50.

32 Brandt L. Nitrous oxide—no laughing matter? *Thoracic Cardiovasc Surg* 1990;38:79–80.

33 Hadzic A, Glab K, Sanborn KV, Thys DM. Severe neurological deficit after nitrous oxide anaesthesia. *Anesthesiol* 1995;83:863–6.

34 Logan M, Farmer JG. Anaesthesia and the ozone layer. *Br J Anaesth* 1989;63:645–6.

35 Keeling PA, Rocke DA, Ninn JF, Monk SJ, Lumb MJ, Halsey MJ. Folinic acid protection against nitrous oxide teratogenicity in the rat. *Br J Anaesth* 1986;58:1469–70.

36   Lane GA, Nahrwold ML, Tait AR, Taylor-Busch M, Cohen PJ, Beaudoin AR. Anesthetics as teratogens: nitrous oxide is fetotoxic, xenon is not. *Science* 1980;210:899–901.

37   Hawkins JL. Anesthesia for the pregnant patient undergoing non-obstetric surgery. In: Annual Refresher Course Lectures, American Society of Anesthesiologists, 1997, p. 235.

38   Myles PS, Leslie K, Silbert B, Paech MJ, Peyton P. A review of the risks and benefits of nitrous oxide in current anaesthesia practice. *Anesth Intensive Care* 2004;32:165–72.

39   Vote BJ, Hart RH, Worsely DR, Borthwick JH, Laurent S, McGeorge AJ. Visual loss after nitrous oxide gas with general anaesthetic in patients with intraocular gas still persistent up to 30 days after vitrectomy. *Anesthesiology* 2002;9:1305–8.

40   Tarkkila P, Rosenberg PH. Perioperative analgesia with non-steroidal analgesics. *Curr Opin Anaesthesiol* 1998;11:407–10.

41   *Guidelines for the Use of Non-steroidal Anti-inflammatory Drugs in the Perioperative Period.* Issued by The Royal College of Anaesthetists, January 1998.

42   Mashford ML, Andreoli T, Cosolo W et al. *Therapeutic Guidelines: Analgesic,* 3rd edn. Therapeutic Guidelines Limited, 1997, p. 14.

43   McManus P, Henry DA, Birkett DJ. Recent changes in the profile of prescription NSAID use in Australia. *Med J Aust* 2000;172:188.

44   Cryer B. Nonsteroidal anti-inflammatory drug gastrointestinal toxicity. *Current Opin Gastroenterology* 2001;17:503–12.

45   Ahmad SR, Kortepeter C, Brinker A, Chen M, Beitz J. Renal failure associated with the use of celecoxib and rofecoxib. *Drug Safety* 2002;25:537–44.

46   Guidelines 2000 for cardiopulmonary resuscitation and emergency cardiovascular care. *Circulation* 2000;102 (suppl I):1–131.

O

1   Benumof JL. Sleep apnoea and the obese patient. *Audio Digest: Anesthesiology* 2000;42.

2   Boushra NN. Review article: Anaesthetic management of patients with sleep apnoea syndrome. *Can J Anaesth* 1996;43:599–616.

3   Kerr P, Shoenut JP, Millar T, Buckle P, Kryger MH. Nasal CPAP reduces gastroesophageal reflux in obstructive sleep apnea syndrome. *Chest* 1992;101:1539–44.

4   Loadsman JA, Hillman DR. Review article: Anaesthesia and sleep apnoea. *Br J Anaesth* 2001;86:254–66.

5   Watcha MF, White PF. Postoperative nausea and vomiting—its aetiology, treatment and prevention. *Anesthesiology* 1992;77:162–84.

6   Tramér MR, Reynolds DJM, Moore RA, McQuay HJ. Efficacy, dose response and safety of ondansetron in prevention of post-operative nausea and vomiting: A quantitative systematic review of randomized placebo-controlled trials. *Anesthesiology* 1997;87:1277–89.

7   Brodsky JB, Macario A, Cannon WB, Mark JBD. Blind placement of plastic left double-lumen tubes. *Anaesth Intensive Care* 1995;23:583–6.

8   Benumof JL, Alfery DD. Anesthesia for thoracic surgery. In: Miller RD (ed.). *Anesthesia*, 3rd edn. Churchill Livingstone, New York, 1990, pp. 1517–1603.

9   Russell W. A blind guided technique for placing double lumen endotracheal tubes. *Anaesth Intensive Care* 1992;20:71–4.

10 Campos JH. Current techniques for perioperative lung isolation in adults. *Anesthesiology* 2002;97:1295–301.

11 Slinger P, Triolet W, Wilson S. Improving arterial oxygenation during one lung ventilation. *Anesthesiology* 1988;68:291–5.

12 Eastwood J, Mahajan R. One-lung anaesthesia. *Brit J Anaesth CEPD Reviews* 2002;3:83–7.

13 Philbin DM. Opioids. *Balliere's Clinical Anaesthesiology* 1989;3:1:205–14.

14 Wilkinson DJ. Opioid agonist/antagonists in general anaesthesia. *Br J Hosp Med* 1987;Aug:130–2.

15 Mather LE. Pharmacology of opioids—part 1. Basic aspects. *Med J Aust* 1986;144:424–7.

16 Mashford ML, Andreoli T, Cosolo W et al. *Therapeutic Guidelines: Analgesic*, 3rd edn. Therapeutic Guidelines Limited, 1997, p. 15.

P

1   Trakina M. Pacemakers. In: Faust RJ, Cucchiara RF, Rose SH, Spackman TN, Wedel DJ, Wass CT (eds.). *Anesthesiology Review*, 3rd edn. Churchill Livingstone, Philadelphia, 2002, pp. 340–1.

2   Bryan CS et al. Endocarditis related to transvenous pacemakers: syndromes and surgical implications. *J Thorac Cardiovasc Surg* 1978;75:758.

3   Bloomfield P, Bowler MR. Anaesthetic management of the patient with a permanent pacemaker. *Anaesthesia* 1989;44:42–6.

4   Kam PCA. Anaesthetic management of a patient with an automatic implantable cardioverter defibrillator in situ. *Br J Anaesth* 1997;78:102–6.

5   Otto CW. Clinical utilisation of pacemakers and defibrillators for the anesthesiologist. 48th Annual Refresher Course Lectures, American Society of Anesthesiologists, 1997;216:1–6.

6   Cooper J. What's new in temporary pacing? *Br J Hosp Med.* 1994;52:9:437–8.

7   Szafranski JS, Obberoi MP, Chetty PK, Dabiri MD. Use of transesophageal atrial pacing during electroconvulsive therapy. *Anesthesiology* 1996;84:211–14.

8   Sasada MP, Smith SP. *Drugs in Anaesthesia and Intensive Care*, 2nd edn. Oxford University Press, Oxford, 1997, p. 282.

9   Peutrell JM, Wolf AR. Pain in children. *Br J Hosp Med* 1992;47:4:289–93.

10 Pusch F, Freitag H, Weinstabl C, Obwegeser R, Huber E, Wilding E. Single-injection paravertebral block compared to general anaesthesia in breast surgery. *Acta Anaesthesiol Scand* 1999;43:770–4.

11 Richardson J, Sabanathan S. Thoracic paravertebral anaesthesia. *Acta Anaesthesiol Scand* 1995;39:1005–15.

12 Noveck R, Laurent A, Kuss M, Talwalker S, Hubbard RC. Parecoxib sodium does not impair platelet function in healthy elderly and non-elderly individuals. *Clin Drug Invest* 2001;21:465–76.

13 Harris SI, Kuss M, Hubbard RC. Upper gastrointestinal safety evaluation of parecoxib sodium, a new parenteral cyclooxygenase-2-specific inhibitor, compared with ketorolac, naproxen, and placebo. *Clin Ther* 2001;23:1422–8.

14 Errington DR, Severn AM, Meara J. Parkinson's disease. *Brit J Anaesth CEPD Reviews* 2002;2:69–73.

15 Nicholson G, Pereira AC, Hall GM. Parkinson's disease and anaesthesia (Review Article). *Brit J Anaesth* 2002;89:904–16.

16 Gravlee GP. Succinylcholine-induced hyperkalaemia in a patient with Parkinson's disease. *Anesth Analg* 1980;59:444–6.

17 Muzzi DA, Black S, Cucchiara RF. The lack of effect of succinylcholine on serum potassium in patients with Parkinson's disease. *Anesthesiology* 1989;71:322.

18 Anderson BJ, Marks PV, Futter ME. Propofol-contrasting effects in movement disorders. *Br J Neurosurg* 1994;8:387–8.

19 Golden WE, Lavender RC, Metzer WS. Acute postoperative confusion and hallucinations in Parkinson's disease. *Ann Intern Med* 1989;111:218–22.

20 Toussaint S, Maidl J, Schwagmeier R, Striebel HW. Patient-controlled intranasal analgesia: effective alternative to intravenous PCA for postoperative pain relief. *Can J Anesth* 2000;47:299–302.

21 Volmanen P, Akural EI, Raudaskoski T, Alahuhta S. Remifentanil in obstetric analgesia: a dose-finding study. *Anesth Analg* 2002;94:913–7.

22 Cooper MG. *The New Children's Hospital Acute Pain Treatment Manual*, 2nd edn, revised June 1996.

23 Serour F, Mori J. Optimal regional anaesthesia for circumcision. *Anesth Analg* 1994;79:129–31.

24 Brown TCK, Weidner NJ, Bouwmeester FW. Dorsal nerve of the penis block—anatomical and radiological studies. *Anaesth Intensive Care* 1989;17:34–8.

25 Irwin M, Cheng W. Comparison of subcutaneous ring block of the penis with caudal epidural block for post-circumcision analgesia in children. *Anaesth Intensive Care* 1996;24:365–7.

26 Burke D, Joypaul V, Thomson MF. Circumcision supplemented by dorsal penile nerve block with 0.75% ropivacaine: a complication. *Regional Anaesthesia and Pain Medicine* 2000;25:424–7.

27 Berens R, Pontus SP. A complication of circumcision and dorsal nerve block of the penis. *Reg Anesth* 1990;15:309–10.

28 George LM, Gatt SP, Lowe S. Peripartum cardiomyopathy: four case histories and a commentary on anaesthetic management. *Anaesth Intensive Care* 1997;25:292–6.

29 Browa G, O'Leary M, Douglas J, Herkes R. Perioperative management of a case of severe peripartum cardiomyopathy. *Anaesth Intens Care* 1992;20:80–3.

30 McCarroll CP, Paxton LD, Elliott P, Wilson DB. Use of remifentanil in a patient with peripartum cardiomyopathy requiring Caesarean section. *Brit J Anaesth* 2001;86:135–8.

31 Pirlet M, Baird S, Pryn S, Jones-Ritson M, Kinsella SM. Low dose combined spinal-epidural anaesthesia for caesarean section in a patient with peripartum cardiomyopathy. *Internat J Obstetric Anesth* 2000;9:189–92.

32 Sasada MP, Smith SP. *Drugs in Anaesthesia and Intensive Care,* 2nd edn. Oxford University Press, Oxford, 1997, p. 288.

33 Wood M. Opioid Agonists and Antagonists. In: Wood M, Wood A (eds.). *Drugs and Anaesthesia,* 2nd edn. Williams and Wilkins, Baltimore, 1990, p. 146.

34 Gaensler EA, McGowan JM, Henderson FF. A comparative study of the action of demoral and opium alkaloids in relation to biliary spasm. *Surgery* 1947;22:211–20.

35 Latta KS, Ginsberg B, Barkin RL. Meperidine: a clinical review. *American J Therapeutics* 2002;9:53–68.

36 Ngan Kee WD. Epidural Pethidine: pharmacology and clinical experience. *Anaesth Intensive Care* 1998;26:247–55.

37 Jasani NB, O'Connor RE, Bouzoukis JK. Comparison of hydromorphone and meperidine for ureteral colic. *Acad Emerg Med* 1994;1:539–43.

38 Singh G, Kam P. An overview of anaesthetic issues in phaeochromocytomas. *Annals Academy of Medicine* 1998;27:843–8.

39 Whalley DG. Anaesthetic management of the patient with phaeochromocytoma. *Audio-Digest Anesthesiology*;37:22.

40 Roizen MF, Harrigan RW, Koike M. A prospective randomized trial of four anaesthetic techniques for resection of phaeochromocytoma. *Anaesthesiology* 1982;57:A43.

41 Watson VF, Vaughan RS. Magnesium and the anaesthetist. *Brit J Anaesth CEPD Reviews* 2001;1:16–20.

42 Breslin DS, Farling PA, Mirakhur RK. Case report: The use of remifentanil in the anaesthetic management of patients undergoing adrenalectomy: A report of three cases. *Anaesthesia* 2003;58:358–62.

43 Davies MJ, McGlade DP, Banting SW. A comparison of open and laparoscopic approaches to adrenalectomy in patients with phaeochromocytoma. *Anaesth Intensive Care* 2004;32:224–9.

44 Tauzin-Fin P, Hilbert L, Krol-Houdek M, Gosse P, Maurette P. Mydriasis and acute pulmonary oedema complicating laparoscopic removal of phaeochromocytoma. *Anaesth Intensive Care* 1999;27:646–9.

45 Roizen MF. Endocrine abnormalities and anaesthesia. ASA Refresher Course Lectures. San Francisco: American Society of Anesthesiologists, 1985, pp. 253–65.

46 Apgar V, Papper EM. Phaeochromocytoma—anaesthetic management during surgical treatment. *Arch Surg* 1951;62:634–48.

47 Foo M, Burton BJL, Ahmed R. Phaeochromocytoma. *Brit J Hosp Med* 1995;54:318–21.

48 Read JA, Cotton DB, Miller FC. Placenta accreta: changing clinical aspects and outcome. *Obstet Gynecol* 1980;56:31–4.

49 Litwin MS, Loughlin KR, Benson CB, Droega GF, Richie JP. Placenta percreta invading the bladder. *Br J Urol* 1989;64:283–6.

50 Lerner JP, Deane S, Timor-Tritsch IE. Characterization of placenta accreta using transvaginal sonography and color Doppler imaging. *Ultrasound Obstet Gynecol* 1995;5:198–201.

51 Paull JD, Smith J, Williams L, Davison G, Devine T, Holt M. Balloon occlusion of the abdominal aorta during Caesarean hysterectomy for placenta percreta. *Anaesth Intensive Care* 1995;23:731–4.

52 Clark SL, Koonings P, Phelan JP et al. Placenta praevia/accreta and prior Caesarean section. *Obstet Gynecol* 1985;66:89–92.

53 Parekh N, Husaini SWU, Russell IF. Caesarean section for placenta praevia: a retrospective study of anaesthetic management. *Brit J Anaesth* 2000;84:725–30.

54 Kam PCA, Nethery CM. Review article: The thienpyridine derivatives (platelet adenosine diphosphate receptor antagonists), pharmacology and clinical developments. *Anaesthesia* 2003;58:28–35.

55 Kam PCA, Egan MK. Platelet glycoprotein IIb, IIIa antagonists. *Anesthesiology* 2002;96:1237–49.

56 Sreeram GM, Sharma AD, Slaughter TF. Platelet glycoprotein IIb/IIIa antagonists: perioperative implications. *J Cardithoracic Vascular Surg* 2001;15:237–40.

57 Tcheng JE. Clinical challenges of platelet glycoprotein IIb/IIIa receptor inhibitor therapy: Bleeding, reversal, thrombocytopaenia and retreatment. *Am Heart J* 2000;139:S38–45.

58 Australian Red Cross Circular of Information, May 1994.

59 American Society of Anesthesiologists task force on blood component therapy. Practice guidelines for blood component therapy. *Anesthesiology* 1996;84:732–47.

60 Hardy JF, Belisle S, Robitaille D. Blood products: when and how to use them. *Can J Anaesth* 1994;41:5:R52–R60.

61 Mulroy MF. *Regional Anesthesia: An Illustrated Procedural Guide,* 2nd edn. Little, Brown and Company, Boston, 1989, pp. 209–10.

62 Konrad C, Jöhr M. Blockade of the sciatic nerve in the popliteal fossa: a system for standardization in children. *Anesth Analg* 1998;87:1256–8.

63 Jensen NF, Fiddler DS, Striepe V. Anesthetic considerations in porphyrias. *Anesth Analg* 1995;80:591–9.

64 Ashley EMC. Anaesthesia for porphyria. *Br J Hosp Med* 1996;56(1):37–42.

65 Stoelting RK, Dierdorf SF. *Anesthesia and Co-existing Disease,* 3rd edn. Churchill Livingstone, New York, 1993, pp. 375–8.

66 Elcock D, Norris A. Elevated porphyrins following propofol anaesthesia in acute intermittent porphyria. *Anaesthesia* 1994;49:957–8.

67 Moore MR, International review of drugs in acute porphyrias—1980. *Int J Biochem* 1980;12:1089–97.

68 Brown K. FANZCA Part II Exam Short Course Lectures, Melbourne, July 1996.

69 Thomas C, Madej T. Obstetric emergencies and the anaesthetist. *Brit J Anaesth CEPD Reviews* 2002;2:174–7.

70 Riley DP, Burgess RW. External aortic compression: A study of a resuscitation manoeuvre for postpartum haemorrhage. *Anaesth Intensive Care* 1994;22:571–5.

71 Bowen LW, Beeson JH. Use of a large Foley catheter balloon to control postpartum haemorrhage resulting from low placental implantation. A report of two cases. *J Reprod Med* 1985;30(8):623–5.

72 Worthley L. IG Fluid and Electrolyte Therapy. In: Oh TE, Bersten A, Soni N (eds.). *Oh's Intensive Care Manual.* Butterworth-Heinemann, UK, 2003, pp. 891–2.

73 Tetzlaff JE, Walsh MT. (Review article) Potassium and anaesthesia. *Can J Anaesth* 1993;40:3:227–46.

74 Consensus Statement of the Australasian Society for the Study of Hypertension in Pregnancy. Management of hypertension in pregnancy: executive summary. *Med J Aust* 1993;158:700–2.

75 Brown MA, Hague WM, Higgins J, Lowe S, McCowan L, Oats J, Peek MJ, Rowan JA, Walters BNJ. Consensus Statement: The detection, investigation and management of hypertension in pregnancy: executive study. *Aust NZ J Obstet Gynaecol* 2000;40:139–55.

76 Cheng AY, Kwan A. Perioperative management of intra-partum seizure. *Anesth Intens Care* 1997;25:535–8.

77 Boxer LM, Malinow AM. Pre-eclampsia and eclampsia. *Curr Opin Anaesthesiol* 1997;10:3:188–97.

78 Weinstein L. Syndrome of hemolysis, elevated liver enzymes, and low platelet count: a severe consequence of hypertension in pregnancy. *Am J Obstet Gynecol* 1989;142:159–67.

79 Crosby ET. Obstetrical anaesthesia for patients with the syndrome of haemolysis, elevated liver enzymes and low platelets. *Can J Anaesth* 1991;38:2:227–33.

80 Malinow AM. Obstetric anaesthesia revisited: Anesthetic considerations for the pre-eclamptic patient. *Audio-Digest Anesthesiology* 1995;37.

81 James MFM. Magnesium in obstetric anesthesia. *International J Obstetric Anesth* 1998;7:115–23.

82 Allen RW, James MFM, Uys PC. Attenuation of the pressor response to tracheal intubation in hypertensive proteinuric pregnant patients by lignocaine, alfentanil and magnesium sulphate. *Br J Anaesth* 1991;66:216–23.

83 Engelhardt T, MacLennan FM. Fluid management in pre-eclampsia. *Internation J Obstet Anesthesia* 1999;8:253–9.

84 Schindler M, Gatt S, Isert P, Morgans D, Cheung A. Thrombocytopenia and platelet functional defects in pre-eclampsia: implications for regional anaesthesia. *Anaesth Intensive Care* 1990;18:169–74.

85 Hood DD, Curry R. Spinal versus epidural anesthesia for caesarean section in severely preeclamptic patients. *Anesthesiology* 1999;90:1276–82.

86 Santos AC. (Editorial) Spinal anaesthesia in severely preeclamptic women. *Anesthesiology* 1999;90:1252–4.

87 Morrison DH. Anaesthesia and preeclampsia. *Can J Anaesth* 1987;34:4:415–22.

88 Blass N. Non-obstetric Surgery During Pregnancy. In: Datta S (ed.). *Obstetric Anesthesia*, 2nd edn. Mosby, St Louis, 1995, pp. 427–38.

89 Griffiths C, Agarwal R. Hypotension. In: Duke J, Rosenberg SG (eds.). *Anesthesia Secrets*. Hansley & Belfus, Inc, Philadelphia, Mosby, St Louis, 1996, pp. 196–7.

90 Blass N. Non-obstetric Surgery During Pregnancy. In: Datta S (ed.). *Obstetric Anesthesia*, 2nd edn. Mosby, St Louis, 1995, pp. 427–38.

91 Hawkins JL. Anesthesia for the Pregnant Patient Undergoing Nonobstetric surgery. In: 48th Annual Refresher Course Lectures, American Society of Anesthesiologists, 1997, p. 235.

92 Trissel LA. *Injectable Drugs Handbook*, 12th edn. American Society of Health System Pharmacists, 2003, p. 273.

93 Borgeat A, Wilder-Smith OHG, Suter PM. The nonhypnotic therapeutic applications of propofol. *Anesthesiology* 1994;80:3:642–54.

94 Leslie K. Diprivan-based anaesthesia using Diprifusor™ TCI. Zeneca product literature, October 1998.

95 Myles PS, Hendrata M, Bennett AM, Langley M, Buckland MR. Postoperative nausea and vomiting. Propofol and thiopentone: Does choice of induction agent affect outcome? *Anaesth Intensive Care* 1996;24:355–9.

96 Sutherland MJ, Burt P. Propofol and seizures. *Anaesth Intensive Care* 1994;22:733–7.

97 Harwood TN. Optimizing outcome in the very elderly surgical patient. *Curr Opin Anaesthesiol* 2000;13:327–32.

98 Parke TJ, Stevens JE, Rice AS et al. Metabolic acidosis and fatal myocardial failure after propofol infusion in children; five case reports. *Br Med J* 1992;305:613–16.

99 Douglas MJ. New drugs, old drugs and the obstetric anaesthetist (Refresher Course Outline). *Can J Anaesth* 1995;42:5:R3–R8.

100 Douglas MJ, Farquharson DR, Ross PL et al. Cardiovascular collapse following an overdose of prostaglandin F$_2$ α : A case report. *Can J Anaesth* 1989;36:466.

101 Mukadam ME, Pritchard P, Riddington D et al. Case conference: Case 7 2001 Management during cardiopulmonary bypass of patients with presumed fish allergy. *J Cardiothorac Vasc Anesth* 2001;4:512–19.

102 Kong R, Singer M. Insertion of a pulmonary artery flotation catheter: how to do it. *Br J Hosp Med* 1997;57:9:432–5.

103 Bouchard RJ, Gault JH, Ross J Jr. Evaluation of pulmonary arterial end-diastolic pressure as a measurement of left ventricular end-diastolic pressure in patients with normal and abnormal left ventricular performance. *Circulation* 1971;44:1072–9.

104 Lehr S. Pulmonary Artery Catheterization. In: Parsons P, Wiener-Kronish JP (eds.). *Critical Care Secrets.* Mosby, St Louis, 1992, pp. 53–8.

105 Bowyer MW. Invasive Cardiac Monitoring. In: Parsons P, Wiener-Kronish JP (eds.). *Critical Care Secrets.* Mosby, St Louis, 1992, pp. 15–20.

106 McGrath B, Fletcher SJ. Intensive care management of pulmonary embolism. *Anaesth Intensive Care* 2001;2:347–52.

107 McConnell MV, Solomon SD, Ryan ME et al. Regional right ventricular dysfunction detected by echocardiography in acute pulmonary embolism. *Am J Cardiol* 1996;78:469–73.

108 Capellier G, Jacques T, Balvay P et al. Inhaled nitric oxide in patients with pulmonary embolism. *Intensive Care Med* 1997;23:1089–92.

109 Webb SA, Stott S, van Heerden PV. The use of inhaled aerosolized prostacyclin (IAP) in the treatment of pulmonary hypertension secondary to pulmonary embolism. *Intensive Care Med* 1996;22:353–5.

110 Smedstad KG, Morison DH. Pulmonary hypertension and pregnancy: a series of eight cases. *Can J Anaesth* 1994;41:6:502–12.

111 Stoelting RK, Dierdorf SF. *Anesthesia and Co-existing Disease*, 3rd edn.

Churchill Livingstone, New York, 1993, p. 103.

112 Myles PS. Anaesthetic management for laparoscopic sterilization and termination of pregnancy in a patient with severe primary pulmonary hypertension. *Anaesth Intensive Care* 1994;22:465–9.

113 Roessler P, Lambert TF. Anaesthesia for Caesarean section in the presence of primary pulmonary hypertension. *Anaesth Intensive Care* 1986;14:317–20.

114 Slomka F, Salmeron S, Zetlaoui P et al. Primary pulmonary hypertension and pregnancy: anaesthetic management for delivery. *Anesthesiology* 1988;68:959–61.

115 Cheng DCH, Edelist G. Isoflurane and primary pulmonary hypertension. *Anaesthesia* 1988;43:22–4.

116 Mason R. *Anaesthesia Databook—A Perioperative and Peripartum Manual.* Greenwich Medical Media Limited, London, 2001, pp. 419–23.

117 Mangano DT. Anesthesia for the Pregnant Cardiac Patient. In: Schnider SM, Levinson G (eds.). *Anesthesia for Obstetrics,* 2nd edn. Williams and Wilkins, Baltimore, 1987, pp. 123–41.

118 Smedstad KG, Cramb R, Morison DH. Pulmonary hypertension and pregnancy: a series of eight cases. *Can J Anaesth* 1994;41:502–12.

119 Roberts NV, Keast PJ. Pulmonary hypertension and pregnancy—a lethal combination. *Anaesth Intensive Care* 1990;18:366–74.

120 Takeuchi T, Nishii O, Okamura T, Yaginuma T. Primary pulmonary hypertension in pregnancy. *Int J Gynecol Obstet* 1998;26:145–50.

121 Lapinsky SE, Mount DB, Mackey D, Grossman R. Management of acute respiratory failure due to pulmonary edema with nasal positive pressure support. *Chest* 1994;105:229–31.

122 Rizk NW, Murray JF. PEEP and pulmonary oedema. *Am J Med* 1982;72:381–3.

123 Boon NA, Fox AA. Diseases of the Cardiovascular System. In: Edwards CRW, Bouchier IAD, Haslett C, Chilvers ER (eds.). *Davidson's Principles and Practice of Medicine,* 17th edn. Churchill Livingstone, Edinburgh 1995, pp. 294–5.

124 Ransom D, Leicht C. Continuous spinal analgesia with sufentanil for labour and delivery in a parturient with severe pulmonary stenosis. *Anesth Analg* 1995;80:418–21.

R

1 Gabbott DA. Recent advances in airway technology. *Br J Anaesth CEPD Reviews* 2001;1:76–80.

2 Martinowitz U, Kenet G, Segal E et al. Recombinant activated factor VII for adjunctive haemorrhage control in trauma. *J Trauma Injury Infection Crit Care* 2001;51:431–9.

3 Svartholm E, Annerhargen V, Länne T. Treatment of bleeding in severe necrotizing pancreatitis with recombinant factor VIIa. *Anesthesiology* 2002;96:1528.

4 Tobias JD. Synthetic factor VIIa to treat dilutional coagulopathy during posterior spinal fusion in two children. *Anesthesiology* 2002;96:1522–5.

5 Lovric VA. Alterations in blood components during storage and their clinical significance. *Anesth Intensive Care* 1984;12:246–51.

6 Monk TG. Altenatives to allogenic blood transfusions (Refresher Course Outline). *Can J Anesth* 1999;46:R3–R6.

7 Thompson JP, Rowbotham DJ. Editorial. Remifentanil—an opioid for the 21st century. *Br J Anaesth* 1996;76:3:341–2.

8 Barclay K, Kluger MT. Effect of bolus dose of remifentanil on haemodynamic response to intubation. *Anaesth Intensive Care* 2000;28:403–7.

9 Elliott P, O'Hare R, Moyna Bill K, Phillips AS, Gibson FM, Mirakhur RK. Severe cardiovascular depression with remifentanil. *Anesth Analg* 2000;91:58–61.

10 Servin FS, Raeder JC, Merle JC et al. Remifentanil sedation compared with propofol during regional anaesthesia. *Acta Anaesthesiol Scand* 2002;46:309–15.

11 Rabey P. Anaesthesia for renal transplantation. *Br J Anaesth CPED Reviews* 2001;1:24–7.

12 Moote CA. Anesthesia for renal transplantation. *Anesth Clin Nth America* 1994;12:4:691–711.

13 Apps MCP. A guide to lung function tests. *Br J Hosp Med* 1992;48:7:396–401.

14 Glass GD, Olsen GN. Preoperative pulmonary function testing to predict postoperative morbidity and mortality. *Chest* 1986;89:127–35.

15 Benumof JL, Alfery DD. Anesthesia for Thoracic Surgery. In: Miller RD (ed.). *Anesthesia*, 3rd edn. Churchill Livingstone, New York, 1990, pp. 1520–1.

16 Hung OR, Al-Qatari. Light-guided retrograde intubation. *Can J Anaesth* 1997;44:877–82.

17 Hung OR. Airway adjuncts and alternative techniques of endotracheal intubation. (Refresher Course Outline) *Can J Anaesth* 1995;42:R31–R34.

18 Epemolu O, Bom A, Hope F, Mason R. Reversal of neuromuscular blockade and simultaneous increase in plasma rocuronium concentration after intravenous infusion of the novel reversal agent Org 25969. *Anesthesiology* 2003;3:632–7.

19 Pühringer FK. Hemodynamic Effects of Rocuronium. In: Crul JF (ed.). *Clinical Aspects of Rocuronium Bromide*. Organon Teknika, Turnhout, Belgium, 1996, pp. 37–44.

20 Pollard BJ. Drug focus: Rocuronium and cisatracurium. *Br J Hosp Med* 1997;57:346–8.

21 Patel N, Smith CE, Pinchak AC. Emergency surgery and rapid sequence intubation: rocuronium vs succinylcholine. *Anesthesiology* 1995;83:A914.

22 Heier T, Guttormsen AB. Anaphylactic reactions during induction of anaesthesia using rocuronium for muscle relaxation: a report of 3 cases. *Acta Anaesthesiol Scand* 2000;44:775–81.

23 Laake JH, Røttingen JA. Rocuronium and anaphylaxis—a statistical challenge. *Acta Anaesthesiol Scand* 2001;45:1196–203.

24 McClure JH. Ropivacaine. *Br J Anaesth* 1996;76:300–7.

25 McNamee DA, McClelland AM, Scott S, Milligan KR, Westman L, Gustafsson U. Spinal anaesthesia: a comparison of plain ropivacaine 5 mg mL^{-1} with bupivacaine 5 mg mL^{-1} for major or orthopaedic surgery. *Br J Anaesth* 2002;89:702–6.

26 Morton C. Ropivacaine. *Br J Hosp Med* 1997;58:97–8.

27 Chazalon P, Tourtier JP, Villevieille T, Giraud D, Saissy JM, Mion G, Benhamou D. Ropivacaine-induced cardiac arrest after peripheral nerve block: Successful resuscitation. *Anesthesiology* 2003;99:1449–51.

28 Huet O, Eyrolle IJ, Mazoit JX, Ozier YM. Cardiac arrest and plasma concentration after injection of ropivacaine for posterior lumbar plexus blockade. *Anesthesiology* 2003;99:1451–3.

S

1   Shann F. Drug Doses, 9th edn. Collective Pty Ltd, Melbourne, 1996, pp. 50–1.

2   Brinsmead M. Fetal and neonatal effects of drugs administered in labour. *Med J Aust* 1987;146:481–5.

3   Comfort K, Lang SA and Ray W. Saphenous nerve anaesthesia—a nerve stimulator technique. *Can J Anaesth* 1996;43:8:852–7.

4   Mulroy M. *Regional Anaesthesia: An Illustrated Procedural Guide,* 2nd edn. Little, Brown and Company, Boston, 1996, pp. 223–7.

5   Arkoosh VA. Neonatal resuscitation in the obstetric suite: what you need to know. In: 48th Annual Refresher Course Lectures. American Society of Anaesthetists 1997;236:1–7.

6   Mulroy MF. *Regional Anesthesia: An Illustrated Procedural Guide,* 2nd edn. Little, Brown and Company, Boston, 1996, pp. 201–27.

7   Smith I, Nathanson M, White PF. Sevoflurane—a long awaited volatile anaesthetic. *Br J Anaesth* 1996;76:435–45.

8   Goff MJ, Arain SR, Ficke DJ, Uhrich TD, Ebert TJ. Absence of bronchodilation during desflurane anaesthesia. *Anesthesiology* 2000;93:404–8.

9   Frink EJ. Toxicologic potential of desflurane and sevoflurane. *Acta Anaesthesioloca Scandinavica* 1995;120–1.

10 Patel S, Goa KL. Sevoflurane: A review of its pharmacodynamic and pharmacokinetic properties and its clinical use in general anaesthesia. *Drugs* 1996;51:658–700.

11 Apfelbaum JL. Pharmacology for ambulatory anaesthesia. *Audio-Digest Anesthesiology* 1996;38:21.

12 Mazze RI, Jamison R. Renal effects of sevoflurane. *Anesthesiology* 1995;83:443–5.

13 Kleinsasser A, Kuenszberg E, Loekinger A et al. Sevoflurane, but not propofol, significantly prolongs the Q-T interval. *Anesth Analg* 2000;90:25–7.

14 Abe K, Takada K, Yoshiya I. Intraoperative torsade de pointes ventricular tachycardia and ventricular fibrillation during sevoflurane anesthesia. *Anesth Analg* 1998;86:701–2.

15 Kleinsasser A, Loeckinger A, Lindner KH et al. Reversing sevoflurane-associated Q-Tc prolongation by changing to propofol. *Anaesthesia* 2001;56:248–71.

16 Beskow A, Westrin P. Sevoflurane causes more postoperative agitation in children than does halothane. *Acta Anaesthesiol Scand* 1999;43:536–41.

17 Eger E. Volatile anaesthetics for the new millennium. *Audio-Digest Anesthesiology* 2000;42:15.

18 Horn E-P. Postoperative shivering: aetiology and treatment. *Current Opinion in Anaesthesiology* 1999;12:449–53.

19 Mahajan RP, Grover VK, Sharma SL, Singh H. Intraocular pressure changes during muscular activity after general anesthesia. *Anesthesiology* 1988;66:419–21.

20 Horn E-P, Standl T, Sessler DI, von Knobelsdorf G, Buchs C, Esch JS. Physostigmine prevents postanesthetic shivering as does meperidine or clonidine. *Anesthesiolology* 1998;88:108–13.

21 Bamigbade TA, Langford RM. The clinical use of tramadol hydrochloride. *Pain Reviews* 1998;5:155–82.

22 Bhatnagar S, Saxena A, Kannan TR, Punj J, Panigrahi M, Mishra S. Tramadol for postoperative shivering: a double-blind comparison with pethidine. *Anaesth Intensive Care* 2001;29:149–54.

23 Mason R. *Anaesthesia Databook: A Perioperative and Peripartum Manual*, 3rd edn. Greenwich Medical Media Limited, London, 2001, pp. 218–24.

24 Embury SH. The clinical pathophysiology of sickle cell disease. *Ann Rev Med* 1986;36:361–76.

25 Vijay V, Cavenagh JD, Yate P. The anaesthetist's role in acute sickle cell crisis. *Br J Anaesth* 1998;80:820–8.

26 Stein RE, Urbaniak J. Use of the tourniquet during surgery in patients with sickle cell haemoglobinopathies. *Clin Orthopaed Related Research* 1980;151:231–3.

27 Al-Ghamdi AA. Bilateral total knee replacement with tourniquets in a homozygous sickle cell patient. *Anesth Analg* 2004;98:543–4.

28 Brajtbord D, Johnson D, Ramsay M et al. Use of the cell saver in patients with sickle cell trait. *Anesthesiology* 1989;70:878.

29 Koshy M, Weiner SJ, Miller ST et al. Surgery and anaesthesia in sickle cell disease. *Blood* 1995;86:3676–84.

30 Denzer BI, Birnbach DJ, Thys DM. Anesthesia for the parturient with sickle cell disease. *J Clin Anesth* 1996;8:598–602.

31 Chiron B, Laffon M, Ferrandiére M, Pittet J-F. Postdural puncture headache in a parturient with sickle cell disease: use of an epidural colloid patch. *Can J Anaesth* 2003;50:812–4.

32 Steinberg MS. Management of sickle cell disease. *Drug Therapy* 1999;340:1021–30.

33 Bernini JC, Rogers ZR, Sandler ES et al. Beneficial effects of intravenous dexamethasone in children with mild to moderate severe acute chest syndrome complicating sickle cell disease. *Blood* 1998;92:3082–9.

34 Sasada MP, Smith SP. *Drugs in Anaesthesia and Intensive Care*, 2nd edn. Oxford University Press, Oxford, 1997, pp. 334–5.

35 Friedrich JA, Butterworth JF. Sodium nitroprusside: twenty years and counting. *Anesth Analg* 1995;81:152–62.

36 Weekes JWN. Poisoning and Drug Intoxication. In: Oh TE (ed.). *Intensive Care Manual*, 4th edn. Butterworth-Heinemann, Oxford, 1997, p. 667.

37 Donovan KD, Hockings BEF. Antiarrhythmic Drugs. In: Oh TE (ed.). *Intensive Care Manual*, 4th edn. Butterworth-Heinemann, Oxford, 1997, p. 101.

38 Ho DS, Zecchin RP, Richards DAB, Uther JB, Ross DL. Double-blind trial of lignocaine versus sotalol for acute termination of spontaneous sustained ventricular tachycardia. *Lancet* 1994;344:18–23.

39 Reynolds F. Case report: Damage to the conus medullaris following spinal anaesthesia. *Anaesthesia* 2001;56:235–47.

40 Stoelting RK, Dierdorf SF. *Anesthesia and Co-existing disease*, 4th edn. Churchill Livingstone, New York, 2002, p. 427.

41 Wall RT. Unusual endocrine problems. *Anesth Clin North Am* 1996;14:3:471–93.

42 Nicholson G, Burrin JM, Hall GM. Review article: Peri-operative steroid supplementation. *Anaesthesia* 1998;53:1091–104.

43 Yang H. Intraoperative automated ST segment analysis: a reliable 'black box'? *Can J Anaesth* 1996;43:1041–51.

44 Pippa P, Barbagli R, Rabassini M, Doni L, Rucci FS. Postspinal headache in Taylor's approach: A comparison between 21 and 25 gauge needles in orthopaedic patients. *Anesth Intensive Care* 1995;23:560–3.

45 Sparkes CJ, Perndt H, Agiomea K, Fa'Arondo J. Spinal anaesthesia for caesarean section in the Solomon Islands. *Anaesth Intensive Care* 1994;22:187–91.

46 Yeh H-M, Chen L-K, Lin C-J et al. Prophylactic intravenous ondansetron reduces the incidence of intrathecal morphine-induced pruritis in patients undergoing cesarean delivery. *Anesth Analg* 2000;91:172–5.

47 Glynn CJ. Intrathecal and epidural administration of opiates. *Bailliere's Clinical Anaesth* 1987;1:4:915–32.

48 Dahl JB, Jeppesen SI, Jørgensen H et al. (Review article) Intraoperative and postoperative analgesic efficacy and adverse effects of intrathecal opioids in patients undergoing Caesarean section with spinal anaesthesia. *Anesthesiology* 1999;91:1919–27.

49 Nguyen Thi TV, Orliaguet G, Ngu TH, Bonnet F. Spinal anesthesia with meperidine as the sole agent for caesarean delivery. *Reg Anesth* 1994;19:386–9.

50 Ross AW, Greenhalgh C, McGlade DP et al. The Sprotte needle and post dural puncture headache following Caesarean section. *Anaesth Intensive Care* 1993;21:280–3.

51 Gielen MJM. Postdural puncture headache (PDPH): a review. *Regional Anesthesia* 1989;14:101–6.

52 Spencer HC. Postdural puncture headache: what matters is technique. *Regional Anesthesia and Pain Medicine* 1998;23:374–9.

53 Cook TM. Combined spinal epidural anaesthesia: a new technique. *International J Obstet Anesth* 1989;8:3–6.

54 Lifschitz R, Jedeikin R. Spinal epidural anaesthesia; a new combination system. *Anaesthesia* 1992;47:503–5.

55 Eldor J. Metallic particles in the spinal-epidural technique. *Reg Anesth* 1994;19:219.

56 Levy DM. Anaesthesia for Caesarean section. *Brit J Anaesth* 2001;6:162–7.

57 Collis RE, Baxandall ML, Srikantharajah ID et al. Combined spinal epidural (CSE) analgesia: technique, management, and outcome of 300 mothers. *International Journal of Obstetric Anesthesia* 1994;3:75.

58 Maccarthur A. Management of controversies in obstetric anesthesia. *Can J Anesth* 1999;46:R111–R116.

59 Holloway J, Seed PT, O'Sullivan GO, Reynolds F. Paraesthesia and nerve damage following combined spinal epidural anaesthesia: a pilot survey. *International J Obstetric Anesthesia* 2000;9:151–5.

60 Burnell S, Byrne AJ. Continuous spinal anaesthesia. *Brit J Anaesth CEPD Review* 2001;1:134–7.

61 Løvstad RZ, Granhus G, Hetland S. Bradycardia and asystolic cardiac arrest during spinal anaesthesia: a report of five cases. *Acta Anaesthesiol Scand* 2000;44:48–52.

62 Greaves JD. Serious spinal cord injury due to haematomyelia caused by spinal anaesthesia in a patient treated with low-dose heparin. *Anaesthesia* 1997;52:150–68.

63 Tryba M. Epidural regional anaesthesia and low molecular weight heparin: pro (German). *Anaesthesia Intensivmed Notfallmed Schmerzther* 1993;28:179–81.

64 Jenkins K, Baker AB. Review Article: Consent and anaesthetic risk. *Anaesthesia* 2003;58:962–84.

65 Monk JP, Beresford R, Wand A. Sufentanil: a review of its pharmacological properties and therapeutic use. *Drugs* 1988;36:286–313.

66 Ransom D, Leicht C. Continuous spinal analgesia with sufentanil for labour and delivery in a parturient with severe pulmonary stenosis. *Anesth Analg* 1995;80:418–21.

67 Guidelines 2000 for cardiopulmonary resuscitation and emergency cardiovascular care. *Circulation* 2000;102:(suppl) I112–28.

68 Sanghavi S, Rayner-Klein J. Management of pre-arrest arrhythmia. *Br J Anaesth CEPD Reviews* 2002;4:104–12.

69 Donovan KD, Hockings BEF. Cardiac Arrhythmias. In: Oh TE (ed.). *Intensive Care Manual*, 4th edn. Butterworth-Heinemann, Oxford, 1997, pp. 73–81.

70 Chauhan VS, Krahn AD, Klein GJ et al. Supraventricular tachycardia. *Med Clin North Am* 2001;85:193–223.

71 Whittaker M. Plasma cholinesterase variants and the anaesthetist. *Anaesthesia* 1980;35:174–97.

72 Stern R. *Drugs, Diseases and Anaesthesia*. Lippincott-Raven, Philadelphia, 1997, p. 457.

73 Sullivan M, Thompson WK. Succinylcholine-induced cardiac arrest in children with undiagnosed myopathy. *Can J Anaesth* 1994;41:497–501.

T

1 Sasada M, Smith S. *Drugs in Anaesthesia and Intensive Care*, 2nd edn. Oxford University Press, Oxford, 1997, pp. 362–4.

2 Myles PS, Hendrata M, Bennett AM, Langley M, Buckland MR. Postoperative nausea and vomiting—propofol or thiopentone: Does choice of induction agent affect outcome? *Anaesth Intensive Care* 1996;24:355–9.

3 Gelman S. The pathophysiology of aortic cross-clamping and unclamping. *Anesthesiology* 1995;82:1026–60.

4 Safi HJ, Miller C. Spinal cord protection in descending thoracic and thoracoabdominal aortic repair. *Ann Thorac Surg* 1999;67:1937–9.

5 Safi HJ, Miller CC, Carr C et al. The importance of intercostal artery reattachment during thoracoabdominal aneurysm repair. *J Vasc Surg* 1998;27:58–68.

6 Kouchoukos NT, Rokkas CK. Hypothermic cardiopulmonary bypass for spinal cord protection: rationale and clinical results. *Ann Thorac Surg* 1999;67:1940–2.

7 Mallett SV, Cox DJA. Thromboelastography. *Br J Anaesth* 1992;69: 307–13.

8 Oster DL, Chang S-P B. Thyrotoxicosis. In: Yao FSF and Artusio JF (eds.). *Anesthesiology: Problem-Orientated Patient Management*, 4th edn. Lippincott-Raven, Philadelphia, 1998, pp. 571–83.

9 Viertiö-Oja H, Maja V, Särkela M et al. Description of the Entropy™ algorithm as applied in the Datex-Ohmeda S/5™ Entropy Module. *Acta Anaesthesiol Scand* 2004;48:154–61.

10 Vakkuri A, Yli-Hankala A, Talija P. Time-frequency balanced spectral entropy as a measure of anesthetic drug effect in central nervous system during sevoflurane, propofol, and thiopental anesthesia. *Acta Anaesthesiol Scand* 2004;48:145–53.

11 Mason R. *Anaesthesia Databook: A Perioperative and Peripartum Manual*, 3rd edn. Greenwich Medical Media Limited, London, 2001, pp. 491–3.

12 Weiner KL. Cardiac Dysrhythmias. In Duke J (ed.). *Anaesthesia Secrets*, 2nd edn. Hanley and Belfus, Philadelphia, 2000, pp. 169–77.

13 Kleinsasser A, Kuenszberg E, Loekinger A et al. Sevoflurane, but not propofol, significantly prolongs the Q-T interval. *Anesth Analg* 2000;90:25–7.

14 *Cardiovascular Drug Guidelines,* 2nd edn. VMPF Therapeutics Committee, Melbourne, 1995, p. 124.

15 Pleym H, Bathen J, Spigset O, Gisvold SE. Ventricular fibrillation related to reversal of the neuromuscular blockade in a patient with a long QT syndrome. *Acta Anaesthesiol Scand* 1999;43:352–5.

16 Lim HJ, Miller GM, Rainbird A. Airway fire during elective tracheostomy. *Anaesth Intensive Care* 1997;25:150–2.

17 Lewis KS, Han NH. Clinical Review. Tramadol: a new centrally acting analgesic. *Am J Health-Syst Pharm* 1997;54:643–52.

18 Sasada M, Smith S. *Drugs in Anaesthesia and Intensive Care*, 2nd edn. Oxford University Press, Oxford, 1997, pp. 370–1.

19 Delikan AE, Vijayan R. Forum: Epidural tramadol for post-operative pain relief. *Anaesthesia* 1993;48:328–31.

20 Bamigbade TA, Langford RM. The clinical use of tramadol hydrochloride. *Pain Reviews* 1998;5:155–82.

21 Broome IJ, Robb HM, Raj N, Girgis Y, Wardall GJ. The use of tramadol following day case surgery. *Anaesthesia* 1999;54:289–92.

22 Medical mishaps: serotonin syndrome. *Australian Prescriber* 2002;25:19.

23 Cossmann M, Kohnen C. General tolerability and adverse profile of tramadol hydrochloride. *Rev Contemp Pharmacother* 1995;246–9.

24 Horrow JC, Van Ripper DF, Strong MD, Brodsky I, Parmet JL. Hemostatic effects of tranexamic acid and desmopressin during cardiac surgery. *Circulation* 1991;84:2063–70.

25 Levy JH. Novel pharmacologic approaches to reduce bleeding. *Can J Anesth* 2003;50:S26–S30.

26 Horrow JC, Van Ripper DF, Strong MD, Grunewald KE. The dose response relationship of tranexamic acid. *Anesthesiology* 1995;82:383–92.

27 Mebust WK, Holtgrewe HL, Crockett ATK et al. Transurethral prostatectomy: immediate and postoperative complications. A co-operative study of thirteen participating institutions evaluating 3885 patients. *J Urol* 1989;141:243–7.

28 Monk TG. Anesthesia for urological procedures. *Audio-Digest Anesthesiology* 1998;40:5.

29 Hatch PD. Surgical and anaesthetic considerations in transurethral resection of the prostate. *Anaesth Intensive Care* 1987;15:203–11.

30 Hahn RG. The transurethral resection syndrome. *Acta Anaesthesiol Scand* 1991;35:557–67.

31 Jensen V. The TURP syndrome. *Can J Anaesth* 1991;38:1:90–7.

32 Quinney N, Lomas I. Treatment of priapism during transurethral resection of the prostate. *Br J Hosp Med* 1995;54(8):393–4.

33 Costello TG, Crowe H, Costello AJ. Laser prostatectomy versus transurethral resection of the prostate for benign prostatic hypertrophy: comparative changes in haemoglobin and serum sodium. *Anaesth Intens Care* 1997;25:493–6.

34 Stoelting RK, Dierdorf SF. *Anesthesia and Co-Existing Disease*, 4th edn. Churchill Livingstone, Philadelphia, 2002, pp. 25–44.

35 Groves ER, Groves JB. Epidural analgesia for labour in a patient with Ebstein's anomaly. *Can J Anaesth* 1995;42:77–9.

36 Mason R. *Anaesthesia Databook: A Perioperative and Peripartum Manual*, 3rd edn. Greenwich Medical Media Limited, London, 2001, pp. 155–6.

37 Donnelly JE, Brown JM, Radford DJ. Pregnancy outcome and Ebstein's anomaly. *Br Heart J* 1991;66:368–71.

38 Linter SPK, Clarke K. Caesarean section under extradural analgesia in a patient with Ebstein's anomaly. *Br J Anaesth* 1984;56:203.

39 Mostellar JR. Deliberate Hypotension. In: Duke J, Rosenberg SG (eds.). *Anesthesia Secrets*. Hanley & Belfus, Philadelphia, Mosby, St Louis, 1996, p. 465.

U

1 Dawson NJ, Gabbott DA. Use of sublingual glyceryl trinitrate as a supplement to volatile inhalational anaesthesia in a case of uterine inversion. *International Journal of Obstetric Anaesthesia* 1997;6:135–7.

2 Peng ATC, Gorman RS, Shulman SM, DeMarchis E, Nyunt K, Blancato LS. Intravenous nitroglycerin for uterine relaxation in the postpartum patient with retained placenta (letter). *Anesthesiology* 1989;71:172–3.

3 Axemo P, Fu X, Lindberg B, Ulmsten U, Wessen A. Intravenous nitroglycerine for rapid uterine relaxation. *Acta Obstet Gynecol Scand* 1998;77:50–3.

4 Lynch JC, Pardy J. Survey: Uterine rupture and scar dehiscence. A five-year survey. *Anesth Intensive Care* 1996;24:699–704.

5 Yap OW, Kim ES, Laros RK Jr. Maternal and neonatal outcomes after uterine rupture in labour. *Am J Obstet Gynecol* 2001;184:1576–81.

V

1 Wesley RC, Rash W, Zimmerman D. Reconsiderations of the routine and preoperational use of lidocaine in the emergent treatment of ventricular arrhythmias. *Crit Care Med* 1991;19:1439–41.

2 *Cardiovascular Drug Guidelines*, 2nd edn. Victorian Medical Postgraduate Foundation Therapeutics Committee, Melbourne, 1995, p. 133.

3 Sanghavi S, Rayner-Klein J. Management of pre-arrest arrhythmia. *Br J Anaesth CEPD Reviews* 2002;4:104–12.

4 Ho DSW, Zecchin RP, Richards DA, Uther JB, Ross DL. Double blind trial of lignocaine versus sotalol for acute termination of spontaneous ventricular tachycardia. *Lancet* 1994;44:18–22.

5 Holt A. Management of Cardiac Arrhythmias. In: Oh TE, Bersten AD, Soni N (eds.). *Oh's Intensive Care Manual*, 5th edn. Butterworth-Heinemann, Oxford, 2003, pp. 157–205.

6 *Cardiovascular Drug Guidelines*, 2nd edn. Victorian Medical Postgraduate Foundation Therapeutics Committee, Melbourne, 1995, p. 119.

7   *Cardiovascular Drug Guidelines*, 2nd edn. Victorian Medical Postgraduate Foundation Therapeutics Committee, Melbourne, 1995, p. 108.

8   Willis C. Acute Dysrhythmias. In: Parsons PE, Wiener-Kronish JP (eds.). *Critical Care Secrets*. Hanley and Belfus, Inc, Philadelphia, Mosby, St Louis, 1992, pp. 126–35.

9   Sambrook A, Small R. Antiarrhythmic drugs; antihypertensive drugs in pregnancy. *Anaesthesia and Intensive Care Medicine* 2003;4:266–72.

W

1   Gallo J. Brodifacoum (letter). *Anaesth Intensive Care* 1998;26:708–9.

2   Gerstenfeld EP, Beaudette SP, Mittleman RS, Becker RC. Supraventricular Tachycardias. In: Irwin RS, Rippe JM (eds.). *Manual of Intensive Care Medicine*, 3rd edn. Lippincott Williams and Wilkins, Philadelphia, 2000, pp. 240–52.

3   McGovern B. Precipitation of cardiac arrest by verapamil in patients with WPW syndrome. *Ann Intern Med* 1986;104:791.

4   Willis C. Acute Dysrhythmias. In: Parsons PE, Wiener-Kronisch JP (eds.). *Critical Care Secrets*. Hanley and Belfus, Philadelphia, 1992, pp. 126–35.

5   Delaunay L, Chelly JE. Blocks at the wrist provide effective anesthesia for carpal tunnel release. *Can J Anesth* 2001;48:656–60.

6   Bridenbaugh LD. The Upper Extremity: Somatic Blockade. In: Cousins MJ, Bridenbaugh PO (eds.). *Neural Blockade in Clinical Anesthesia and Management of Pain*, 2nd edn. JB Lippincott Company, Philadelphia, 1988, pp. 387–416.

X

1   Boomsma F, Rupneht J, Veld AJ et al. Haemodynamic and neurohumoral effects of xenon anaesthesia. *Anaesthesia* 1990;45:273–8.

2   Lynch C, Baum J, Tenbrinck R. Xenon anaesthesia. *Anesthesiology* 2000;3:865–8.

3   Kennedy RR, Stokes JW, Downing P. Review: Anaesthesia and the 'inert' gases with special reference to xenon. *Anaesth Intensive Care* 1992;20:66–70.

4   Shaw AD, Morgan M. Editorial: Nitrous oxide: time to stop laughing? *Anaesthesia* 1998;53:213–5.